Nanomanufacturing Techniques in Sustainable Healthcare Applications

The text begins by discussing the processing and characterization of nano-manufactured resorbable bionanocomposites and presents the latest advances in carbon-based polymer nanocomposite materials for sensing applications. It further presents different characterization techniques such as scanning electron, transmission electron, atomic force microscopy, and powder X-ray diffraction for the identification of bionanocomposites.

This book:

- Introduces nano-manufactured processed composites for biomedical application, processing, and characterization of bionanocomposites.
- Presents biobased nano-manufactured processed composites for imaging, tissue repairing, and drug-delivery applications.
- Explains future trends of nano-manufactured composites in 3D bio-implants and fluorescent bioimaging.
- Highlights the challenges and perspectives of polymeric nano-manufactured composites for biomedical applications.
- Covers multifunctional nano-manufactured bio-composites, and advances in polymeric membranes for healthcare applications.

It is primarily written for senior undergraduates, graduate students, and academic researchers in the fields of manufacturing engineering, biomedical engineering, materials science and engineering, mechanical engineering, and production engineering.

Advances in Manufacturing, Design and Computational Intelligence Techniques

Series Editor-Ashwani Kumar- *Senior Lecturer, Mechanical Engineering, at Technical Education Department, Uttar Pradesh, Kanpur, India*

The book series editor is inviting edited, reference and text book proposal submission in the book series. The main objective of this book series is to provide researchers a platform to present state of the art innovations, research related to advanced materials applications, cutting edge manufacturing techniques, innovative design and computational intelligence methods used for solving nonlinear problems of engineering. The series includes a comprehensive range of topics and its application in engineering areas such as additive manufacturing, nanomanufacturing, micromachining, biodegradable composites, material synthesis and processing, energy materials, polymers and soft matter, nonlinear dynamics, dynamics of complex systems, MEMS, green and sustainable technologies, vibration control, AI in power station, analog-digital hybrid modulation, advancement in inverter technology, adaptive piezoelectric energy harvesting circuit, contactless energy transfer system, energy efficient motors, bioinformatics, computer aided inspection planning, hybrid electrical vehicle, autonomous vehicle, object identification, machine intelligence, deep learning, control-robotics-automation, knowledge based simulation, biomedical imaging, image processing and visualization. This book series compiled all aspects of manufacturing, design and computational intelligence techniques from fundamental principles to current advanced concepts.

Hybrid Metal Additive Manufacturing: Technology and Applications
Edited by Parnika Shrivastava, Anil Dhanola, and Kishor Kumar Gajrani

Thermal Energy Systems: Design, Computational Techniques, and Applications
Edited by Ashwani Kumar, Varun Pratap Singh, Chandan Swaroop Meena, Nitesh Dutt

https://www.routledge.com/Advances-in-Manufacturing-Design-and-Computational-Intelligence-Techniques/book-series/CRCAIMDCIT?publishedFilter=alltitles&pd=published,forthcoming&pg=1&pp=12&so=pub&view=list?publishedFilter=alltitles&pd=published,forthcoming&pg=1&pp=12&so=pub&view=list

Nanomanufacturing Techniques in Sustainable Healthcare Applications

Edited by
Arbind Prasad and
Pramod Kumar

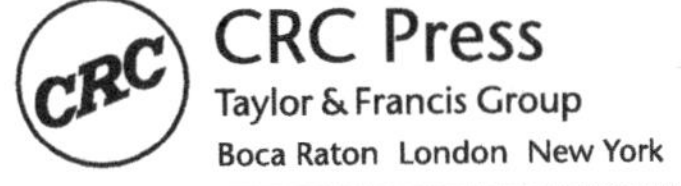

CRC Press
Taylor & Francis Group
Boca Raton London New York

CRC Press is an imprint of the
Taylor & Francis Group, an **informa** business

Designed cover image: shutterstock

First edition published 2025
by CRC Press
2385 NW Executive Center Drive, Suite 320, Boca Raton FL 33431

and by CRC Press
4 Park Square, Milton Park, Abingdon, Oxon, OX14 4RN

CRC Press is an imprint of Taylor & Francis Group, LLC

© 2025 selection and editorial matter, Arbind Prasad and Pramod Kumar; individual chapters, the contributors

ISBN: 978-1-032-74364-6 (hbk)
ISBN: 978-1-032-74672-2 (pbk)
ISBN: 978-1-003-47031-1 (ebk)

DOI: 10.1201/9781003470311

Typeset in Sabon
by Deanta Global Publishing Services, Chennai, India

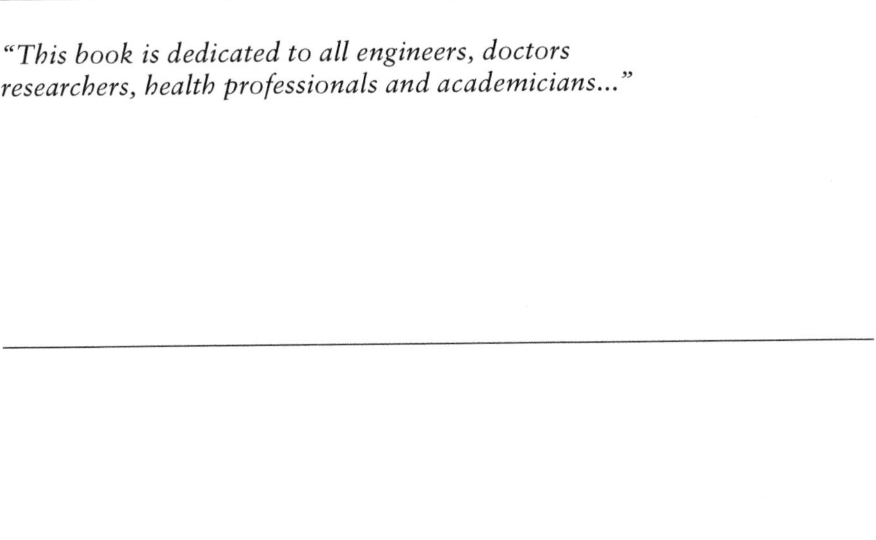

"This book is dedicated to all engineers, doctors researchers, health professionals and academicians..."

Contents

Preface   x
Introduction   xiii
About the Editors   xvi
Contributors   xviii
Acknowledgments   xxiii

1   Introduction to Bio-based Polymers and
    Their Advancements   1
    SIDDHARTH MOHAN BHASNEY, SHUBHRANSHU RANJAN DAS,
    ARBIND PRASAD, PRAMOD KUMAR, AND BIDYANAND MAHTO

2   Processing and Characterization of Bionanocomposites   25
    MANJEETA KUMARI, MANISHA CHADHA, AND SHIWANI BERRY

3   Bio-based Nanocomposites for Imaging, Tissue Repairing,
    and Drug Delivery Applications   39
    PURNIMA JUSTA, NANCY JASWAL, VIJAY BAHADUR,
    MANOJ K. SINGH, DEVENDRA KUMAR GANGWAR,
    MOHAN BHUSHAN KALHANS, AND PRAMOD KUMAR

4   Carbon Nanocomposites: A Good Candidate for Sensing
    and Detection of Neurotransmitters   57
    NEERAJ GUPTA, VISHAL BHARATI JARYAL, SAHIL, AND ABHISHEK SONI

5   Bioinspired Nanocomposites: Multifunctional Materials
    towards Sustainable Alternatives   78
    NIPUN JAIN, YUSUF OLATUNJI WAIDI, RANJIT BARUA, SAMIR DAS,
    VILAY VANNALADSAYSY, ARBIND PRASAD, AND SUDIPTO DATTA

6   Bio-based Starch Blends in Active Food Packaging
    Applications   94
    SHAZIA HUSSAIN, PRIYA, AND SHIWANI BERRY

7   Smart and Self-healing Hydrogels for Biomedical
    Applications   110
    YUSUF OLATUNJI WAIDI, NIPUN JAIN, RANJIT BARUA, VILAY
    VANNALADSAYSY, SAMIR DAS, ARBIND PRASAD, AND SUDIPTO DATTA

8   High-Energy Beam-Based Surface Texturing on Advanced
    Engineering Materials Used in Bioimplants   131
    D. CHINMOYEE, T.N. DEEPU KUMAR, R.R. RAVI, AND D.S. SRINIVASU

9   Nanocomposites in Cytotoxicity and Targeted Drug
    Delivery Applications   168
    JITENDER KUMAR, HEMANT KUMAR, RAJESH KUMAR,
    AND PRAMOD KUMAR

10 Polymer-based Bionanocomposites: Smart
    Adsorbents for Detection and Removal of Metal
    Contaminants from Water   195
    POOJA KUMARI, TABASSUM NIKE, DEEPIKA KAUSHAL,
    VIVEK SHEEL JASWAL, VINAY CHAUHAN, AND MANISH KUMAR

11 Biomimetic Nanocomposites for Orthopedic Applications   215
    MILAD HEIDARI, SIVASAKTHIVEL THANGAVEL, AND ASHWANI KUMAR

12 Functional Nano-manufactured
    Bio-composite in Healthcare Applications   233
    FRANCIS LUTHER KING M, THILLIKKANI S, RAJA K, AND SRINIVASAN V

13 Degradation Studies of Resorbable Materials for
    Biomedical Applications   258
    VISHNUVARTHANAN MAYAKRISHNAN AND PREETHI ARUL MURUGAN

14 Nanobiocomposites in Wound Healing   278
    DIVYA THAKUR, DEEPIKA KAUSHAL, RAJENDER KUMAR,
    VINAY CHAUHAN, AND MANISH KUMAR

15 Nanocomposites in 3D Bioimplants and Fluorescent
    Bioimaging   296
    NANCY JASWAL, VIJAY BAHADUR, ALI RAZA, ARBIND PRASAD,
    AND PRAMOD KUMAR

16 Challenges and Perspectives of Polymeric Nanocomposites
for Biomedical Applications   317
MILAD HEIDARI, SULAIMAN AL HASANI, SIVASAKTHIVEL THANGAVEL, AND
ASHWANI KUMAR

Index   341

Preface

Nanomanufacturing Techniques in Sustainable Healthcare Applications elaborates on the design, development, synthesis, and applications of various biobased nanocomposites derived from natural and synthetic sources, which are used in the medical industry. Sustainable bio-based nano-manufactured composites are the central theme of this book. Effectively, sixteen chapters presented in this book are quite interesting and up-to-date with the scope of future research work. This has the strong potential to be valuable to researchers in engineering and material-related disciplines. The background information and the literature review provided in each chapter are an in-depth analysis of the topic covered in the chapter.

In origin, sustainable bio-based nano-manufactured composites can come from nature or can be synthesized in the laboratory with a variety of approaches that use metals, polymers, ceramics, or other filler materials.

These renewable nanocomposite materials consist of nontoxic compounds that are capable of biological degradation by several soil microorganisms. This emerging concept will help in the reduction of environmental damage due to petrochemical dependence. For nanocomposites that comprise synthetic polymers and inorganic reinforcements, the distribution of silicates or hydroxyapatite in a biopolymer matrix initiates the "tortuous" pathway, leading to a reduction in the gas diffusion property of nanohybrid materials. In addition to silicates, several different inorganic solids have been added as reinforcements to biopolymer materials; for example, the distribution of sepiolite in natural rubber improves the mechanical properties of rubber. Sustainable bio-based nano-manufactured composites are used in many healthcare applications, namely nanocarrier applications (diabetes diagnosis and treatment, cancer diagnosis and treatment, smart delivery of pesticides, ophthalmic drug delivery systems, food processing applications (active microbial packaging, oxygen-scavenging films), biomedical applications (3D bio-implant, fluorescent bioimaging), point of care smart devices (DNA biosensors, enzyme biosensors), all of which are discussed in this book. In this book, Chapter 1 deals with the introduction to biobased composites for biomedical applications, authors have covered different biomass-derived carbon-based nanomaterials that have potential biomedical applications and their advancements. Chapter 2 deals with the processing and characterization of bio nanocomposites which describes a large number of characterization techniques such as optical, scanning electron, transmission electron, and atomic force microscopy; small-angle X-ray scattering; and powder X-ray diffraction used for the detailed identification of bio nanocomposites. Chapter 3 introduces the reader to applications of bio-based nano-manufactured composites in imaging, tissue repairing, and drug-delivery applications. Here, the tendency of bio-based nanostructured material to interface with human cells and tissues makes them perfect for the construction of biomedical applications including polysaccharides (chitin, chitosan, and cellulose), polylactic acid, poly-caprolactone, poly(γ-glutamic acid) and natural bioceramics is discussed extensively. Chapter 4 comprises a brief introduction to carbon nanocomposite: Promising materials for sensing and detection. This chapter provides an overview of recent developments in the field of carbon-based polymer nanocomposite materials for sensing applications. Furthermore, the various nanocomposite materials systems as well as their sensing properties along with applications for sensing heavy metals and body fluids have been discussed in detail. Chapter 5, Bio-inspired Nano-manufactured Composites: Multifunctional Materials towards Sustainable Alternatives, and Chapter 6 deal with a biobased starch blend in active food packaging applications, commonly used nanoparticle formulations are ZnO, CuO, MgO, and AgNPs with starch, gelatine, PVA chitosan, proteins, and other biopolymers. It provides a detailed description of the role of biobased starch blends in active food packaging applications and the role of food packaging in waste management, circular packaging design, bio-origin plastic, and circular economy of food packaging. Chapter 7 aims at self-healing materials for biomedical applications discussing the classification of biocomposites and their significance in sensor applications. It also explains the sensing mechanism of biodegradable nanocomposites and deals with matrix-based biodegradable composites for sensing environmental toxins and for sensing certain chemicals in clinical research. Chapter 8 highlights the high-energy beam-based surface texturing for bioimplants. Surface texture plays a vital role especially where cellular interaction is held. These are explained in this chapter. Chapter 9 talks about nano-manufactured composites in cytotoxicity and targeted drug delivery applications. In this chapter, various strategies and procedures for nanocomposite synthesis-suited drug delivery applications are addressed, along with a brief explanation of possible cytotoxicity. Additionally, the most popular ways of linking the nanocomposites to pharmaceuticals are highlighted, and methods for their toxicity are briefly addressed. Chapter 10 highlights the advances in polymeric membranes for healthcare applications. Chapter 11 deals with the biomimetic nano-manufactured composites for orthopedic applications. The rheological investigation is much more important in this case as the melt strength of the composites determines the properties such as castability, deformation, and loadbearing properties. Chapter 12 presents some of the most multifunctional nano biocomposites in healthcare applications, This chapter discusses the utilization of various multifunctional bio-nano manufactured composites in biomedical and healthcare applications. The healthcare applications of these multifunctional nanocomposites are multitudinous including wound healing and dressing, medical textiles, dental application, osteoporosis, cancer therapy, drug delivery, and tissue engineering. It focuses on the nanocomposites based on different biomaterials as well as depicts the striking potential of these materials in the healthcare industry. Chapter 13 deals with degradation studies of the resorbable materials and their behaviors. Chapter 14 deals with nanocomposites in wound healing applications. Chapter 15 emphasizes the Future trends of nano-manufactured composites in 3D bio-implants and fluorescent bio-imaging. This chapter describes the emerging field of biotechnology which involves a wide variety of biomedical applications such as tissue engineering, biosensors, drug delivery, and wound healing. In this chapter, we focus on fluorescent nanocomposites showing magnetic behavior particularly due to their wide range of applications in fluorescent imaging along with the various types of bioimplants that can be printed with additive manufacturing. Chapter 16 deals with the challenges and perspectives of polymeric nano-manufactured composites for biomedical applications. Thus this book will have a great impact among stakeholders.

Editors
Dr. Arbind Prasad and
Dr. Pramod Kumar

Introduction

The huge demand for bio-based materials and their nanomanufacturing techniques usage are in increasing trends. Researchers and professionals are looking for nanotechnologies for sustainable healthcare and other applications in biomedical applications. Metallic biomaterials have many limitations such as stress shielding, leaching of ions, underlying bone damage, and corrosion of the implants. The alternative solution is bioabsorbable biobased polymeric materials, which have many unique features to replace the metallic bioimplants. In this era, every patient is looking for comfort and a painless solution; in this regard, nanomanufacturing-based sustainable biobased nanocomposites can come from nature or can be synthesized in the laboratory with a variety of approaches that use metals, polymers, ceramics, or other filler materials.

These renewable nano-manufactured composite materials consist of nontoxic compounds that are capable of biological degradation by several soil microorganisms. This emerging concept will help in the reduction of environmental damage due to petrochemical dependence. Nano-manufactured composites that comprise synthetic polymers and inorganic reinforcements, the distribution of silicates or hydroxyapatite in a biopolymer matrix initiates the "tortuous" pathway, leading to a reduction in the gas diffusion property of nanohybrid materials. In the book *Nanomanufacturing Techniques in Sustainable Healthcare Applications*, Chapter 1 deals with the introduction to biobased composites for biomedical applications, authors have covered different biomass-derived carbon-based nanomaterials that have potential biomedical applications and their advancements. Chapter 2 deals with the processing and characterization of bio nanocomposites which describes a large number of characterization techniques such as optical, scanning electron, transmission electron, and atomic force microscopy; small-angle X-ray scattering; and powder X-ray diffraction used for the detailed identification of bio nanocomposites. Chapter 3 introduces the reader to the applications of biobased nano-manufactured composites in imaging, tissue repairing, and drug-delivery applications. Here, the tendency of biobased nanostructured material to interface with human cells and tissues makes them perfect for the construction of biomedical applications including polysaccharides (chitin, chitosan, and cellulose), polylactic acid, polycaprolactone, poly(γ-glutamic acid) and natural bioceramics is discussed extensively. Chapter 4 comprises a brief introduction to carbon nanocomposite: Promising materials for sensing and detection. This chapter provides an overview of recent developments in the field of carbon-based polymer nanocomposite materials for sensing applications. Furthermore, the various nanocomposite materials systems as well as their sensing properties along with applications for sensing heavy metals and body fluids have been discussed in detail. Chapter 5, Bio-inspired Nano-manufactured Composites: Multifunctional Materials towards Sustainable Alternatives, and Chapter 6 deal with a biobased starch blend in active food packaging applications, commonly used nanoparticle formulations are ZnO, CuO, MgO, and AgNPs with starch, gelatine, PVA chitosan, proteins, and other biopolymers. It provides a detailed description of the role of biobased starch blends in active food packaging applications and the role of food packaging in waste management, circular packaging design, bio-origin plastic, and circular economy of food packaging. Chapter 7 aims at self-healing materials for biomedical applications discussing the classification of biocomposites and their significance in sensor applications. It also explains the sensing mechanism of biodegradable nanocomposites and deals with matrix-based biodegradable composites for sensing environmental toxins and for sensing certain chemicals in clinical research. Chapter 8 highlights the high-energy beam-based surface texturing for bioimplants. Surface texture plays a vital role especially where cellular interactions are held. This is explained in this chapter. Chapter 9 talks about nano-manufactured composites in cytotoxicity and targeted drug delivery applications. In this chapter, various strategies and procedures for nanocomposite synthesis-suited drug delivery applications are addressed, along with a brief explanation of possible cytotoxicity. Additionally, the most popular ways of linking the nanocomposites to pharmaceuticals are highlighted, and methods for their toxicity are briefly addressed. Chapter 10 highlights the advances in polymeric membranes for healthcare applications. Chapter 11 deals with the Biomimetic nano-manufactured composites for orthopedic applications. The rheological investigation is much more important in this case as the melt strength of the composites determines the properties such as castability, deformation, and loadbearing properties. Chapter 12 presents some of the most Multifunctional nano biocomposites in healthcare applications, This chapter discusses the utilization of various multifunctional bio-nano manufactured composites in biomedical and healthcare applications. The healthcare applications of these multifunctional nanocomposites are multitudinous including wound healing and dressing, medical textiles, dental application, osteoporosis, cancer therapy, drug delivery, and tissue engineering. It focuses on the nanocomposites based on different biomaterials as well as depicts the striking potential of these materials in the healthcare industry. Chapter 13 deals with degradation studies of the resorbable materials and their behaviors. Chapter 14 deals with nanocomposites in wound healing applications. Chapter 15 emphasizes the Future trends of nano-manufactured composites in 3D bio-implants and fluorescent bio-imaging. This chapter describes the emerging field of biotechnology which involves a wide variety of biomedical applications such as tissue engineering, biosensors, drug delivery, and wound healing. In this chapter, we focus on fluorescent nanocomposites showing magnetic behavior particularly due to their wide range of applications in fluorescent imaging along with the various types of bioimplants that can be printed with additive manufacturing. Chapter 16 deals with the challenges and perspectives of polymeric nano-manufactured composites for biomedical applications.

In addition to silicates, several different inorganic solids have been added as reinforcements to biopolymer materials; for example, the distribution of sepiolite in natural rubber causes improvement in mechanical properties. Sustainable Biobased Nano manufactured composites used in many healthcare applications which constitute nanocarrier applications are also discussed.

Editors
Dr. Arbind Prasad and
Dr. Pramod Kumar

About the Editors

Arbind Prasad earned his PhD (mechanical engineering) from the Indian Institute of Technology Guwahati, Assam, India. He is a gold medalist in his MTech. He is currently working as an assistant professor and head (mechanical engineering) in the Department of Science, Technology and Technical Education, Government of Bihar, at Katihar Engineering College, Katihar, Bihar, India. He holds four granted patents in his research work. He has 15 international journal papers, edited 9 books (Wiley, Elsevier, AAP, De Gruyter, and CRC Press (Taylor & Francis) USA), 35 book chapters, and 15 reputed international conference papers to his credit. Dr. Prasad has obtained various prestigious awards such as the Sponsored Research Industrial Consultancy (SRIC) award from IIT Kanpur, Best Oral Presentation from the American Chemical Society, and Best Paper awards from IIT Guwahati during Research Conclave. He has completed numerous projects funded by the State Government. He is an associate editor for the *International Journal of Materials, Manufacturing and Sustainable Technologies (IJMMST)* and an early career editor for the *International Journal of Mathematical, Engineering and Management Sciences (IJMEMS)* indexed in Emerging Sources Citation Index/Scopus and Directory of Open Access Journals. He is an editorial board member of various international journals and acts as an active review board member of ten prestigious (indexed in Science Citation Index/Science Citation Index Expanded/Scopus) and guest editor in special issues of international journals with high impact factor i.e. Bioengineering, Journal of Design, Materials, Journal of functional materials, Molecules, etc. His main areas of research include resorbable polymers, recycling of biodegradable polymers, healthcare devices, Implants, biomaterials, materials processing, design, and manufacturing techniques of biomedical implants. He is also a lifetime member of the Society for Polymer Science India, the Materials Research Society of India, the Society for Biomaterials and Artificial Organs of India, the Asian Polymer Association, and the Indian Society for Technical Education.

Pramod Kumar received his PhD degree from the University of Delhi, India. He served as an assistant professor at the Department of Chemistry, at Ramjas College, University of Delhi (2014–2020). His research interests include nanomedicine, specializing in the use of inorganic-based and gold nanoparticles for applications in targeted drug delivery, non-viral gene delivery, photodynamic therapy, photothermal therapy, in vitro diagnostics, and multimodal diagnostic imaging. Current research interests include hybrid nanoparticles, hydrogel nanoparticles, and quantum dots for triggered drugs, bioimaging/biosensors, and gene delivery for the treatment of cancer, respiratory and neurological diseases. His teaching areas are nanomaterials and nanocomposites, quantum mechanics, atomic structure and spectroscopy, chemical kinetics and reaction dynamics, group theory, photochemistry, electrochemistry, principles of instrumentation of NMR/ESR/Mössbauer and nuclear quadrupole resonance spectroscopy. He has been awarded a National Eligibility Test – Junior Research Fellowship in Chemical Science and Graduate Aptitude Test in Engineering Fellowship in Chemistry. He has published more than 25 articles in leading scientific journals. Currently, he is an assistant professor of the Department of Chemistry and Chemical Sciences, at the Central University of Himachal Pradesh (India) and has supervised 18 dissertations to date. Along with these, four students are pursuing their PhDs under his supervision.

Contributors

Vijay Bahadur
Department of Science
Alliance University
Bengaluru, India

Ranjith Barua
Centre for Healthcare Science and
Technology
Indian Institute of Engineering
Science and Technology
Howrah, India

Shiwani Berry
Central University of Himachal
Pradesh
Shahpur Parisar
Shahpur, Kangra, India

Siddharth Mohan Bhasney
Manager (R&D)
Machino Polymers Limited
Gurugram, India

Manisha Chadha
Central University of Himachal
Pradesh
Shahpur Parisar
Shahpur, Kangra, India

Vinay Chauhan
School of Advanced Chemical
Sciences
Shoolini University
Solan, India

D. S. Srinivasu
Indian Institute of Technology
Madras
Chennai, India

Samir Das
Biomaterials and Tissue
Engineering Lab
School of Medical Science and
Technology
Indian Institute of Technology
Kharagpur, India

Shubhranshu Ranjan Das
Machino Polymers Limited
Gurugram, India

Chinmoyee Datta
Indian Institute of Technology
Madras
Chennai, India

Sudipto Datta
Department of Materials
Engineering
Indian Institute of Science
Bangalore, India

Devendra Kumar Gangwar
Department of Chemistry
Vardhaman College
Bijnor
M. J. P. Rohilkhand University
Bareilly, India

Neeraj Gupta
Department of Chemistry and
  Chemical Sciences
Central University of Himachal
  Pradesh
Dharamshala, India

Sulaiman Al Hasani
Mechanical Engineering Department
Global College of Engineering and
  Technology
Muscat, Oman

Milad Heidari
Mechanical Engineering Department
Global College of Engineering and
  Technology
Muscat, Oman

Shazia Hussain
Department of Chemistry and
  Chemical Science
Central University of Himachal
  Pradesh
Shahpur, India

Nipun Jain
Department of Materials
  Engineering
Indian Institute of Science
Bangalore, India

Vishal Bharati Jaryal
Department of Chemistry and
  Chemical Sciences
Central University of Himachal
  Pradesh
Dharamshala, India

Nancy Jaswal
Department of Chemistry &
  Chemical Science
School of Physical & Material
  Sciences
Central University of Himachal
  Pradesh
Dharamshala, India

Vivek Sheel Jaswal
Department of Chemistry and
  Chemical Sciences
Central University of Himachal
  Pradesh
Dharamshala, Kangra, India

Purnima Justa
Department of Chemistry &
  Chemical Science
School of Physical & Material
  Sciences
Central University of Himachal
  Pradesh
Dharamshala, India

K Raja
Department of Mechanical
  Engineering
Sri Jayaram Institute of Engineering
  and Technology
Gummidipoondi, India

Mohan Bhushan Kalhani
Department of Chemistry
Bareilly College Bareilly
M. J. P. Rohilkhand University
Bareilly, India

Deepika Kaushal
Department of Chemistry
Sri Sai University
Palampur, India

Ashwani Kumar
Technical Education Department
Kanpur, India

Hemant Kumar
Department of Chemistry
Ramjas College
University of Delhi
Delhi, India

Jitender Kumar
Department of Chemistry
University of Delhi
Delhi, India

Manish Kumar
Department of Chemistry and
  Chemical Sciences
Central University of Himachal
  Pradesh
Dharamshala, Kangra, India

Manjeeta Kumar
Central University of Himachal
  Pradesh
Kangra, India

Pramod Kumar
Department of Chemistry &
  Chemical Science
School of Physical & Material
  Sciences
Central University of Himachal
  Pradesh
Dharamshala, India

Rajender Kumar
Department of Chemistry and
  Chemical Sciences
Central University of Himachal
  Pradesh
Dharamshala, Kangra, India

Rajesh Kumar
Department of Chemistry
Himachal Pradesh University
Shimla, India

Pooja Kumari
Department of Chemistry and
  Chemical Sciences
Central University of Himachal
  Pradesh
Dharamshala, Kangra, India

M Francis Luther King
Department of Mechanical
  Engineering
Swarnandhra College of
  Engineering and Technology (A)
Narsapur, India

Bidyanand Mahto
Government Engineering College,
  Vaishali (Under Department
  of Science, Technology
  and Technical Education,
  Government of Bihar)
Vaishali, India

Vishnuvarthanan Mayakrishnan
Department of Materials Science
  and Engineering
Indian Institute of Technology Delhi
New Delhi, India

Preethi Arul Murugan
Department of Chemical
  Engineering
Indian Institute of Technology
  Bombay
Mumbai, India

Tabassum Nike
Department of Chemistry and
  Chemical Sciences
Central University of Himachal
  Pradesh
Dharamshala, Kangra, India

Dileep Pathote
Department of Materials
  Engineering
Indian Institute of Science
Bangalore, India

Sahil Patial
Department of Chemistry and
  Chemical Sciences
Central University of Himachal
  Pradesh
Dharamshala, India

Arbind Prasad
Mechanical Engineering
  Department
Katihar Engineering College
  (Under Department of Science,
  Technology and Technical
  Education, Government of
  Bihar)
Katihar, India

R. R. Ravi
Indian Institute of Technology
  Madras
Chennai, India

Ali Raza
Department of Criminal Justice
College of Professional Studies
Bowie State University
MD, USA

S Thillikkani
Department of Mechanical
  Engineering
Akshaya College of Engineering
  and Technology
Coimbatore, India

Manoj K. Singh
Energy Conversion & Storage Lab
Department of Applied Science &
  Humanities
Rajkiya Engineering College
Banda, India

Abhishek Soni
Department of Chemistry and
  Chemical Sciences
Central University of Himachal
  Pradesh
Dharamshala, Kangra, India

T. N. Deepu Kumar
Indian Institute of Technology
  Madras
Chennai, India

Divya Thakur
Department of Chemistry and
  Chemical Sciences
Central University of Himachal
  Pradesh
Dharamshala, Kangra, India

Sivasakthivel Thangavel
Mechanical Engineering
  Department
Global College of Engineering and
  Technology
Muscat, Oman

V Srinivasan
Department of Manufacturing
  Engineering
Faculty of Engineering and
  Technology
Annamalai University
Chidambaram, India

Vilay Vannaladsaysy
Department of Mechanical
  Engineering
Faculty of Engineering
National University of Laos
Vientiane, Laos

Yusuf Olatunji Waidi
Department of Materials
   Engineering
Indian Institute of Science
Bangalore, India

Priya
Department of Chemistry and
   Chemical Science
Central University of Himachal
   Pradesh
Shahpur, India

Acknowledgments

We express our gratitude to CRC Press (Taylor & Francis Group) and the editorial team for their suggestions and support during completion of this book. We are grateful to all contributors and reviewers for their illuminating views on each book chapter presented in *Nanomanufacturing Techniques in Sustainable Healthcare Applications.*

Editors
**Dr. Arbind Prasad and
Dr. Pramod Kumar**

Introduction to Bio-based Polymers and Their Advancements

Siddharth Mohan Bhasney, Shubhranshu Ranjan Das, Arbind Prasad, Pramod Kumar, and Bidyanand Mahto

1.1 INTRODUCTION

Polymers are a combination of two or more monomers. The monomers are linked in tandem to form a long molecular chain, hence the name polymer Polymers are also called macromolecules. Polymers can be of various types according to their origin, functionality, thermal response, polarity, polymerization, and crystallinity. The term polymer was first introduced in 1833 by a Swedish chemist Jöns Jacob Berzelius. Leo Baekeland invented the first synthetic polymer in 1907. Bio-based polymers are a subset of natural polymers and thus a viable alternative to synthetic polymers. Bio-based polymers can be biodegradable and non-biodegradable according to its origin and properties.

Bio-based polymers still hold many usages in the global market. Right now, biopolymers share less than 1% of the overall showcase [1]. Biomaterials have picked up engaging quality within the final decades due to both biological and financial concerns [2]. The around the world intrigued in bio-based polymers has quickened in later a long time due to crave of non-fuel-based polymers. There are two different ways are used to obtain bio-based polymers. By (bio)chemical polymerization bio-based monomers are converted into polymers [3]. The first generation of bio-based polymers focused on deriving the monomers from agricultural feedstocks like potatoes, corn starches, vegetable oils, sugarcanes, and other feedstocks. Natural bio-based polymers are the other class of bio-based polymers which are found naturally, such as proteins, nucleic acids, and polysaccharides [4]. These polymers have shown enormous growth in recent years in the technological developments and their commercial applications [2]. By utilizing biomass as feedstock, bio-based polymers contribute less to greenhouse gas emissions and offer a more sustainable life cycle. There are three principal ways to produce bio-polymers using renewable resources: i) partial modification of natural polymers; ii) fermentation process; iii) formation of bio-based polymers directly by bacteria (polyhydroxyalkanoates) [3]. These bio-based polymers influence by their production routes after degradation [4]. Bio-based polymer production methods supply a lasting and also eco pleasant method to polymer manufacturing making use of sustainable biomass

DOI: 10.1201/9781003470311-1

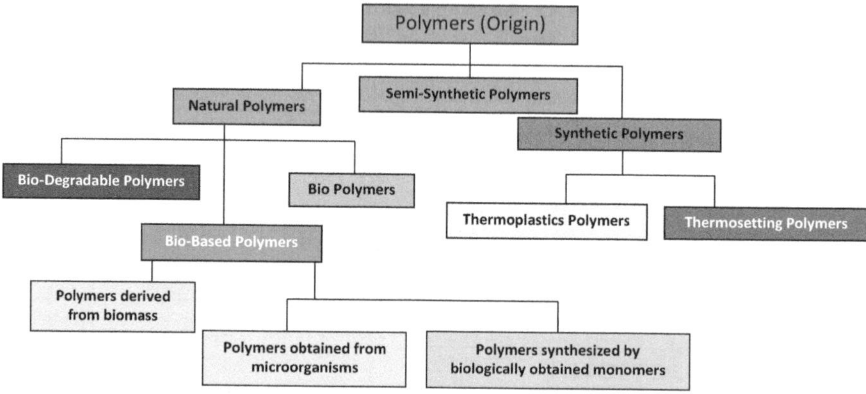

Figure 1.1 Classification of polymers.

sources coupled with lowering dependence on non-renewable fuel sources. From biomass pre-treatment as well as fermentation to polymerization handling, as well as surface area alteration, these strategies make it possible for the reliable conversion of biomass right into bio-based polymers with varied residential or commercial properties plus applications (Figure 1.1).

1.2 A SUB-SET OF NATURAL POLYMERS

Natural polymers: These types of polymers commonly occur in nature and can be extracted. Natural polymers are formed by addition polymerization or condensation polymerization. Some of the examples are starch, cellulose, chitin, latex, silk, collagen, and gelatin. Bio-based polymers and biodegradable polymers can be made from natural biopolymers.

Biopolymers: Biopolymer encompasses both natural polymers and synthetic polymers derived from biological resources. Mainly, biopolymers are produced by living organisms. Biopolymers consists of monomeric units that are covalently bonded in chains to form larger molecules [5]. The combination of water molecules with biopolymers was found to alter the internal structure. Biopolymer may be bio-based or may not be and, also varies in degradability such as proteins, nucleic acids, proteins, carbohydrates, lipids, and polysaccharides.

Biodegradable polymers: The polymers which can decompose in a few days are decomposed by the action of microorganisms and are known as biodegradable polymers. Biodegradable polymers can be of any origin (natural, synthetic, or bio-based). Examples are PLA, PHA, and cellulose acetate. They find applications in packaging, agriculture, medical devices, and textiles.

Bio-based polymers: Bio-based polymers are derived from renewable biological resources, providing an eco-friendly alternative to traditional, petroleum-based polymers. By bacterial fermentation process bio-based polymers synthesized and build into new blocks [4]. From packaging to automotive and in many sectors are being used that holds a good position in the market. Clinically available camptothecins like irinotecan and topotecan act as antitumor agents which are made from bio-based polymers. Examples are Bio-PE, PBS, PTT, and starch-based polymers.

1.3 OVERVIEW OF BIO-BASED POLYMERS

Bio-based polymers (also called bio-based plastics or bioplastics) are a promising milestone in the search for sustainable materials. Unlike traditional polymers that are derived from fossil fuels, bio-based polymers are derived from renewable resources such as plants, microorganisms, and agricultural by-products [6]. The transition to bio-based alternatives is being driven by growing awareness of the environmental issues associated with traditional plastics, such as pollution, depletion of non-renewable resources, and greenhouse gas emissions. One of the main advantages of bio-based polymers is their low environmental impact. Consequently, it leads to reduced carbon emissions compared to petroleum-based polymers. This is in line with global efforts to mitigate climate change and transition to a more sustainable circular economy. It can be classified into different types such as polylactic acid (PLA), which is derived from fermented plant sugars such as corn starch that is most commonly used bioplastics [7]. It is compostable and often used in packaging, disposable cutlery, and textile products. Another notable example is polyhydroxyalkanoates (PHA), which are produced by bacteria through a fermentation process. PHA is biodegradable and is used in packaging materials and medical devices. Cellulose biopolymers derived from plant cell walls are also attracting attention [8]. Cellulose acetate is used in film manufacturing and cigarette filters. These materials have excellent mechanical properties and serve as useful replacements for traditional plastics in a variety of applications [9]. Researchers are exploring advanced technologies such as genetically engineering microorganisms to improve yields and developing new raw materials to ensure a diverse and sustainable supply chain [10].

However, challenges remain regarding cost competitiveness and scalability. The production of bio-based polymers can be more expensive than the production of traditional plastics, primarily due to the cost of raw materials and manufacturing processes [11]. As the industry matures and economies of scale are achieved, these costs are expected to decrease and bio-based polymers would become more economical [12]. Government policies and consumer preferences play an important role in promoting the adoption of bio-based polymers. Many countries have introduced regulations and incentives to promote the use of sustainable materials, encouraging industry to invest in research and development of bio-based alternatives [13]. In summary, bio-based polymers offer a promising means to address the environmental issues associated with traditional plastics. Due to their renewable nature, reduced carbon footprint and biodegradability potential, they play an important role in the transition to a more sustainable and circular economy [14]. As research and innovation continue to advance the field, bio-based polymers are poised to play a key role in reshaping the materials landscape across a variety of industries [15].

Polylactic Acids (PLA): PLA, which is otherwise known as polylactide, is a bio-based polymer which is found from natural resources like corn starch, sugarcane, or cassava. It is produced by the fermentation of starches from plant sources and prepared by a direct polycondensation reaction or a ring-opening polymerization of lactide which is the cyclic dimer of the basic repeating unit. Its chemical formula is $(C_3 H_4 O_2)n$ or "$[-C(CH3) HC(=O) O-]$ n".

Since 1990, PLA has been commercialized. It belongs to the family of polyester groups having aliphatic carbon compound with the basic constitutional unit. The recycling code is 7. The monomer of lactic acid is hydroxyl carboxylic acid which can be obtained by bacterial fermentation (Figure 1.2). Some characteristics are: melting point-:130–180°C; density: 1.24 g/cm^3; T_g: 60–65°C; Young's modulus: 2.7–16 GPA. In addition, PLA has some excellent properties such as good mechanical strength, non-toxicity, easy availability, environment-friendly nature, biocompatibility, and good processability. Because of high Tg which makes it brittle. There are two types of lactic acid (L -lactic acid and D -lactic acid) is obtained by fermentation process [4, 16]. Hydrolysis, glycolysis, pyrolysis and alcoholysis like steps are followed for the depolymerization and recycling techniques.

Processing: PLA is the most manufactured bio-based Polymer because of the compatibility and varying processing techniques. Lactic acid is the synthetic factor by ring-opening polymerization or poly-condensation reaction. Due to water formation in the condensation reaction for PLA it is difficult to obtain a high molecular weight. In this process, pre-polymer lactide dimers are formed which is a low-molecular weight compound. In the next step, via ring-opening polymerization with compatible catalysts pre-polymers are converted into high molecular weight [17]. In summary, the steps are as follows:

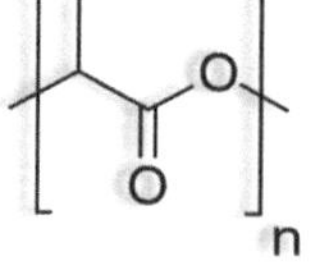

Figure 1.2 Poly(lactic acid) (PLA).

Raw Material Sourcing and Preparation: material is prepared from corn kernels or sugarcane; undergo processing to extract the starch. This starch is then fermented by microorganisms to produce lactic acid.

Lactic Acid Purification: It is then purified through filtration and distillation process to remove impurities and achieve the desired purity level.

Polymerization: The purified lactic acid undergoes condensation polymerization and ring-opening polymerization process to form long chains of PLA polymer.

Surface Finishing: Depending on the application, PLA products may undergo surface finishing processes such as polishing, coating, or printing to improve their appearance or functionality.

Palletization: The PLA polymer is cooled and pelletized into small beads or pellets. Then, it goes for Extrusion process for desired size and mass production.

Quality Control: Throughout the manufacturing process, quality control measures are implemented to ensure that the PLA products meet the required specifications and standards. This involves testing for mechanical properties, dimensions, and visual appearance.

These steps describe specific techniques and parameters may vary depending on factors such as the intended application, equipment used, and quality standards enforced by manufacturers [18, 19].

Polyhydroxy alkanoates (PHA): PHA is a family of polyesters which are prepared by microorganisms like bacteria, fungi, algae, and archaea. Mainly, there are two processes to prepare PHA (Figure 1.3), namely, bacterial fermentation and chemical synthesis, two hydroxy fatty acids are synthesized from two bacteria, *Aeromonas hydrophila* and *Thiococcus pfennigi* [6]. The chemical formula of PHA is shown in Figure 1.3.

Characteristics: melting point: 40–180°C; density: 1.2–1.4 g/cm^3; Tg: –20°C; impact strength: 20–100 kJ/m^2. There are various types of PHA as per its monomers like PHB (polyhydroxy butyrate) and PHBV (polyhydroxy butyrate-co-hydroxybutyrate). It can be recycled to nutrients by living organisms through full biodegradation. The various recycling methods are biodegradation, mechanical recycling, and chemical recycling [20].

Processing: In summary, there are some steps followed to process PBS.

Choice of Microorganism: Numerous sorts of microbes such as germs, yeast, as well as algae can create PHA. The selection of the microorganism relies on variables such as the preferred homes of the PHA coupled with the substratum readily available for fermentation.

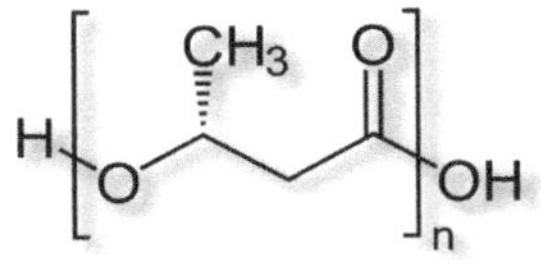

Figure 1.3 Polyhydroxy alkanoates (PHA).

Substratum Selection: PHA-producing microbes normally use eco-friendly carbon resources such as sugars, starches, or fats as substratum for fermentation. The selection of substratum relies on aspects such as expense, accessibility plus compatibility with the picked microorganism.

Fermentation: The chosen microorganism is cultured in a fermenter controlled. Throughout fermentation, the microorganism eats the substratum plus transforms it right into PHA as an intracellular storage space substance [7]. Different criteria such as temperature level, pH, and oxygen focus plus excitement price are maximized to take full advantage.

Celebration: Once the fermentation procedure is full as well as the microorganism has actually collected PHA intracellular, the biomass requires to be gathered [21]. This normally entails separating cells from the fermentation broth, making use of methods such as centrifugation, purification, or flocculation.

Cell Disruption (Optional): In some instances, relying on the microorganism utilized and also the PHA removal approach, cell disruption might be needed to launch the intracellular PHA [22]. Cell interruption strategies consist of mechanical approaches (e.g., grain milling, ultrasonication) or chemical techniques (e.g., enzymatic treatment, solvent removal).

PHA Extraction: After collecting the biomass, PHA is removed from the cells making use of solvents or various other removal techniques. Typical solvents utilized for PHA removal consist of chloroform, chloroform/methanol mixtures or warm water. The selection of removal technique relies on variables such as the kind of PHA created, the pureness demands and also ecological factors to consider.

Improvement: The drawn-out PHA might go through improvement enter to remove contaminations such as recurring biomass, solvent, or various other results. Improvement strategies might consist of rainfall purification or chromatography.

Drying out: The cleansed PHA is commonly dried out to eliminate any type of continuing to be dampness and also get a completely dry powder or granular kind appropriate for more handling or usage in applications.

Handling: The dried out PHA can be more refined right into numerous kinds such as pellets, films, fibers, or built items making use of strategies such as extrusion, shot moulding, compression moulding, or film spreading.

Quality assurance: Throughout the production procedure, quality control steps are applied to make certain that the PHA items fulfil the preferred requirements as well as criteria [5]. This might entail examining the physical, chemical, and also mechanical residential properties of the PHA along with guaranteeing conformity with regulative demands.

Product packaging and also Distribution: Once the PHA items have actually been produced as well as passed quality control checks, they are packaged and also dispersed to clients or end-users for usage in numerous applications.

Key applications: packaging, agriculture, textile, cosmetic and personal care products, water treatment, biodegradable mulch film, etc.

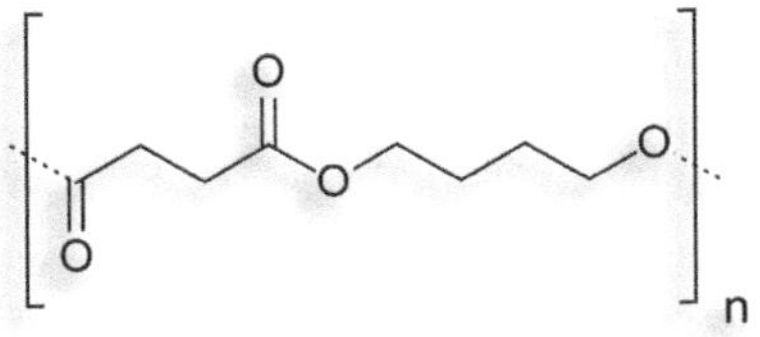

Figure 1.4 Polybutylene succinate (PBS).

Polybutylene succinate (PBS): It is aliphatic polyester with having similar properties of PET. It is sometimes called as polytetramethylene succinate is a bio-based polymer with repeating $C_8H_{12}O_4$ units. In 1863, a Portuguese professor, A. V. Lourenco, described about PBS. There are two types of process which redirects to PBS synthesis, i.e., trans-esterification process and direct esterification process. The characteristics are: melting point: 115°C; density: 1.26 g/c.m^3; glass transition temperature: 60–65°C. PBS is insoluble in water. Bio-based PBS is revolutionary in its two-fold bio properties. The structure of PBS is given in Figure 1.4.

1.4 PROCESSING

Succinic acid is direct esterified with 1,4-butanediol to produce PBS. It consists of two processes, i.e., an excess of diol is esterified with diacid for the formation of PBS oligomers with elimination of water. Then, high molar mass formed by oligomers trans-esterification. Titanium, zirconium, tin, or germanium derivatives are used as catalysts.

Producing PBS entails a number of actions from the manufacturing of basic materials to the last item (Figure 1.5). A review of the production procedure follows:

1.4.1 Raw Material Preparation

Succinic Acid: The key basic material for PBS manufacturing is succinic acid. Succinic acid can be created via different techniques consisting of chain reaction from maleic anhydride or fermentation of renewable resource such as sugar.

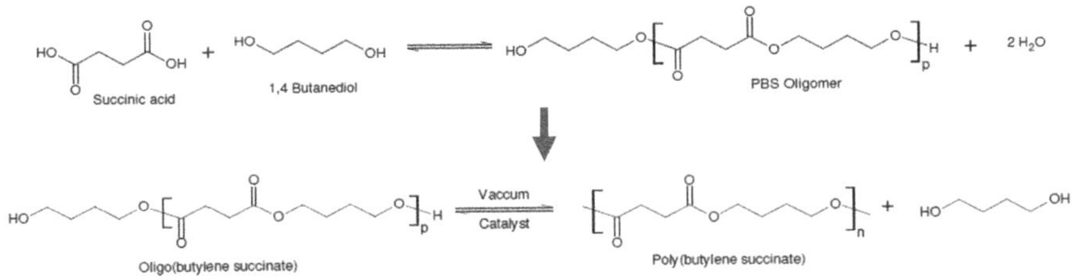

Figure 1.5 Chemical reaction for PBS.

1,4-Butanediol (BDO): Another vital basic material is 1,4-butanediol which is commonly stemmed from petrochemical resources with procedures like hydroformylation of propylene or fermentation of sugars.

Catalysts as well as Additives: Catalysts along with additives might additionally be included in the basic materials to help with the polymerization procedure plus improve the residential or commercial properties of the end PBS product.

Polymerization: The polymerization of succinic acid plus 1,4-butanediol happens via a condensation response developing PBS polymer chains [23]. This response is generally catalysed by certain stimulants under regulated temperature level and also stress problems. Various polymerization methods can be utilized consisting of set, semi-batch, or continual procedures relying on the range of manufacturing along with preferred homes of the PBS polymer [4].

Polymer Processing: PBS polymers can be made into pellets, granules, or powders, via techniques such as extrusion, palletization, or grinding [24]. The polymers might undergo fringe benefit actions such as drying out to get rid of wetness as well as boost storability.

Compounding: PBS might be intensified with ingredients such as plasticizers, stabilizers, fillers, or supports to customize its buildings and also satisfy certain efficiency demands. Compounding procedures entail blending PBS polymers with ingredients utilizing tools such as twin-screw extruders s[25].

Moulding as well as Forming: The cooled PBS material is then built or developed into end products, making use of methods such as shot moulding, extrusion moulding, impact moulding, or thermoforming [26]. The choice of the moulding method relies on the consistency of the item, preferred household or commercial properties as well as manufacturing quantity [27].

Cooling as well as Finishing: After moulding PBS items are cooled down and also solidified to preserve their form and also framework [28]. Additional completing procedures such as cutting, machining, or surface area treatment might be carried out to boost the look plus capability of the end products.

Quality Control: Throughout the production procedure quality assurance steps are carried out to make certain the uniformity, efficiency, and also safety and security of the PBS items [29]. Quality control might entail checking the physical, mechanical, and also thermal characteristics of the polymer and also end products, in addition to adherence to governing criteria and also requirements.

Packaging as well as Distribution: The resulting PBS items are packaged according to the particular needs of clients or end-users and are disseminated for circulation.

In general, polybutylene succinate (PBS) has various applications across different industries due to its biodegradability, mechanical properties, and processability, such as packaging, mulching films, disposable cutlery and tableware, textiles and nonwovens, automotive components, medical devices, biodegradable films and coatings, and 3D printing filaments [27].

Bio-polyethylene: Polyethylene is a type of synthetic polymer made from fossil fuels. It is a thermoplastics polymer exhibit a large number of advantageous properties. Mostly, it is used for commodity applications. By free radical polymerization ethylene monomers are converted into polyethylene in the presence of catalysts. High-pressure processes and steam cracking are used for this purpose. Owing to the increase in oil prices, microbial polyethylene or green polyethylene is now manufactured from dehydration of ethanol produced by microbial fermentation [3]. Currently, bio-ethanol is produced from sugarcane which is used industrially. Sugar cane juice is extracted and anaerobically fermented to produce ethanol. Then, distillation is carried out to remove water and the azeotropic mixture of ethanol,. In the next step, ethanol is dehydrated at a high temperature over a catalyst and Bio-PE is made. Some characteristics of Bio-PE are: melting point 230°C; density 0.94–0.965 g/cm^3; and Young's modulus 750 MPa.

The processing steps of bio-based polyethylene (Bio-PE) are as follows:

1. *Raw Material Sourcing:* Bio-PE is collected from eco-friendly biomass resources such as sugarcane, sugar beet, or corn. The primary step in making Bio-PE is to collect or sourcing these basic materials.
2. *Feedstock Preparation:* The collected biomass is refined to remove the sugars or starches that will certainly work as the feedstock for Bio-PE manufacturing. This might entail squashing, milling, or enzymatic treatment to break down the biomass and also launch the sugars.
3. *Fermentation:* The drawn-out sugars are then fermented by microorganisms such as bacteria or yeast to produce ethanol. This fermentation procedure usually happens in large bioreactors under regulated conditions of temperature level, pH, and oxygen levels.
4. *Dehydration:* The ethanol generated from fermentation undertakes a dehydration procedure to transform it right into ethylene which is the foundation for polyethylene manufacturing. Dehydration is normally accomplished via procedures such as catalytic dehydration or molecular screens.
5. *Polymerization:* The ethylene acquired from dehydration is after that polymerized to create polyethylene. This polymerization procedure might include either high-pressure or low-pressure polymerization strategies depending upon the wanted residential properties of the Bio-PE item.
6. *Additive Incorporation*: Additives such as anti-oxidants, stabilizers, or pigments might be included right into the Bio-PE throughout the polymerization procedure to boost its buildings or look.
7. *Extrusion as well as Forming:* The polymerized Bio-PE is after that expelled with a pass away to create pellets or various other forms appropriate for additional handling or usage. These pellets can be

additional refined utilizing methods such as shot moulding, impact moulding, or extrusion to create end products such as containers, product packaging products or films.

8. *Quality Control:* Throughout the production procedure quality assurance steps are executed to make certain that the Bio-PE items fulfil the preferred requirements as well as criteria. This might include evaluating the mechanical residential or commercial properties, thermal security together with biodegradability of the Bio-PE [30].

9. *Packaging as well as Distribution:* Once the Bio-PE items have actually been made as well as passed quality assurance checks then, they are ready to circulate to consumers or end-users.

Bio-based polyethylene has similar properties to traditional polyethylene but offers the advantage of being derived from renewable sources. The applications are packaging, agricultural films, disposable products, personal care products, medical devices, automotive components and construction materials, etc.

Bio-polypropylene: Bio-based polypropylene (Bio-PP) may be of polypropylene begun from eco-friendly biomass assets such as sugarcane, corn or different other plant items [8]. By utilizing renewable asset sources Bio-PP helps lower reliance on restricted non-renewable fuel source sources as well as diminishes nursery gas depletes related to standard polypropylene fabricating. Bio-PP finds applications completely different markets comprising of item bundling, vehicle, textures as well as strong merchandise. In the vehicle sector, Bio-PP is utilized in indoor components such as entryway boards, control board trim, additionally situate paddings. Its light-weight nature helps diminish vehicle weight upgrading gas adequacy as well as minimizing carbon releases. Bio-PP is expected to play a progressively significant role in the near future.

Processing: The production procedure of Bio-PP includes a number of actions listed below:

Raw Material Sourcing: The primary step in making Bio-PP is to resource eco-friendly biomass feedstocks. These feedstocks can consist of different plant-based products such as sugarcane, corn, or various other biomass plants. These products are selected for their capacity to be exchanged the required chemical parts for polymer manufacturing.

Feedstock Preparation: Once the biomass feedstocks are sourced, they go through handling to remove the wanted elements required for Bio-PP manufacturing. This might include squashing, milling or various other mechanical procedures to break the basic materials right into an appropriate type for more handling.

Chemical Conversion: The drawn-out biomass parts are after that chemically exchanged monomers that can be made use of to manufacture polypropylene [31]. This conversion procedure typically includes a number of actions such as hydrolysis, fermentation, coupled with chain reactions to change the biomass right into propylene monomers.

Polymerization: The propylene monomers acquired from the chemical conversion action are after that polymerized to create Bio-PP polymer chains. Polymerization can be attained with different techniques such as bulk polymerization or gas-phase polymerization, making use of stimulants to start the polymerization response [32].

Purification: After polymerization the Bio-PP polymer undertakes filtration to eliminate any kind of pollutants or unreacted monomers. This action is necessary to guarantee the last Bio-PP item fulfils quality control plus has the wanted buildings.

Processing right into Products: Once cleansed the Bio-PP polymer can be refined right into numerous items making use of strategies such as extrusion, shot moulding, blow moulding or thermoforming [33]. These procedures form the polymer right into end products such as product packaging products, auto elements, fabrics or various other applications.

Quality Control: Throughout the production procedure quality assurance steps are executed to keep an eye on plus guarantee the uniformity and also high quality of the Bio-PP items. This might entail evaluating the mechanical residential or commercial properties, thermal security, molecular weight circulation as well as various other qualities of the polymer [34].

Packaging along with Distribution: Once made as well as quality-tested the Bio-PP items are packaged together with planned for circulation to clients or end-users [35]. Generally, the production procedure of Bio-PP includes comparable actions to standard polypropylene manufacturing with the vital distinction being the usage of eco-friendly biomass feedstocks as opposed to non-renewable fuel sources as the basic material resource.

Starch: it is the end product of photosynthesis in plants and consists of the linear polysaccharide amylose and the highly branched polysaccharide amylopectin. Glass transition temperature lies between $-50°C$ and $110°C$.

The molecular formula of starch is $(C_6H_{10}O_5)n$. Some characteristics are: melting point: $256–258°C$; molar mass: 342.295; density: $1.5–1.8$ g/cm^3; tensile strength: 45 Mpa. Some properties of starch are being insoluble in cold water due to the presence of hydrogen bonds, being non-toxic and biodegradable, texture modification, shear stability, etc.

Processing: Starch production normally includes a number of actions from sourcing basic materials to handling and also improving their properties [36]:

Raw Material Sourcing: Starch can be sourced from different basic materials consisting of corn, wheat, potatoes, cassava, and also rice.

Cleaning plus Washing: The resources undergo cleansing coupled with cleaning to get rid of dust, particles, and also contaminants.

Milling or Grinding: After cleansing, the resources is crushed or based on a great pulp or slurry. This procedure breaks the basic material right into smaller sized bits promoting succeeding handling actions [24].

Separation: The crushed slurry is after that based on splitting up strategies to separate the starch from various other parts such as healthy protein, fiber, as well as lipids [37]. Usual splitting up techniques consist of centrifugation sieving along with hydrocycloning.

Liberation: In this action, the starch granules are freed from the mobile framework of the basic material. This is usually attained with steeping, where the slurry is taken in water to soften the cell wall surfaces as well as launch the starch granules [38].

Wet Processing: The released starch granules are divided from the staying slurry via cleaning together with testing. The starch slurry is after that focused to raise the starch web content as well as get rid of excess water.

Out: The focused starch slurry is dried out to minimize its wetness material and also get the preferred starch powder or granules. Drying out approaches consist of air drying out drum drying out, as well as spray drying out relying on the attributes of the starch as well as the preferred output.

Refining: Depending on the application the starch might undertake refresher courses procedures to boost its pureness, structure, or practical residential properties. This might consist of procedures such as lightening, enzymatic treatment or alteration.

Packaging and also Storage: The dried-out starch is packaged right into bags or containers for circulation coupled with storage space. Correct product packaging aids keep the high quality along with shelf-life of the starch item.

Quality Control: Throughout the production procedure, quality control steps are executed to make certain that the starch satisfies the called for requirements as well as requirements. This might entail screening for specifications such as wetness web content, pureness, bit dimension circulation as well as thickness.

By-product Utilization: Some results created throughout starch production, such as protein-rich deposits or fiber, might be used for pet feed or various other applications to decrease waste and also make best use of source effectiveness.

Some applications are: food industry, textile industry, papermaking, adhesives, pharmaceuticals, personal care products, oil and gas industry etc.

Cellulose: it is a type of biopolymer which is found in trees, cotton, algae and even some bacteria. When sugar molecules (glucose) are linked together by beta-1, 4 glycosidic bonds then cellulose is formed. Cellulose was first discovered in 1838 by the great chemist Anselme Payen. Cellulose has no taste, odourless and hydrophilic in nature. Cellulose chemical formula is $(C_{12}H_{20}O_{10})$.

The properties of this bio-based polymer are high tensile strength, insolubility in the presence of water, biodegradability, good thermal stability, etc. Characteristics: melting point: 260–2700°C; density: 1.5 g/cm^3; glass transition temperature: –3200°C; tensile strength: 1–2 GPa.

Processing: Cellulose is an all-natural polymer discovered in the cell wall surfaces of. Right here are the basic actions associated with production cellulose:

1. *Harvesting:* Cellulose is stemmed from plant resources, mainly trees and also cotton. The very first step in producing cellulose is gathering the raw plant product. (38) For wood-based cellulose trees are commonly harvested from lasting woodlands while cotton-based cellulose includes gathering cotton bolls from cotton plants.
2. *Pulping:* The collected plant product undergoes a pulping procedure to divide the cellulose fibers from various other elements such as lignin, hemicellulose, and pectin. There are numerous approaches:

Mechanical Pulping: In this approach the plant product is mechanically shredded or based on simplify the fibers.

Chemical Pulping: Chemicals such as salt hydroxide (destructive soft drink) as well as salt sulphide are made use of liquefy lignin coupled with various other non-cellulosic elements leaving cellulose fibers.

Semi-Chemical Pulping: This approach integrates mechanical together with chemical refines to break down the plant product right into cellulose fibers.

Washing plus Screening: After pulping and also bleaching the cellulose fibers are cleaned to get rid of any kind of recurring chemicals as well as contaminations.

Drying: The cleaned as well as evaluated cellulose fibers are dried out to decrease their wetness material and also prepare them for more handling [39]. This can be done utilizing approaches such as air drying out or mechanical drying out.

Finishing and also processing: The dried out cellulose fibers might go through added handling actions depending upon their designated usage. As an example:

Packaging as well as Distribution: Once the cellulose items have actually been made, they are packaged and also dispersed to consumers or end-users for usage in their corresponding applications [20].

These are the basic processing steps associated with making cellulose, yet details methods as well as procedures might differ depending upon the sort of plant product made use of (e.g., timber, cotton, bamboo) along with the designated end-use of the cellulose item.

1.5 PROCESSING TECHNIQUES OF BIO-BASED POLYMERS

The production of bio-based polymers includes different methods that intend to effectively transform biomass right into polymer products [13]. Here, the production strategies made use of in the manufacturing of bio-based polymers, highlighting their sustainability and also possible applications.

Biomass Sourcing and Also Pre-treatment: This is the first step in bio-based polymer production is the sourcing of renewable resource biomass products. These can consist of farming deposits, forestry results, specialized power plants, or algae biomass [6]. As soon as it is sourced, the biomass undegoes pre-treatment procedures to eliminate contaminants and also improve its viability for polymer manufacturing. Pre-treatment techniques might consist of milling, grinding, cleaning, as well as enzymatic or chemical processing to break down complex carbohydrates into less complex sugars.

Fermentation plus Bioprocessing: After pre-treatment, the biomass undergoes fermentation or bioprocessing strategies to transform sugars right into monomers or polymer precursors [40]. Microbes such as bacteria, yeast, or fungi are utilized in fermentation procedures to create bio-based monomers such as lactic acid, succinic acid or 3-hydroxypropionic acid. These monomers act as foundation for bio-based polymers like polylactic acid (PLA), polyhydroxyalkanoates (PHA) or polybutylene succinate (PBS).

Polymerization: Polymerization is the vital action in transforming bio-based monomers right into polymer products. As example

Ring-opening Polymerization: Used for PLA coupled with PHA manufacturing, where cyclic monomers are opened up as well as polymerized right into straight chains under regulated problems [2].

Condensation Polymerization: Employed for polyesters such as PBS where monomers with practical teams respond to develop polymer chains along with launch little particles like water or alcohol as by-products.

Polymerization Catalysts: Catalysts such as enzymes, , or organometallic substances are frequently utilized to regulate polymerization kinetics, thus producing with preferred molecular weights plus frameworks.

Extrusion together with Moulding: As soon as polymerized, bio-based polymers are refined right into end products utilizing strategies such as extrusion moulding and then injection moulding, compression moulding are made use of to form molten polymer right into certain geometries consisting of containers, containers, product packaging as well as vehicle parts [41]. Extrusion is a broadly made utilize of dealing with approach for bio-based polymers [42]. Bio-based polymers such as PLA and PHA can be extruded right into fibers, sheets, or motion picture films for applications in item bundling and 3D printing [8].

Injection Moulding: Injection moulding is another popular processing technique, particularly for the production of complex three-dimensional parts. In this process, the polymer resin is melted and injected into a mould cavity under high pressure. Once cooled and solidified, the moulded part is ejected from the mould. Bio-based polymers such as polyethylene (PE) and polypropylene (PP) can be injection moulded into a wide range of products, including automotive components, consumer goods, and medical devices [43–46].

Blow Moulding: Blow moulding is commonly used to produce hollow plastic products such as bottles, containers, and tanks. In this process, a hollow tube or parison of molten polymer is extruded and clamped into a mould cavity. Compressed air is then introduced into the parison, causing it to expand and take the shape of the mould. Bio-based polymers such as polyethylene terephthalate (PET) and bio-based polyethylene (Bio-PE) are often used due to their excellent strength and barrier properties.

Thermoforming: It is a versatile processing method for shaping bio-based polymers into various products such as trays, cups, and packaging inserts [17]. In thermoforming, a sheet of thermoplastic material is heated to its softening point and then formed into a specific shape using a mould or vacuum forming equipment. Bio-based polymers can be thermoformed into the products for food packaging and disposable tableware.

Compression Moulding: It is a cost-effective processing method, particularly for low-volume production runs. In this process, the polymer resin is placed in a heated mould cavity and compressed under high pressure until it takes the shape of the mould [47]. Once cooled, the moulded part is removed from the mould. It is commonly used for producing parts with complex geometries, such as automotive interior components and electrical enclosures [48].

Additive Manufacturing (3D Printing): It is also known as 3D printing, is revolutionizing the way bio-based polymers are processed and used. In this layer-by-layer manufacturing process, a digital model is sliced into thin cross-sectional layers, and successive layers of material are deposited to build up the final part. Bio-based polymers are widely used in 3D printing due to their biodegradability and ease of processing [6]. This technology enables rapid prototyping, customization, and on-demand production for various applications [49].

In conclusion, processing methods play a critical role in converting bio-based polymers into functional products for diverse applications [29]. From extrusion and injection moulding to blow moulding and additive manufacturing, these processing techniques offer versatility, efficiency, and sustainability in the production of bio-based polymer materials.

Surface Modification plus Functionalization: Surface area adjustment methods are used to improve the residential properties with performances of bio-based polymer products for certain applications [50] Surface area treatment such as plasma treatment, chemical grafting, or layer deposition can boost bonding, of bio-based polymers [41]. Functionalization approaches present useful teams or ingredients right into polymer chains to give wanted residential or commercial properties such as antimicrobial activity, UV resistance, or fire resistance [51].

Quality Control plus Certification: Throughout the production procedure, rigorous quality assurance actions are executed to ensure the uniformity, pureness, and efficiency of bio-based polymer items. Quality assurance examinations might consist of molecular weight evaluation, thermal along with mechanical inherent characteristics as well as biodegradability analyses such as ASTM D6866, EN 13432, or USDA.

1.6 IMPORTANCE OF BIO-BASED POLYMERS

Bio-based polymers play a substantial duty in dealing with ecological, financial as well as social difficulties related to conventional petroleum-based plastics. Their significance hinges on a number of vital factors:

Environmental Sustainability: Perhaps one of the most vital elements of bio-based polymers is their payment to ecological sustainability. Unlike petroleum-based plastics, which are lessened from limited non-renewable fuel source plus add to greenhouse gas [40].

Biodegradability coupled with Compostability: Many bio-based polymers are naturally degradable or compostable under ideal conditions, implying they can break down right into all-natural substances such as water, CO_2 as well as biomass via microbial activity [17].

Resource Conservation: It can be sustainably collected and also stored unlike non-renewable fuel sources, which are limited in supply. By using farming waste, or power plants bio-based polymers aid save all-natural deposits and also advertise biodiversity by minimizing stress on land and also water sources.

Reduced Environmental Footprint: The manufacturing of bio-based polymers commonly needs less power inputs as well as creates reduced greenhouse gas exhausts in contrast to standard petroleum-based plastics.

Diversification of Feedstock: A large variety of feedstocks can be used for producing biopolymers, including non-food biomass resources such as farming waste, algae, or effluents. This diversity of feedstocks minimizes competitors with food manufacturing as well as garbage disposal problems. [52].

Market Innovation and also Job Creation: The introduction of bio-based polymers has actually promoted development and also financial investment in eco-friendly innovations, bio-refineries, and also bio-based markets. This development has actually developed brand-new financial possibilities, produced work in countryside and also city locations as well as promoted partnerships between organizations.

Consumer Preference and also Corporate Responsibility: As customers end up being extra eco aware as well as need eco-friendly choices bio-based polymers provide a lasting option for business looking for to fulfil consumer assumptions plus improve brand name online reputation.

Policy Support as well as Market Incentives: Government plus regulative companies worldwide are applying plans; rewards joined with requirements to advertise the fostering of bio-based polymers and also boost market need. These steps consist of eco-friendly power required, carbon prices systems, eco-friendly purchase plans that sensitize and drive market change in the direction of a round bioeconomy. Finally, utilizing sustainable biomass sources, decreasing plastic contamination as well as promoting technology in scientific research, an encouraging path in the direction of an extra lasting coupled with durable future.

1.6 LIMITATIONS OF BIO-BASED POLYMERS

While bio-based polymers supply various benefits they additionally encounter specific constraints and also difficulties that require to be dealt with for prevalent fostering and also business success. A few of the crucial constraints consist of:

Contending Land Use: The farming of biomass feedstock for bio-based polymers might take on food manufacturing, biodiversity preservation, or various other land usages, cause land disputes as well as ecological worries. Cautious land administration and also lasting sourcing techniques are required to alleviate these influences and also make certain the accountable manufacturing of bio-based polymers.

Limited Feedstock Availability: The schedule and also supply of appropriate biomass feedstock for bio-based polymers might be restricted by aspects such as location, environment, dirt top quality, as well as land schedule. Additionally changes in plant returns, seasonal variants, and contending needs for biomass sources can impact the dependability plus scalability of bio-based polymer manufacturing.

Processing Complexity plus Cost: The conversion of biomass right into bio-based polymers typically includes intricate handling strategies such as fermentation, enzymatic hydrolysis, plus polymerization which can be energy-intensive and also costly [39].

Performance and also Durability: Some bio-based polymers might display substandard mechanical, thermal, or obstacle homes contrasted to typical petroleum-based plastics, restricting their viability for sure applications. Enhancements in polymer chemistry, solution, and also handling are required to boost the efficiency, sturdiness, as well as useful residential properties of bio-based polymers plus expand their market approval.

Biodegradability and also Disposal: Not all bio-based polymers are easily naturally degradable under usual ecological problems, and also their deterioration kinetics, by-products, and also ecological influences might differ relying on variables such as polymer structure, handling approach plus disposal atmosphere [19].

Scale-Up and also Commercialization: The laboratory-scale research to commercial manufacturing can be testing because of technological, regulative as well as market unpredictability. Elements such as economic situations of range, manufacturing prices, market need, governing conformity with supply chain logistics should be meticulously thought about to make sure the effective release of bio-based polymer modern technologies.

Performance Consistency as well as Quality Control: Achieving constant item top quality coupled with efficiency requirements throughout various sets of bio-based polymers can be challenging because of variants in biomass structure, handling problems, and also polymer residential properties. Durable quality assurance steps, logical methods plus criteria are important to make certain item integrity, traceability plus conformity with governing needs.

Market Competition and also Consumer Acceptance: It encounter competitors about price, efficiency and market approval. Customer assumptions, choices, together with readiness to spend for lasting items might likewise affect the fostering plus infiltration of bio-based polymers in the market. Education and learning, awareness-building plus advertising initiatives is required to advertise the advantages of bio-based polymers [17].

Finally, while bio-based polymers use appealing options to ecological as well as sustainability obstacles they are not without restrictions with compromises. Attending to these restrictions calls for interdisciplinary partnership, technology, plan assistance coupled with market incentives to conquer obstacles as well as understand the complete capacity of bio-based polymers as a lasting option to traditional plastics.

1.7 APPLICATIONS OF BIO-BASED POLYMERS

Automotive: Bio-based products provide appealing options to improve sustainability in the automobile industry.

Inside parts: Bio-based polymers are made use of different indoor elements of cars to minimize weight, boost longevity as well as enhance cabin air high quality. Bio-based polyurethane froths stemmed from renewable resources such as soybean oil or castor oil is utilized in seat paddings, headliners as well as door panels. *Outside parts:* Bio-based compounds are progressively made use of exterior elements of cars to boost wind resistant, gas performance, as well as recyclability. Bio-based polyesters such as PLA and PHA are used in outside panels, bumpers, and also trim parts. These products supply light-weight, impact-resistant and also corrosion-resistant residential properties, making them appropriate for usage in automobile applications. *Architectural components:* Bio-based compounds are used in architectural parts of cars to boost toughness, tightness as well as crashworthiness while minimizing weight plus ecological effect. All-natural fiber-reinforced compounds such as hemp, flax or kenaf fibers installed in bio-based material floor coverings are made use of in body panels, framework parts as well as indoor supports. *Insulation plus acoustic materials:* Bio-based products are used in insulation together with acoustic applications to lower sound, resonance along with cruelty (NVH) degrees in automobiles while boosting convenience and also power effectiveness. Bio-based froths such as soy-based polyurethane foam or cellulose-based acoustic panels are made use of in headliners, door panels, along with flooring floor coverings. These products use sound-absorbing, thermal-insulating plus moisture-resistant buildings, boosting the indoor convenience plus peacefulness of automobiles. ***Bio-based lubricants and also fluids:*** Bio-based lubricating substances as well as liquids stemmed from renewable resource like veggie oils or bioethanol are made use of in vehicle applications to minimize rubbing, wear as well as exhausts while boosting efficiency as well as durability. Bio-based engine oils, transmission liquids along with hydraulic liquids provide lubrication residential properties similar to traditional petroleum-based equivalents while reducing ecological influence as well as conference regulative criteria. ***Lasting manufacturing practices:*** Bio-based products are used in vehicle production procedures to decrease power intake, waste generation, plus carbon exhausts [15]. Bio-based materials, adhesives, coupled with coverings are utilized in bonding, securing as well as completing procedures to minimize unpredictable natural substance exhausts as well as enhance air high quality in production centres.

Household Sectors: ***Product Packaging and also Containers and Cleaning Products:*** Bio-based polymers are included right into family cleansing items to enhance their ecological account as well as decrease using unsafe chemicals. Naturally degradable surfactants together with polymers acquired from renewable resources such as plant oils, sugars, or starches are utilized in dishwashing cleaning agents washing cleaning agents along with surface area cleansers. These bio-based components use reliable cleansing efficiency while decreasing ecological influence and also advertising more secure choices for household usage [10].

Textiles as well as Fabrics: Bio-based polymers are used in the manufacturing of environmentally friendly fabrics as well as materials for household uses.

Furniture as well as Home Decor: Bio-based polymers are incorporated right into furnishings and also house layout items to boost sustainability together with reduced ecological influence. Bio-based products such as bio-based polyethylene (Bio-PE) along with bio-based polyurethane (Bio-PUR) are used in manufacturing chairs, tables, couches with cushions. These products are known for their durability and convenience along with visual appeal while reducing dependence on non-renewable fuel sources and also promoting the use of renewable resources in home furnishings.

Food Storage as well as Preservation: Bio-based polymers are used in home food storage areas and conservation products to prolong shelf life, reduce food waste, and lessen environmental impact. Fruits, vegetables, leftovers, and snacks are packaged in biodegradable and naturally degradable food covers, bags, and containers manufactured of bio-based polymers like PLA, PHA, and starch-based plastics. These products are safe for food contact, environmentally friendly, and feature superior barrier structures against moisture and oxygen.

Home Appliances as well as Electronics: Bio-based polymers are progressively used in family devices and also electronic devices to enhance sustainability and also lower carbon impact. Bio-based plastics such as PLA, Bio-PE, and also bio-based polycarbonate (Bio-PC) are made use of in the manufacturing of housings, panels, as well as parts for devices such as fridges, cleaning makers, along with little digital gadgets.

Building and Construction: Bio-based polymers discover applications in the structure and building market for creating lasting structure products, insulation, coverings, and composites. Bio-based polyurethane (Bio-PUR) along with bio-based epoxy materials are used to make eco-friendly insulation products, bio-composite panels, adhesives, sealers, and coverings. These products provide thermal insulation, wetness resistance plus resilience while lowering ecological impact.

Agricultural Films as well as Mulches: Bio-based polymers are made use of in farming for creating naturally degradable films as well as mulches to enhance plant return, dirt wellness, and also water preservation. Bio-based polymers such as PLA and PHA coupled with starch-based plastics are used to produce compostable films, greenhouse films, bursey pots as well as plant product packaging products [11]. These products supply advantages such as weed reductions, dirt dampness retention, and also biodegradability advertising lasting farming techniques.

Clinical coupled with Healthcare: In the clinical as well as healthcare field, bio-based polymers are used in different applications such as clinical gadgets, medication distribution systems, scaffolds design along with injury treatment items. Bio-based polymers such as PLA and PHA, along with bio-based polyesters, are used to create naturally degradable and also biodegradable implants, sutures medical mesh, drug-eluting stents, and also injury dressings.

1.8 CONCLUSION

In sum, production of bio-based polymers holds an encouraging opportunity for a lasting growth in different markets. Via cutting-edge modern technologies as well as procedures these polymers stemmed from renewable resources, considerable possibilities to minimize ecological effect coupled. Additionally, the innovation of bio-based polymer handling methods boosts product homes, offering options that satisfy the strenuous requirements of modern-day applications while sticking to environmentally friendly concepts. Nevertheless, obstacles such as scalability, economical as well as efficiency optimization remain to be resolved via recurring studies coupled with advancement initiatives.

Diverse Applications of Bio-based Polymers – Among the crucial benefits of bio-based polymers is their convenience in applications throughout several sectors. In addition, bio-based polymers are being discovered for usage in the vehicle market, where they can be made use of to make light-weight elements that add to sustain effectiveness as well as decreased discharges. In the biomedical field bio-based polymers have actually revealed terrific possibility for numerous applications, consisting of substance distribution systems, cells design scaffolds along with clinical implants. These products are naturally degradable, suggesting that they are well-tolerated by the body plus can break down normally over time, lessening the requirement for added surgical procedures or treatments.

Driving Innovation for a Sustainable Future – Innovations in bio-based polymer handling as well as applications are evidence to the recurring initiatives to create lasting products that can attend to pushing ecological issues.

Finally, the advancements in bio-based polymers provide possible services to the difficulties positioned by conventional petroleum-based plastics adding to decreased carbon impact as well as boosted eco-friendliness. Furthermore, the functional applications of bio-based polymers in different markets such as product packaging, vehicle plus biomedical sectors highlight their possibility to drive development plus resolve pressing ecological issues. As research and development progresses, bio-based polymers are poised to play a crucial role in forming a much more lasting and also eco-friendly future for product scientific research plus design.

REFERENCES

1. Rosenboom, J.G.; Langer, R.; Traverso, G. Bioplastics for a Circular Economy. *Nat Rev Mater.* **2022**, *7*(2), 117–137. https://doi.org/10.1038/s41578-021-00407-8. Epub 2022 Jan 20. PMID: 35075395; PMCID: PMC8771173.

2. Babu, R.P.; O'Connor, K.; Seeram, R. Current Progress on Bio-Based Polymers and Their Future Trends. *Prog Biomater.* **2013** Mar 18, 2(1), 8. https://doi.org/10.1186/2194-0517-2-8. PMID: 29470779; PMCID: PMC5151099.

3. Berezina, N.; Martelli, S. Bio-based Polymers and Materials. *RSC Green Chemistry.* **2014**, 1–28. https://doi.org/10.1039/9781782620181-00001.

4. Okolie, O.; Kumar, A.; Edwards, C.; Lawton, L.A.; Oke, A.; McDonald, S.; Thakur, V.K.; Njuguna, J. Bio-Based Sustainable Polymers and Materials: From Processing to Biodegradation. *J. Compos. Sci.* **2023**, *7*(6), 213. https://doi.org/10.3390/jcs7060213

5. Lu, D.R.; Xiao, C.M.; Xu, S.J. Starch-Based Completely Biodegradable Polymer Materials. *Express Polym. Lett.* **2009**, *3*, 366–375.

6. Winkworth-Smith, C.; Foster, T.J. General Overview of Biopolymers: Structure, Properties, and Applications. In Sabu Thomas, Dominique Durand, Christophe Chassenieux, and Jyotishkumar (Eds.), *Handbook of Biopolymer-Based Materials: From Blends and Composites to Gels and Complex Networks.* Wiley-VCH: Weinheim, Germany, **2013**; pp. 7–36. ISBN 9783527328840.

7. Rinaudo, M. Chitin and Chitosan: Properties and Applications. *Prog. Polym. Sci.* **2006**, *31*, 603–632.
8. Narayan, R.; Tran, T.P. *Sustainable Biopolymer Nanocomposites: Advanced Processing, Properties, and Applications.* Springer: Germany, **2019**.
9. Mohanty, A.K.; Misra, M.; Hinrichsen, G. (Eds.). *BioFiber Reinforcements in Composite Materials.* Woodhead Publishing: United Kingdom, **2017**.
10. Rinaudo, M. (Ed.). *Chitin and Chitosan: Properties and Applications.* John Wiley & Sons: USA, **2019**.
11. Singh, R.; Gautam, S.; Sharma, B.; Jain, P.; Chauhan, K.D. *Biopolymers and Their Classifications*; Elsevier Inc.: New Delhi, India, **2021**; ISBN 9780128192405.
12. Di Donato, P.; Taurisano, V.; Poli, A.; Gomez, G.; Nicolaus, B.; Malinconinco, M.; Santagata, G. Vegetable Wastes Derived Polysaccharides as Natural Eco-Friendly Plasticizers of Sodium Alginate. *Carbohydr. Polym.* **2020**, *229*, 115427.
13. Wang, W.; Meng, Q.; Li, Q.; Liu, J.; Zhou, M.; Jin, Z.; Zhao, K. Chitosan Derivatives and Their Application in Biomedicine. *Int. J. Mol. Sci.* **2020**, *21*, 487.
14. Gupta, R. K.; Sharma, A.K. *Biopolymer-Based Materials for Sustainable Development and Biomedical Applications.* CRC Press: USA, **2019**.
15. Plackett, D.; Berglund, L. (Eds.). *Biopolymers: New Materials for Sustainable Films and Coatings.* John Wiley & Sons: USA, **2019**.
16. Du, Y.; Li, S.; Zhang, Y.; Rempel, C.; Liu, Q. Treatments of Protein for Biopolymer Production in View of Processability and Physical Properties: A Review. *J. Appl. Polym. Sci.* **2016**, *133*, 43351.
17. Bastiaens, L.; Soetemans, L.; Hondt, E.D.; Elst, K. Sources of Chitin and Chitosan and Their Isolation. *Chitin Chitosan Prop. Appl.* **2019**, 1–34.
18. Jones, R.; Petrie, E.M. (Eds.). *Biopolymer Processing Technologies.* CRC Press: USA, **2018**.
19. Gautam, K.; Vishvakarma, R.; Sharma, P.; Singh, A.; Kumar, V.; Varjani, S.; Kumar, J. Production of Biopolymers from Food Waste: Constrains and Perspectives. *Bioresour. Technol.* **2022**, *361*, 127650.
20. Chen, Q.; Roethe, J.A.; Boccaccini, A.R. Tissue Engineering Scaffolds from Bioactive Glass and Composite Materials. *Top. Tissue Eng.* **2008**, 4, 1–27.
21. Jiang, G.; Hou, X.; Zeng, X.; Zhang, C.; Wu, H.; Shen, G.; Li, S.; Luo, Q.; Li, M.; Liu, X.; et al. Preparation and Characterization of Indicator Films from Carboxymethyl-Cellulose/Starch and Purple Sweet Potato (*Ipomoea Batatas* (L.) Lam) Anthocyanins for Monitoring Fish Freshness. *Int. J. Biol. Macromol.* **2020**, *143*, 359–372.
22. Olatunji, O. *Natural Polymers: Industry Techniques and Applications.* Springer: Cham, Switzerland, **2015**; pp. 1–370.
23. Salit, M.S.; Jawaid, M.; Yusoff, N.B.; Hoque, M.E. *Manufacturing of Natural Fibre Reinforced Polymer Composites.* Springer: Cham, Switzerland, **2015**; pp. 1–383.
24. Djagny, K.B.; Wang, Z.; Xu, S. Gelatin: A Valuable Protein for Food and Pharmaceutical Industries: Review. *Crit. Rev. Food Sci. Nutr.* **2001**, *41*, 481–492.
25. Koller, M.; Mukherjee, A. A New Wave of Industrialization of PHA Biopolyesters. *Bioengineering* **2022**, *9*, 74.

26. Chen, G.Q.; Patel, M.K. Plastics Derived from Biological Sources: Present and Future: A Technical and Environmental Review. *Chem. Rev.* **2012**, *112*, 2082–2099.

27. Cooper, W.J.; Krasicky, P.D. Dissolution Rates of Poly (Methyl Methacrylate) Films in Mixed Solvents. *J. Appl. Polym. Sci.* **1986**, *31*, 65–73.

28. Wang, L.; Auty, M.A.E.; Rau, A.; Kerry, J.F.; Kerry, J.P. Effect of PH and Addition of Corn Oil on the Properties of Gelatin-Based Biopolymer Films. *J. Food Eng.* **2009**, *90*, 11–19.

29. Lagrain, B.; Goderis, B.; Brijs, K.; Delcour, J.A. Molecular Basis of Processing Wheat Gluten toward Biobased Materials. *Biomacromolecules* **2010**, *11*, 533–541.

30. Papanu, J.S.; Hess, D.W.; Soane (Soong), D.S.; Bell, A.T. Swelling of Poly(Methyl Methacrylate) Thin Films in Low Molecular Weight Alcohols. *J. Appl. Polym. Sci.* **1990**, *39*, 803–823.

31. Cameron, D.J.A.; Shaver, M.P. Aliphatic Polyester Polymer Stars: Synthesis, Properties and Applications in Biomedicine and Nanotechnology. *Chem. Soc. Rev.* **2011**, *40*, 1761–1776.

32. Rhim, J.W.; Ng, P.K.W. Natural Biopolymer-Based Nanocomposite Films for Packaging Applications. *Crit. Rev. Food Sci. Nutr.* **2007**, *47*, 411–433.

33. Ranganathan, S.; Dutta, S.; Moses, J.A.; Anandharamakrishnan, C. Utilization of Food Waste Streams for the Production of Biopolymers. *Heliyon* **2020**, *6*, e04891.

34. Pechová, V.; Gajdziok, J.; Muselík, J.; Vetchý, D. Development of Orodispersible Films Containing Benzydamine Hydrochloride Using a Modified Solvent Casting Method. *AAPS PharmSciTech* **2018**, *19*, 2509–2518.

35. Aaliya, B.; Sunooj, K.V.; Lackner, M. Biopolymer Composites: A Review. *Int. J. Biobased Plast.* **2021**, *3*, 40–84.

36. Baranwal, A.; Kumar, A.; Priyadharshini, A.; Oggu, G.S.; Bhatnagar, I.; Srivastava, A.; Chandra, P. Chitosan: An Undisputed Bio-Fabrication Material for Tissue Engineering and Bio-Sensing Applications. *Int. J. Biol. Macromol.* **2018**, *110*, 110–123.

37. Pattanashetti, N.A.; Heggannavar, G.B.; Kariduraganavar, M.Y. Smart Biopolymers and Their Biomedical Applications. *Procedia Manuf.* **2017**, *12*, 263–279.

38. Mekonnen, T.; Mussone, P.; Khalil, H.; Bressler, D. Progress in Bio-Based Plastics and Plasticizing Modifications. *J. Mater. Chem. A* **2013**, *1*, 13379–13398.

39. George, A.; Sanjay, M.R.; Srisuk, R.; Parameswaranpillai, J.; Siengchin, S. A Comprehensive Review on Chemical Properties and Applications of Biopolymers and Their Composites. *Int. J. Biol. Macromol.* **2020**, *154*, 329–338.

40. Kamal, H.; Foh Le, C.; Salter, A.M.; Ali, A.; Asgar Ali, C. Extraction of Protein from Food Waste: An Overview of Current Status and Opportunities. *Compr. Rev. Food Sci. Food Saf.* **2021**, *20*, 2455–2475.

41. Shariatinia, Z. Pharmaceutical Applications of Chitosan. *Adv. Colloid Interface Sci.* **2019**, *263*, 131–194.

42. Manian, A.P.; Široká, B.; Bechtold, T. Polysaccharide Applications in Textiles and Materials Technologies. *Lezinger Ber.* **2012**, *91*, 98–102.

43. Prasad, A.; Bhasney, S.M.; Prasannavenkadesan, V.; Sankar, M.R.; Katiyar, V. Polylactic Acid Reinforced with Nano-Hydroxyapatite Bioabsorbable Cortical Screws for Bone Fracture Treatment. *J Polym Res.* **2023**, *30*(5), 177.

44. Prasad, A.; Bhasney, S.M.; Prasannavenkadesan, V.; Sankar, M.R.; Katiyar, V. Nano-hydroxyapatite Reinforced Polylactic Acid Bioabsorbable Cancellous Screws for Bone Fracture Fixations. *J Appl Polym Sci.* **2023**, *140*(43), e54577.

45. Prasad, A. Bioabsorbable Polymeric Materials for Biofilms and Other Biomedical Applications: Recent and Future Trends. *Mater Today: Proc.* **2021**, *44*, 2447–2453.

46. Prasad, A. State of Art Review on Bioabsorbable Polymeric Scaffolds for Bone Tissue Engineering. *Mater Today: Proc.* **2021**, *44*, 1391–1400.

47. Bigi, A.; Cojazzi, G.; Panzavolta, S.; Roveri, N.; Rubini, K. Stabilization of Gelatin Films by Crosslinking with Genipin. *Biomaterials* **2002**, *23*, 4827–4832.

48. Valdés, A.; Garrigós, M.C. Carbohydrate-Based Advanced Biomaterials for Food Sustainability: A Review. *Mater. Sci. Forum* **2016**, *842*, 182–195.

49. Thakur, V.K.; Thakur, M.K. *Handbook of Composites from Biorenewable Resources: Processing and Applications.* John Wiley & Sons: USA, **2019**.

50. Agarwal, S. Major Factors Affecting the Characteristics of Starch Based Biopolymer Films. *Eur. Polym. J.* **2021**, *160*, 110788.

51. Ray, S.S.; Bousmina, M. (Eds.). *Biopolymer Nanocomposites: Processing, Properties, and Applications.* John Wiley & Sons: USA, **2017**.

52. Abdelmouleh, M.; Boufi, S.; Belgacem, M.N.; Dufresne, A. Short Natural-Fibre Reinforced Polyethylene and Natural Rubber Composites: Effect of Silane Coupling Agents and Fibres Loading. *Compos. Sci. Technol.* **2007**, *67*, 1627–1639.

Processing and Characterization of Bionanocomposites

Manjeeta Kumari, Manisha Chadha, and Shiwani Berry

2.1 INTRODUCTION

Bionanocomposites is a new emerging area of research. The term "bionanocomposites" refers to two-component bio-based polymers, one of which serves as a reinforcement agent and has dimensions between 1 and 100 nm, and the other acts as a matrix (Sharma *et al.*, 2020). The interface between the dispersed nanoparticles and the polymeric matrix is improved by large surface area of the nanosized particles, which gives bionanocomposites their key functional properties like improved tensile strength, electrical conductivity, heat stability, better barrier properties, electrostatic stability and improved chemical resistance. Nanocomposite materials are made up of biopolymers such as proteins, polysaccharides and lipids exhibit excellent thermal, mechanical, chemical resistance and antimicrobial properties towards moisture, lipids and flavors (Khanzadi *et al.*, 2015; Mahdi *et al.*, 2015). Because of being their biodegradability, availability, economic cost, and capacity to diminish the significant use of fossil fuels, bio-nano-composites are promising basis for their replacement.

Nanofillers are made from a wide variety of materials, for example metals, oxides, polymers, and carbon-based materials. Nanofillers are often used as additives to improve the properties of various materials, including composites, polymers, ceramics, and coatings. They can improve mechanical properties for instance strength, stiffness, and toughness, in addition to electrical and thermal conductivity, and barrier properties. A number of significant studies conducted during last years established that nanoparticles made up of cellulose (Siqueira *et al.*, 2010). Nanofillers can also enhance the optical and magnetic properties of bionanocomposites. Some examples of nanofillers include nanoparticles of silica, alumina, titanium dioxide, carbon nanotubes, graphene, and nanoclay. These materials are commonly used in applications such as automotive parts, electronics, medical devices, and packaging materials, among others. Nanofillers like AgO, ZnO, montmorillonite, SiO_2 biodegradable polymers like, polybutylene succinate, poly-caprolactone, polyhydroxylbutyrate and polylactic acid and TiO_2 can be combined through natural biopolymers like starch and

DOI: 10.1201/9781003470311-2

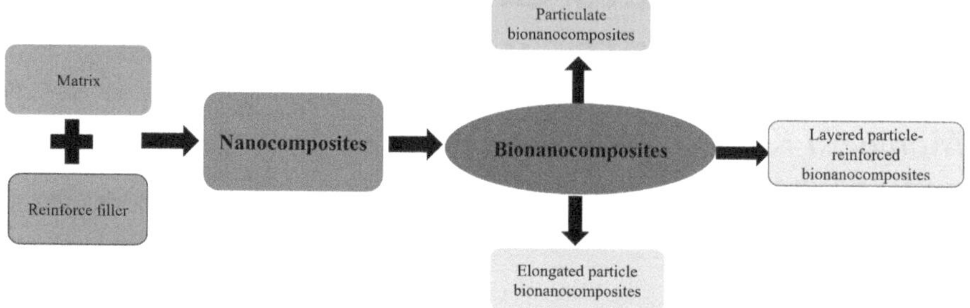

Figure 2.1 Types of Bionanocomposites

chitosan to modify bio-nanocomposites. The development of long-lasting, environmentally friendly food packaging is made possible by the combination of biopolymers and nanofillers. Bionanocomposites are auspicious materials for developing applications, such as biosensor, environmental remediation, biomedicine and photonics.

2.1.1 Constituents of Bionanocomposites

Bionanocomposites are mostly made of cellulose, lignin, and hemicellulose. Bionanocomposites are made up of biomaterials that are found naturally.

Cellulose: Cellulose is mainly present in animals and plants. Cellulose nanofibers are naturally inexpensive, widely available, and easily recyclable through combustion. They also take little energy to produce. Microfibrils and whiskers are the two main types of nano reinforcements that can be produced from cellulose (Azeredo, 2009; Oksman *et al.*, 2016).

Chitosan: Chitosan is a natural polymer contains a large number of OH and NH_2 substituents. It is generally created by deacetylating chitin. It is a linear copolymer with beta (1,4) linkage unit and also consists of 2-amino-2-deoxy-D-glycopyranos and 2-acetamido2-deoxy-D-glucopyranose. Chitosan is used in various medical procedures, including the creation of absorbable sutures and wound dressings.

Chitin: N-acetylglucosamine units are used to create the modified cellulose with a high molecular weight known as chitin. It primarily aids as an efficient binder in dyes and textiles (Mousa *et al.*, 2016).

Poly-lactic acid: PLA also identified as Poly lactide is one of the most extensively fabricated bioplastics. PLA is a thermoplastic unit made from renewable resources like corn. PLA is used for a number of things, including food, packaging, textiles, and medical equipment (Mousa *et al.*, 2016)

Starch: Starch is a polysaccharide that has two components: amylose and amylopectin. In plants and microbes, starch is mostly useful for energy storage. Starch is present in all staple foods, i.e., maize, rice, barley, potatoes, and wheat. They are a good source of energy (Mousa *et al.*, 2016).

Polyhydroxyalkanoates (PHAs): PHAs can be synthesized by various microorganisms, including bacteria, archaea, and some eukaryotic microorganisms. These biopolymers are composed of repeating units of hydroxyalkanoic acids, which can vary in their chain length and degree of saturation. Polyhydroxyalkanoates varies in existing forms which are further utilized by the microorganisms in the interior of the cell by means of light-refracting granules for energy storage (Mousa *et al.*, 2016).

Chitosan has drawn a lot of attention among the polymer-based materials due to its advantageous properties, including its bacteriostatic properties, biosensor applications biodegradability, biocompatibility, and are able to control the leaching as well as delivery of materials nontoxicity, food packaging, lesion-curing properties along with texture correction applications (Hosseinnejad & Jafari, 2016; Jabbari *et al.*, 2019; Kumar & Koh, 2014).

2.1.2 Classification of Bionanocomposite Materials

2.1.2.1 Polyester-based Nanocomposites

Polyester-based nanocomposites are materials that contain a polymer matrix made of polyester and nanoparticles of different materials dispersed throughout the matrix. Thermoplastic and thermoset polymers both benefit from polyesters (Valerio *et al.*, 2018). Polyester-based nanocomposites are created by mixing nanoparticles with polyester resin and then curing the mixture. The resulting composite material has enhanced applications such as increased rigidity, firmness, strength and heat tolerance. Comparing with traditional polyester composites. Good-performance polyester nanocomposites have been created with the help of nanotechnology. Nanoparticles used in these composites can be of different types such as carbon nanotubes, clay, silica, and graphene. The inclusion of nanoparticles to polyester matrix provides a large interfacial area in the middle of matrix and nanoparticles, resulting in enhanced properties. Polyester-based nanocomposites have applications in various fields, including automotive, aerospace, packaging, and construction industries. These materials have excellent mechanical and thermal properties and can be used to exchange traditional materials like ceramics and metals.

2.1.2.2 Polysaccharides-based Nanocomposites

Polysaccharide-based nanocomposites are materials composed of a polymer matrix made of polysaccharides and nanoparticles. Several saccharide units are connected to one another by glycosidic connections to form polysaccharides, which differ from the other families of biopolymers in a number of distinctive ways (Zheng *et al.*, 2015). Polysaccharides are carbohydrates consisting of many monosaccharide units bonded together, like cellulose, chitin, starch, and chitosan. Typically, polysaccharides are much durable than nucleic acids and proteins and do not irreversibly denature when heated. Nanoparticles used in these composites are typically inorganic materials such as silica, clay, or metal oxide nanoparticles. These nanoparticles are dispersed inside the polysaccharide matrix through various procedure , such as solution casting, electrospinning, or extrusion.

The addition of nanoparticles to polysaccharide matrix provides unique properties to resulting nanocomposites, like enhanced mechanical strength, barrier properties and thermal stability. Comparing poly-saccharides based nanocomposites to typical polymers, they may also possess better biocompatibility, antibacterial qualities and biodegradability. Food packaging, drug delivery system and biomedical devices are just a few of the many possible uses for polysaccharide-based nanocomposites. Poly-saccharides based nanocomposites are also being looked into for application in environmentally sustainable materials due to their biocompatibility and biodegradability.

2.1.2.2 Protein-based Nanocomposites

A type of material known as protein-based bionanocomposites mixes proteins and nanoparticles to create a composite material with special features. Due to their potential applications these materials have drawn interest in a number of industries, such as biology and electronics. A naturally occurring protein like silk, collagen, or elastin makes up the bionanocomposite's protein component. Biomedicine is one of the most promising fields in which protein-based bionanocomposites can be used. Protein materials are interesting candidates because of their exceptional and well-developed nanoscale structure and elegant mechanical effects. Protein component or protein-based composites serve as a recognition elements for particular molecule and the nanoparticles can give signal amplification or detecting capabilities which makes them useful in biosensors. In order to produce new kind of electronic devices, protein's unique mechanical and electrical capabilities can be joined with nanoparticles distinctive optical or electronic properties. To make flexible, transparent electrodes for electronics or flexible displays, gold nanoparticles encapsulated in silk fibroin can be employed. Overall, protein-based bionanocomposites offer an exclusive set of properties that make them attractive for a range of applications.

2.2 PROCESSING OF BIONANOCOMPOSITES

The processing of bionanocomposites comprises the merger of nanoparticles into biopolymer to fabricate a single composite material with "nanoscale" particle dispersion. The employed processing regime and technique necessitate taking into account the fact that the processing's main goal is to guarantee proper blend of the particles of nano range in bio-polymer matrices. For example, bionanocomposites containing CNTs, the processing conditions are crucial for achieving well-dispersed nano scale particles while concurrently guaranteeing the structural integrity of the nanoparticles. Degradation should be avoided, and the processing technique and regime should have as little negative impact as possible on the parent polymer. Bionanocomposites are typically made by using three fundamental techniques:

2.2.1 In Situ Polymerization

This technique refers to synthesis of a polymer directly within a material or on its surface, rather than creating the polymer in a separate process and then applying it to the material. In this method, the monomer or monomers are combined with an initiator or catalyst and allowed to react inside the material or on its surface, creating a polymer. For the resulting polymer to have the appropriate qualities and performance, the monomer, catalyst, and reaction conditions must be chosen carefully.

The selection of the monomer, catalyst, and reaction conditions is necessary to achieve the desired performance and effects of the resultant polymer.

2.2.2 Solution Casting Treatment

This treatment is widely used, efficient and straightforward procedure to produce bio nanocomposites in an aqueous media. Through this procedure, the proper blending of polymers and nanofillers is ensured. This approach takes both mixing absorption and duration into account to guarantee uniform filler dispersion in the polymer matrix (Madhumitha *et al.*, 2018).

2.2.3 Melt Procesing Method

Melt processing involves combing nanoparticles and polymers in fused state. In this method, molecules are heated and embedded within the polymers. Because it uses no organic solvents, this method is harmless for the environment (Ojijo & Sinha, 2013). In solution techniques, the polymer matrix is melted with nanoparticles in appropriate solvent, and the solvent is then either evaporated or precipitated. The polymer solvent casting technique is a quick, low-cost method that is frequently used to process flexible biopolymers. The nanoparticles are typically distributed in one solvent while the polymer is typically dissolved in another, and the two components are then combined. A crucial issue that needs to be clarified is the impact of solvent on the processing of films and the properties of materials. The chosen solvent does, in fact, have an impact on the film's qualities in terms of its thermal, mechanical, and surface characteristics (Müller *et al.*, 2017).

2.2.4 Processing Techniques of Polysaccharide-based Nanocomposites

The biosphere's most easily accessible biomolecules are polysaccharides (Chivrac *et al.*, 2009; Dufresne, 2010). The molecules that make up this category of polymers include starch, cellulose, and chitin/chitosan. Solvent intercalation or melt processing are the primary methods used to create nanocomposites (Ojijo & Sinha, 2013). The majority of studies have concentrated on hydro-soluble (or hydro-dispersible) polysaccharide nanoparticles because they produce watery suspensions. Using surfactants or chemical grafting, it is feasible to disperse these nanocrystals in non-aqueous environments, opening up new processing options for nanocomposite materials. The reactive surface that is coated in hydroxyl groups on polysaccharide nanocrystals allows for significant chemical modification (Dufresne, 2010). The reinforcement in first research on cellulose nanocomposites made by solution casting were CNCs, also known as nanowhiskers, and the matrix materials were water soluble like latex or starch (CNWs). Nanocomposites films can be created using a straightforward process and without the use of any specialized tools. Furthermore, by utilizing the common solvent effect, excellent dispersion was typically attained. The creation of 2D framework of nano-crystals or nanofibres in polymer matrix, seen to be advantageous for mechanical properties of these materials, is another well-known benefit of the slow evaporation stage. On the other hand, this gradual evaporation process occasionally caused the nano-crystals in the solution comprising of polymer to settle, resulting in a gradient of concentration in the final nanocomposites and nonhomogeneous distribution of the reinforcements in the matrix. The commonly reported processing methods for the intercalation starch/clay are melt intercalation, in situ intercalative polymerization, and intercalation of polymer. In situ intercalative polymerization, which differs from ion exchange methods in that it uses heat, radiation, or a catalyst to help the clay swell up in the presence of a liquid monomer, is another type of polymerization process. Contrarily, in melt intercalation processes, it has been claimed that during the polymerization process, the solvent molecules are desorbed from the silicate layer, facilitating smooth flow of the incoming polymer. This strategy is regarded as being more environmentally friendly and is very compatible with good environmental practices (Zheng *et al.*, 2015). Chitosan is a perfect material for intercalation in MMT-Na$^+$ via cationic exchange because of the polycationic nature of chitosan in acidic media. In fact, MMTNa$^+$ has been the preferred clay for use in creating chitosan/clay nanocomposites. Chitosan is a readily adsorbed polycation in an acidic medium on the MMT-Na$^+$ surface. Due to Coulombic interactions between the chitosan and the clay molecules, the surface phenomenon is regulated by the detailed description of cationic exchange. In Chitosan structures quantity of clay present has an impact on the nanocomposites' structure and characteristics (Ojijo & Sinha, 2013).

2.2.5 Processing Strategies of Polyester-based Nanocomposites

Unsaturated polyesters (UPEs) are a type of petroleum-based resins that are widely used for their cost-effectiveness, ease of handling, and well-balanced mechanical, electrical, chemical, and fire resistance properties, and are naturally brittle materials (Haq *et al.*, 2009). The integration of nanoparticles into the polymer matrix during the processing of nano-composites based on aliphatic polyester results in a novel material with a nanometric dispersion of the chosen particles. In most cases, obtaining a nano-homogeneous quantity of nanoparticles requires modification of the characteristics of the biopolymer. Nanoparticles are gently mixed with the help of mechanic waves into the polyester, in the melt process-ing technique, to choose a process temperature that is more than the melting temperature (Tm) and considerably lower than the deteriora-tion, it is necessary to know the temperatures at which polymers melt and thermally degrade in an oxidizing environment. Additionally, the temperature at which a nanoparticle begins to degrade thermally, par-ticularly for bio-based nanoparticles, is crucial in deciding the mixing circumstances (Armentano *et al.*, n.d.). The in situ polymerization tech-nique has only been used in a small number of experiments to create PLA/clay nanocomposites. MMT, C25A, and C30B organoclays were produced by using aluminium triisopropoxide as the catalyst in an in situ ring opening polymerization of l-lactide (Ojijo & Sinha, 2013). PHAs are thermally sensitive to the processing circumstances, just like PLA. Despite the fact that in situ polymerization frequently results in nanocomposites with excellent clay dispersion, a number of drawbacks make this method unsuitable for industrial applications. Its commer-cial applications might be constrained by organometallic catalysts, degradation-sensitive monomers, and occasionally the requirement for solvent(s). Additionally, melt intercalation is a method that is favoured in the commercial processing of polymers because it is environmentally friendly. However, it is not always simple to produce exfoliated struc-tures through liquid intercalation. Alternative approaches have there-fore been investigated, such as creating master batches through in situ polymerization prior to melt mixing in a polymer.

2.2.6 Processing Techniques of Protein-based Nanocomposites

For degradable bionanocomposite materials such as dairy products (milk, yogurt, cheese), whey protein, gelatine, egg white, and fish myofibrillar protein are the primary animal-derived sources of protein (Zhao *et al.*, 2008). By using solvent casting, sequential mix and melt extrusion of the two processes, protein/clay nanocomposites have been created (Ojijo & Sinha, 2013). The processing conditions on intercalation and exfoliation have been studied in recent developments in melt intercalation. For twin-screw extrusion, it has been observed that the shear rate is crucial for initially tearing apart layers and residence time is crucial for giving diffusion enough time to completely exfoliate layers (Zhao *et al.*, 2008). Proteins must first unfold and realign before being relaxed by fresh with in the molecule and outside of the source interactions. The assembly of proteins into a larger framework needs basically 3 paths: number on is dissolution of molecule to other molecule interactions which are of low energy keeping the threads of proteins together in a natural state; number two is to systemize polymer chains; and last is the creation of a 3D framework balanced by novel bondings and interactions post the removal of intermolecular bond-breaking agent (Angellier-coussy & Chalier, 2004). Protein nanocomposite films have frequently been created using the solvent casting technique. The nature, kind, and extent of interaction, pH, solvent variety, and plasticizer concentration are determined by the polymers involved (Rhim *et al.*, 2007).

2.3 CHARACTERIZATION TECHNIQUES OF BIONANOCOMPOSITES

Wide angle X-ray diffraction (WAXD) analysis, thermal gravimetric analysis (TGA), small angle X-ray scattering (SAXS), and solid-state nuclear magnetic resonance (NMR), atomic force microscopy (AFM), transmission electron microscopy (TEM), scanning electron microscopy (SEM), a dynamic mechanical thermal tester (DMTA), and other tools can be used to characterize polymer nanocomposites (Fu *et al.*, 2019).

2.3.1 Scanning Electron Microscope

Analyses at the microscopic level are crucial in nanotechnology. One of the most popular analysis tools, electron microscopes uses the interaction of the emission ray of electrons with the sample atoms to produce a magnified picture. Depending on the kind of electrons used to produce them, there are various kinds of electron microscopes (Gashti *et al.*, 2012). SEM uses a concentrated electron beam to scan an area to create images of it (Puggal *et al.*, 2016). Electron microscopy can be used to construct and manipulate nanostructures as well as image their composition and measure their physical properties While the image produced by TEM is more two dimensional and the electrons pass through the sample, the image is not useful for the surface structure investigation, the SEM scans the surface of the sample with a beam of electrons and the resulting image has a three-dimensional appearance that can be helpful for the surface structure investigation. It is the most important and commonly used technique in nanotechnology. The structure and its exterior state were examined using SEM images. To compare the fabrics with and without nano coatings, SEM pictures were employed. SEM images were used to compare the textiles with and without nano coatings (Gashti *et al.*, 2012).

2.3.2 Transmission Electron Microscope

TEM is a method employed in a wide variety of application. It is used to explore the internal structure and has the capacity to run detailed information regarding the ultrastructure. The features of microcrystalline cellulose (MCC), were studied using TEM. Information about particle nucleation, core-shell structure, crystallinity, film thickness, particle shape, nanofiber diameter, distribution of nanoparticle through nanofiber and coating structure are all provided by TEM. Wetzel used the TEM method to see how well nanoparticles dispersed. He created a matrix that contained a few small agglomerates and a homogeneous dispersion of nanoparticles (Puggal *et al.*, 2016). Numerous scholarly publications have examined the shape, distribution and particle size of nanomaterials using TEM imaging.A drop of a colloid solution can be deposited on a grid to create a TEM sample for particles with small dimensions (Gashti *et al.*, 2012).

Additionally to this SEM and TEM shortcoming, both of these methods lack the inherent ability to provide a three-dimensional image of the nanocomposite sample (Saheb *et al.*, 2014).

2.3.3 Solid State NMR Spectroscopy

Solid-state NMR spectroscopy is an analytical method used to investigate dynamics, structure, and the interactions of the molecules in solid state settings, including biological molecules like proteins and nucleic acids. Solid-state nuclear magnetic resonance spectroscopy is a valuable technique for understanding the structure and function of materials and biological systems at the atomic and molecular levels. Solid-state NMR spectroscopy has many applications in materials science, chemistry, and biology. It has been demonstrated that solid-state NMR can identify the behaviour of polymers in the interfacial region, where chain movements are more limited than they are in the bulk and interactions between polymers and fillers frequently result in the formation of an adsorption layer (Bokobza, 2018).

2.3.4 Raman and Infrared Spectroscopy

Infrared (IR) and Raman spectroscopy are two powerful techniques used to study the vibrations of molecules in the solid, liquid, and gas phases. These techniques are based on the interaction of electromagnetic radiation with vibrations of the atoms within a molecule. It has been demonstrated that infrared spectroscopy has the ability to characterise the polymer nanocomposites containing montmorillonites.

Cole used the shift in the clay Si-O band envelope to illustrate his point. It was verified that, form of clay absorption ranges within 1350 and 750 cm^{-1}, most likely as a result of better intercalation and exfoliation. According to Zhang et al.'s study, the Si-O interactions of sodium montmorillonite (NaMMT) and 2(two) organo-clays exhibits four typical parts, and they also use FT-IR spectroscopy to analyze the state of scattered layers of silicates in nanocomposites which are usually of polymers put on poly(hexamethylene isophthalamide) (aPa) and montmorillonite nanoclays.

With the development of carbon nanotubes over the past two decades, Raman spectroscopy is widely used to study the composites which are based on carbon materials. This undamaging technique has been widely utilized to understand the many vibrational modes of various substances which are mainly carbon-based, for example allotropes of carbon such as, diamond, graphene, fullerene, and carbon nanotubes. Despite having a relatively low concentration and being dispersed throughout the polymer matrix, they produce strong, well-defined bands because they exhibit resonance-enhanced Raman scattering effects. As a result, Raman spectroscopy is among the most crucial methods for analysing compounds made of carbon-based materials (Bokobza, 2018).

2.3.5 Fluorescence Spectroscopy

Fluorescence spectroscopy is a powerful technique used to study the interaction of light with fluorescent molecules. In order to conduct fluorescence spectroscopy research, a fluorescent probe must be incorporated into the medium and used at extremely low concentrations so as not to overly the mass. The emitted light can be measured and analyzed to obtain data of the sample. This data is mainly the molecular properties of the substance to be examined. Fluorescence spectroscopy can access the dynamics, structure and bonding of substances under examination in solution or solid form. The probe is selected because it can identify changes in through the alteration in its emission behaviour, its near environment. The majority of the time, fluorescence research used in inspection of polymer composites takes advantage of a particular photophysical phenomenon, such as relocation of energy or fluorescence suppressing (Bokobza, 2018).

2.3.6 Atomic Force Microscopy

AFM is a strong imaging method for examining the surface appearance and characteristics of material at nanoscale. Atomic force microscopy has been effectively used to provide a qualitative analysis of the nano reinforcement distribution in polymer matrix, metal matrix, and ceramic matrix nanocomposites in spite of this architectural flaw (Saheb *et al.*, 2014). It operates by scanning a sharp tip over a sample's surface while measuring the forces between the tip and the surfaces of the sample (usually made of silicon or diamond). The tip is supported by a cantilever, which flexes in response to contact with the sample surface. AFM is widely employed in a number of disciplines including biology, nanotechnology and material research. It can be used to examine the topography and characteristics of surfaces made of a variety of materials, including semiconductor, polymers, metals and biological materials. AFM is an effective tool for nanofabrication and nanomanipulation because it can be used to alter and control a material's properties at the nanoscale.

2.3.7 Small-Angle X-ray and Neutron Scattering

The strong experimental methods, i.e., small-sngle X-ray scattering (SAXS) and small angle neutron scattering (SANS), both are employed in the area of materials science to investigate the nanoscale microstructure of material. The external and internal dimensions of particles with diameter ranging from a few nanometer to a few hundred nanometers can be determined using SANS and SAXS, both are reliable technique. Material that are challenging to examine with X-rays, such as hydrogen-containing materials and materials with low electron density like polymers, proteins and biological membranes can benefit greatly from SAXS and SANS techniques. SAXS is a sensitive technique that uses elastic scattering of X-rays from atoms. SAXS and SANS have an exceptionally high resolution that can detect atomic -scale characteristics. These techniques has been used frequently for qualitative study of the distribution of nanoreinforcement in ceramic matrix nanocomposites and polymer matrix nanocomposites. SAXS is an extremely interesting tool for evaluating the spatial distribution of nano reinforcements, in nanocomposites that are only a few nanometers long (Saheb *et al.*, 2014).

2.4 CONCLUSION

Bionanocomposites are a viable source for replacement because of their biodegradability, potential to replace synthetic plastic films and capability to limit the substantial use of fossil fuels.

Table 2.1 Type and modes of characterization techniques

Characterization techniques	Sample form	Distribution types	Mode of analyses
Atomic Force microscopy	bulk	3D localized	Direct
Scanning Electron microscopy	bulk and powder	2D localized	direct
X-ray mapping	powder and bulk	localized	direct
Raman Confocal microscopy	bulk	localized	direct
Transmission Electron microscopy	bulk	2D localized	direct
Zeta potential measurements	powder	localized	indirect
Ultra-small angle X-ray scattering	bulk and powder	-	indirect
X-ray microcomputed Tomography	bulk	3D localized	direct

Biodegradable natural, synthetic, and inorganic/organic additive-derived bionanocomposites are materials with many functions. The main focus of this chapter is to disseminate information that will encourage more in-depth study in this field. A growing number of studies in the field of cellulose nanocomposites have been developed during the past 15 years. Biopolymers and nanofillers work together to create environmentally friendly, long-lasting food packaging. The majority of biomass in nature is made up of cellulose. This chapter discusses the most popular processing methods for cellulose nanocomposites, such as in situ polymerization, solution casting and melt-processing of thermoplastic cellulose nanocomposites. The production of innovative chitosan-based bionanocomposites for biomedical applications is the focus of this chapter, which also identifies the main research obstacles. Due to its ease of usage, solution casting is by far the most popular technique for creating nanocomposite films nevertheless, the process has not yet been developed for use on a large scale or for industrialization. Recently the use of extrusion to process melts has increased significantly, and several attempts at large scale processing have been made. The different characterization techniques discussed in this chapter conforms the formation of bionanocomposites.

REFERENCES

Angellier-coussy, H., & Chalier, P. (2013). Protein-based nanocomposites for food packaging. *Biopolymer Nanocomposites: Processing, Properties, and Applications, 1,* 613–653.

Armentano, I., Gigli, M., & Martino, S. (n.d.). *Applied Sciences Recent Advances in Nanocomposites Based on Aliphatic Polyesters: Design, Synthesis, and Applications in Regenerative Medicine.* https://doi.org/10.3390/app8091452

Azeredo, H. M. C. D. (2009). Nanocomposites for food packaging applications. *Food Research International, 42*(9), 1240–1253. https://doi.org/10.1016/j.foodres.2009.03.019

Bokobza, L. (2018). *Spectroscopic Techniques for the Characterization of Polymer Nanocomposites : A Review.* https://doi.org/10.3390/polym10010007

Chivrac, F., Pollet, E., & Avérous, L. (2009). Progress in nano-biocomposites based on polysaccharides and nanoclays. *Materials Science and Engineering R: Reports, 67*(1), 1–17. https://doi.org/10.1016/j.mser.2009.09.002

Dufresne, A. (2010). *Processing of Polymer Nanocomposites Reinforced with Polysaccharide Nanocrystals,* 4111–4128. https://doi.org/10.3390/molecules15064111

Fu, S., Sun, Z., Huang, P., Li, Y., & Hu, N. (2019). Nano Materials Science Some basic aspects of polymer nanocomposites: A critical review. *Nano Materials Science, 1*(1), 2–30. https://doi.org/10.1016/j.nanoms.2019.02.006

Gashti, M. P., Alimohammadi, F., Song, G., & Kiumarsi, A. (2012). Characterization of nanocomposite coatings on textiles : A brief review on microscopic technology characterization of nanocomposite coatings on textiles: A brief review on microscopic technology. *Current Microscopy Contributions to Advances in Science and Technology, 2*(December), 1424–1437.

Haq, M., Burgueño, R., Mohanty, A. K., & Misra, M. (2009). Composites : Part A processing techniques for bio-based unsaturated-polyester / clay nanocomposites: Tensile properties, efficiency, and limits. *Composites Part A, 40*(4), 394–403. https://doi.org/10.1016/j.compositesa.2009.01.003

Hosseinnejad, M., & Jafari, S. M. (2016). Evaluation of different factors affecting antimicrobial properties of chitosan. *International Journal of Biological Macromolecules, 85,* 467–475. https://doi.org/10.1016/j.ijbiomac.2016.01.022

Jabbari, F., Hesaraki, S., & Houshmand, B. (2019). The physical, mechanical, and biological properties of silk fibroin/chitosan/reduced graphene oxide composite membranes for guided bone regeneration. *Journal of Biomaterials Science, Polymer Edition, 30*(18), 1779–1802. https://doi.org/10.1080/09205063.2019.1666235

Khanzadi, M., Mahdi, S., Mirzaei, H., Khodaian, F., Maghsoudlou, Y., & Dehnad, D. (2015). Physical and mechanical properties in biodegradable films of whey protein concentrate – pullulan by application of beeswax. *Carbohydrate Polymers, 118,* 24–29. https://doi.org/10.1016/j.carbpol.2014.11.015

Kumar, S., & Koh, J. (2014). Physiochemical and optical properties of chitosan based graphene oxide bionanocomposite. *International Journal of Biological Macromolecules, 70,* 559–564. https://doi.org/10.1016/j.ijbiomac.2014.07.019

Madhumitha, G., Fowsiya, J., Roopan, S. M., & Thakur, V. K. (2018). International journal of polymer analysis and recent advances in starch – clay nanocomposites. *International Journal of Polymer Analysis and Characterization, 23*(4), 331–345. https://doi.org/10.1080/1023666X.2018.1447260

Mahdi, S., Khanzadi, M., Mirzaei, H., & Dehnad, D. (2015). International journal of biological macromolecules hydrophobicity, thermal and micro-structural properties of whey protein concentrate – pullulan – beeswax films. *International Journal of Biological Macromolecules, 80,* 506–511. https://doi.org/10.1016/j.ijbiomac.2015.07.017

Mousa, M. H., Dong, Y., & Davies, I. J. (2016). International Journal of Polymeric Materials and Recent advances in bionanocomposites : Preparation, properties, and applications. *GPOM, 65*(5), 225–254. https://doi.org/10.1080/00914037.2015.1103240

Müller, K., Bugnicourt, E., Latorre, M., Jorda, M., Sanz, Y. E., Lagaron, J. M., Miesbauer, O., Bianchin, A., Hankin, S., Bölz, U., Jesdinszki, M., & Lindner, M. (2017). *Review on the Processing and Properties of Polymer Nanocomposites and Nanocoatings and Their Applications in the Packaging, Automotive and Solar Energy Fields.* https://doi.org/10.3390/nano7040074

Ojijo, V., & Sinha, S. (2013). Progress in Polymer Science Processing strategies in bionanocomposites. *Progress in Polymer Science, 38*(10–11), 1543–1589. https://doi.org/10.1016/j.progpolymsci.2013.05.011

Oksman, K., Aitomäki, Y., Mathew, A. P., Siqueira, G., Zhou, Q., Butylina, S., Tanpichai, S., Zhou, X., & Hooshmand, S. (2016). Review of the recent developments in cellulose nanocomposite processing. *Composites Part A: Applied Science and Manufacturing, 83,* 2–18. https://doi.org/10.1016/j.compositesa.2015.10.041

Puggal, S., Dhall, N., Singh, N., & Litt, M. S. (2016). *A Review on Polymer Nanocomposites : Synthesis, Characterization and Mechanical Properties,* March. https://doi.org/10.17485/ijst/2016/v9i4/81100

Rhim, J., Ng, P. K. W., & Rhim, J. (2007). *Natural Biopolymer-Based Nanocomposite Films for Packaging Applications Natural Biopolymer-Based Nanocomposite Films for Packaging,* 8398. https://doi.org/10.1080/10408390600846366

Saheb, N., Qadir, N. U., Siddiqui, M. U., Fazl, A., Arif, M., Akhtar, S. S., Al-aqeeli, N., & Arabia, S. (2014). *Characterization of Nanoreinforcement Dispersion in Inorganic Nanocomposites: A Review,* 4148–4181. https://doi.org/10.3390/ma7064148

Sharma, R., Mahdi, S., & Sharma, S. (2020). Antimicrobial bio-nanocomposites and their potential applications in food packaging. *Food Control, 112*(January), 107086. https://doi.org/10.1016/j.foodcont.2020.107086

Siqueira, G., Bras, J., & Dufresne, A. (2010). Cellulosic bionanocomposites: A review of preparation, properties and applications. *Polymers, 2*(4), 728–765. https://doi.org/10.3390/polym2040728

Valerio, O., Misra, M., & Mohanty, A. K. (2018). *Poly(glycerol-co-diacids) Polyesters: From Glycerol Biorefinery to Sustainable Engineering Applications, A Review.* https://doi.org/10.1021/acssuschemeng.7b04837

Zhao, R., Torley, Æ. P., & Halley, Æ. P. J. (2008). *Emerging Biodegradable Materials: Starch- and Protein-Based Bio-Nanocomposites,* 3058–3071. https://doi.org/10.1007/s10853-007-2434-8

Zheng, Y., Monty, J., & Linhardt, R. J. (2015). Polysaccharide-based nanocomposites and their applications. *Carbohydrate Research, 405,* 23–32. https://doi.org/10.1016/j.carres.2014.07.016

Bio-based Nanocomposites for Imaging, Tissue Repairing, and Drug Delivery Applications

*Purnima Justa, Nancy Jaswal, Vijay Bahadur,
Manoj K. Singh, Devendra Kumar Gangwar,
Mohan Bhushan Kalhans, and Pramod Kumar*

3.1 INTRODUCTION

Bio-based materials are goods whose primary components are first derived from living organisms. Bio-based materials, which are made from substances produced by living things, are used in a variety of industries, including green technologies, consumer product packaging, technology, transportation, and medicine (1). These bio-based nanocomposites are fascinating materials with intriguing properties. Many industries including medicinal, optical, water conditioning, sensors, fabric, energy conversion, beauty, and electrical could benefit from the application of bio nanocomposites (2). Particularly for biomedical applications like targeted transport (of medicines and genes), bioimaging, and skin and bone tissue regeneration, the properties of nanoparticles have recently made them attractive for the creation of nanocomposites. Biopolymeric nanocomposites control cell propagation, polarity, and relocation, which leads to bone regeneration by giving the cells a more closely resembling structural support to the original bone architecture (3).

Nanomaterials with magnetic properties are highly prized for use in magnetic resonance imaging (4, 5), magnetic hyperthermia for cancer therapy (6), biosensors (7), and targeted drug delivery systems (8). Iron oxide Nanoparticles and zero-valent iron are more hydrophilic and biocompatible after functionalization with gum polysaccharides. Acacia gum/Fe_2O_3 magnetic nanocomposite has the prospect of being used as a cell labeling contrast agent for magnetic resonance imaging (9). An antibacterial nanocomposite is created when silver nanoparticles (Ag NPs) are immersed in carboxymethyl cellulose/cashew gum. Ag-Cu NPs and guar gum solution casting have been combined to create antibacterial guar gum/Ag-Cu bionanocomposite films. These films are excellent lightweight light and oxygen barriers as well as antibacterial against *Listeria monocytogenes* and *Salmonella* Typhimurium (10). This chapter reports the developments of biobased nanocomposites and their execution in imaging, tissue repair, and drug delivery.

DOI: 10.1201/9781003470311-3

3.2 APPLICATION OF BIO-BASED NANOCOMPOSITES IN TISSUE REPAIRING

The goal of tissue engineering, an interdisciplinary discipline, is to repair or boost tissue performance that has been lost or damaged due to various pathological conditions. For such damaged tissues, it uses engineering and life sciences principles, either through the creation of biological replacements or through tissue rebuilding. Tissue engineering facilitates the restoration, maintenance, or enhancement of tissue function by providing insights into the arrangement and function of both healthy and diseased bodily tissues. When surgery is required to treat an illness, tissue engineering aims to create fresh, operative tissues and rebuild tissue both *in vitro* and *in vivo* (11, 12).

3.2.1 Chitosan-based Nanocomposite in Tissue Engineering

Chitosan is a polymer that has profuse qualities, together with biocompatibility, antibacterial capabilities, stimuli responsiveness, biodegradability, water solubility, and adjustable mechanical strength (3). Using in-situ nanoparticle production, melt mixing, and solution casting techniques, chitosan nanocomposite thin films can be created. The most common materials used in solution casting are H_2O, cell culture medium, and occasionally organic solvents. To efficiently spread the nanofillers, ultrasonication is frequently utilized as well (13). In addition to films, chitosan-based hydrogels are intriguing biomaterials since they are highly water soluble, making them compatible with the majority of natural tissues (14, 15).

3.2.2 Chitin-based Nanocomposites in Tissue Engineering

Chitin is a nature-derived biopolymer discovered in the outer skeleton of crustaceans, insects, and fungi's cell walls. Due to its compatibility with living tissue, ecofriendly nature, and non-irritant character, chitin has been explored as a probable biomaterial in the tissue engineering field (16). Nanohydroxyapatite (nHAp) is a popular biomaterial for treating bone defects due to its compliance with natural bone composition, biocompatibility, and osteoconductivity (17). nHAp has also been dispersed in chitin solution to create nanocomposites, which can be crosslinked or not (18). The $nZrO_2$ component of the chitosan/$nSiO_2$/$nZrO_2$ scaffold improved biological degradation, protein assimilation, and bio-mineralization properties while reducing swelling (19).

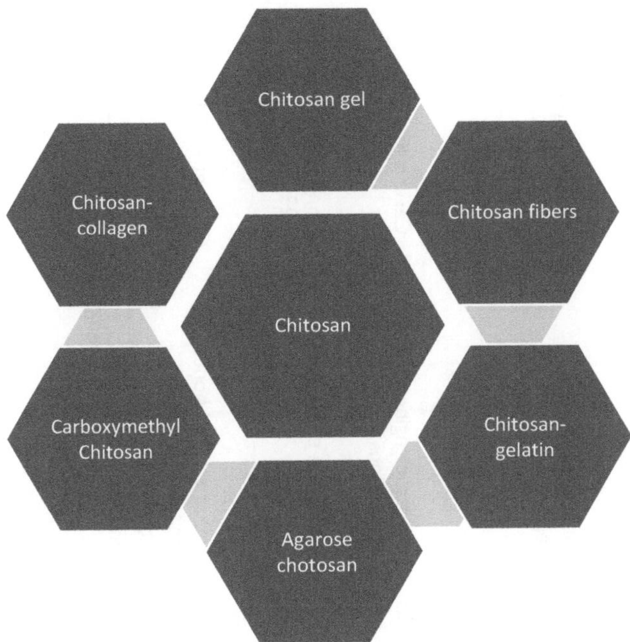

Figure 3.1 Chitosan-based scaffolds in tissue engineering.

3.2.3 Nanocomposites of Nanocellulose in Tissue Engineering

3.2.3.1 Gelatin-based Nanocomposites for tissue engineering

Hydrolysis of native collagen yields gelatin, a fibrous protein with a unique amino acid sequence that breaks intermolecular connections and loses its original helix structure. Gelatin has many useful traits that make it desirable for usage in the food, pharmaceutical, and medical care industries. These qualities include excellent film-forming, gelling, foaming, and emulsifying capabilities, as well as biocompatible and biodegradable properties (32).

Replacement of bones and joints is the first major tissue engineering application for gelatin nanocomposites. A hard mineral that resembles apatite and flexible collagen are the main components of bone and teeth, respectively (33). Lzabella et al. used electrospun polycaprolactone (PCL) and gelatin-modified calcium phosphate nanoparticles to build a scaffold with a three-dimensional bi-layer structure that would improve mineralization and boost the scaffold's binding affinity to the bone tissue (34).

Table 3.1 Bacterial cellulose-based scaffolds in tissue engineering

Nanocomposites	Key aspects	Applications	References
BC-PVA nanocomposites	The mechanical characteristics of cardiovascular tissues, like the aorta and heart valve leaflets, can be adjusted to meet the qualities.	In cardiovascular replacement applications.	Millon and Wan (20)
BC-PVA nanocomposites	In addition to having a high-water content, good visible light transmittance, acceptable UV absorbance, enhanced mechanical strength, and suitable thermal characteristics, the resulting nanocomposites were also suited for corneal replacement.	Suitable for cornea replacement	Wang et al. (21)
BC-Polyethylene glycol (PEG) nanocomposites	Cell adhesion tests employing 3T3 fibroblast cells were used to evaluate the good biocompatibility of the BC-PEG nanocomposite.	Soft tissue engineering applications	Cai and Kim (22)
BC-hydroxyapatite (HAp) nanocomposites	The apatites that contained HAp minerals were carbonate-containing and had low crystallinity and lower crystallite sizes, which were similar to the carbonated Hap present in natural bones.	bone tissue engineering	Hong et al. Fang et al. (23)
BC-HAp nanocomposites	The phosphorylated BC fibers produced HAp crystals, which had tiny nanosized crystallites and carbonate content.	used as artificial bones and scaffolds for tissue engineering	Wan et al. (24)
BC-HAp nanocomposite	When human bone marrow-derived stem cells (hBMSC) were seeded on BC-HAp nanocomposites, they displayed superior adherence and activity in comparison to when they were seeded on pure BC.	Bone tissue engineering	Fang et al. (25)
BC-HAp nanocomposite	The test's use of human embryonic kidney (HEK) cell seeding demonstrated the nanocomposites' exceptional biocompatibility and cell survivability.	Bone tissue engineering	Grande et al. (26)

(Continued)

Table 3.1 Continued

Nanocomposites	Key Aspects	Applications	References
BC-HAp nanocomposite	BC-HAp nanocomposites are a great way to accelerate bone regrowth.	Bone regeneration	Saska et al. (27)
BC-Collagen nanocomposites	The resulting nanocomposites were easier to work with during surgical procedures and exhibited greater flexibility. In vitro, osteoblastic phenotypic development is made possible by these nanocomposites.	Bone regeneration	Saska et al. (28)
BC-CaCO3 nanocomposites	Following microwave radiation, BC-CaCO3 nanocomposites showed increased hardness and water vapour transmission rates.	Bone regeneration	Stoica-Guzun et al. (29)
BC-Gelatin nanocomposites	The BC-Gelatin nanocomposites exhibit fracture strength and elastic modulus nearly identical to articular cartilage, with values in the megaPascal (MPa) range under compressive stress.	Articulate (cartilage) tissue engineering.	Nakayama et al. (30)
BC-PHEMA poly(2-hydroxyethyl methacrylate) nanocomposites	With regard to human adipose-derived mesenchymal stem cells, BC-PHEMA nanocomposites showed excellent biocompatibility, negligible toxicity, and cell adhesion and proliferation.	Tissue regeneration	Figueiredo et al. (31)

3.3 APPLICATION OF BIO-BASED NANOCOMPOSITES FOR BIOIMAGING

Scientists and environmentalists have grown interested in biodegradable materials due to the negative effects that non-biodegradable materials have on people and the environment (35). A recent cancer treatment technique called photothermal therapy (PTT) uses light energy to create heat, which causes thermal ablation and the eventual killing of cancer cells (36). However, because of the non-specific heating caused by the laser during PTT, high temperatures may affect the normal tissues in the vicinity. To enhance the therapeutic effectiveness of photothermal polymer nanoparticles or overcome the negative effects of PTT, an imaging capability is extremely desirable (37).

3.3.1 Porphyrin

Porphyrins are an excellent option for PDT because of their favourable photochemical characteristics, particularly singlet oxygen production. When porphyrin molecules and magnetic resonance delegate are stacked onto a nanocarrier biobased nanocomposites of porphyrin and magnetic resonance imaging serve as a dual-functional theragnostic nanomaterial. To facilitate synergistic sonodynamic therapy and MRI imaging of rat breast carcinoma, an example involves loading of Mn (III)- meso-tetrakis (4- sulphonatophenyl) porphyrin (Mn (III)-TPPS) on hydrophobic polymethyl methacrylate nanoparticles and supplementary modifying their facet by anionic molecules (38).

3.3.2 AIEgen-based Polymer Nanocomposites for Imaging

AIEgens [aggregation-induced emission (AIE)] agents hold great promise for achieving elevated fluorescence intensity within polymer nanoparticles and smoothly and accurately guiding PTT (39). This section will provide an overview of the functions that AIEgens perform as FLI, PAI, or PTI agents in distinct PTT polymer nanoplatforms.

3.3.2.1 Fluorescence Imaging (FLI)

AIEgens are superior fluorescence bioimaging agents for PTT therapy due to their remarkable photostability and very efficient aggregate-state fluorescence. In addition, in 2016 there was an uptick in the number of "Wei" titles. An AIEgen was used as a FLI delegate in this system (40).

3.3.2.2 Photoacoustic Imaging (PAI)

PAI finds widespread application in alive creatures due to its non-intrusive and non-ionizing characteristics, significant perforation depth, and elevated temporal and spatial resolution. The Grüneisen parameter is the efficiency with which heat is converted to sound pressure (41). Using a xenograft 4T1 tumor-bearing mouse model, paramount factors in creating polymer NPs for PAI is their high Grüneisen parameter (42). Liu and Zheng lately created a D-A customized AIEgens with dual NIR-I PAI for PAI and NIR-II FLI functionalities (43).

3.3.2.3 Photothermal Imaging (PTI)

PTI can monitor in real-time *in vivo* execution of photothermal agents to direct the PTT because it is temperature sensitive. PTI is typically used to evaluate the ability of AIEgens to generate heat in living mice and to track the process of temperature raising at the tumor site following intravenous injection. By controlling molecular movements in aggregates, Tang et al. recently discovered a extremely effective PTT nano agent. E.g., Tang & Qian et al. effectively used polymer NPs based on an NIR-emissive AIEgens (TQ-BPN) to image the brain blood arteries of living mice using both fluorescence and thermal microscopic techniques (44).

3.3.3 Graphitic Carbon Nitride-Based Nanocomposites for Imaging

The distinctive optical and catalytic characteristics of graphitic carbon nitride QDs (g-CNs), which are only made of carbon and nitrogen, have gained interest. Because of the chemical composition they possess, minimal toxicity can be used in biological imaging in addition to many other electrical features (44).

3.3.4 Chitosan

Bio nanocomposites based on chitosan are also well-suited as bioimaging tools. Salehi Zadeh's research team created a magnetic core-shell nanocomposite of Fe_2O_3 that has supermagnetic qualities that guarantee magnetic resonance for imaging, and gold nanoparticles, which perform duties as photothermal converters induce optical properties (35, 45).

3.3.5 Carbon Dots of Waste Paper

Most of paper sheets, including A4 white paper, already contain unidentified fluorescent elements. By employing a simple microwave irradiation procedure, many types of garbage can emit strong emissions of light at different wavelengths. Further information on luminous chemical removal procedures may be required when producing CDs from old waste paper. The emission shift may be caused by some complex chemical interactions involving numerous fluorescent compounds (46).

3.3.6 Graphene-Based Nanocomposites in Bioimaging

Graphene and its derivatives have a plethora of biological uses under investigation, such as medication administration, bioimaging, diagnostics, and near-infrared (NIR) light-induced PTT (47). Research and treatment are greatly aided by bioimaging, which makes it possible to observe and study biological processes at all scales, from minute animals to molecules and subcellular structures (48, 49).

3.3.6.1 Optical Imaging

Via the utilization of visible light and the special qualities of photons, optical imaging is a non-destructive technique that create exquisite images of organ, tissues, and even smaller entities like cells and molecules (48). As it is very inexpensive, highly sensitive (109–1012mol/L), non-ionizing radiation, allows for real-time imaging, has a quick accession time, and can multiplex it is considered superior to other modalities (50).

3.3.6.2 Fluorescence Imaging

A non-invasive approach called FL imaging focuses on the photons that emit fluorescent probes (48). The B cell-specific antibody Rituxan (anti-CD20) covalently linked to pegylated nGO (nGO-PEG-Rituxan) was first published by the Dai group as a way to specifically recognise and bind to Raji B cells utilising FL imaging employing an InGaAs detector under 658nm laser excitation. This is because ultrasmall (US) nanographene oxide (nGO) has inherent photoluminescence (51).

3.3.6.3 Radionuclide-Based Imaging

An investigation employed graphene-based nanomaterials as prospective nanoplatforms and 66Ga-labeled nGO-PEG for tumor-targeted PET imaging, (52). PET and SPECT comprise the majority of radionuclide-based imaging.

3.3.6.4 Photoacoustic Imaging

For deep tissue/organ imaging, PAI offers optical absorption contrast with the resolution of ultrasound. Due to its bigger sp^2 domains compared to GOs, rGO plays a crucial function as PA contrast agents in the graphene family of nanomaterials. Additionally, the Cai group found that BSA may decrease and stabilize GOs in a single step, resulting in the nanosized rGO which has great steadiness and minimal cytotoxicity (52).

3.3.6.5 Raman Imaging

In contrast to phonon absorption and emission in FL, Raman spectroscopy studies the inelastic scattering of phonons coming from molecular vibrational excitation states (47). The innately strong D and G peaks that GOs have as Raman tags can be strengthened by collaborating them with metal NPs. Yang et al. verified that folate receptor (FR) positive cancer cells may be imaged with targeted SERS using folic acid conjugated Ag/GO hybrids (53). Using FA-GO-Ag NPs as SERS labels, cancer cells were specifically labelled and imaged. Hela 229 cells treated with Au/GO hybrids show much sturdy Raman signals and more recognizable Raman images than the cells incubated with only GO (54).

3.3.6.6 Multimodal Imaging

Lately, the concept of integrating different imaging modalities for biological utilization has started to gain traction (55). For triple modal FL, PA, and MR imaging, the Liu group developed a probe based on rGO-IONP nanocomposite.

FL imaging can be done using the Cy5-labeled rGO-IONP-PEG. The presence of iron oxide magnetic NPs in rGO-IONP-PEG makes it potentially useful as a T2-weighted MR contrast agent (56). For PDT of tumors, the Chen group created a nano formula of GO-PEG loaded with PS HPPH via stacking (57). This property of the HPPH's FL was utilized for FL imaging. Additionally, copper-64 (^{64}Cu, $t_{1/2}$=12.7 h), a positron-emitting radioisotope, was used to label HPPH for PET imaging (58).

3.3.7 MOF-based Fluorescent Nanocomposites for Bioimaging

Metal-organic frameworks, often known as MOFs, are a type of absorptive functional material that self-assembles from metal ions or metal clusters and organic ligands to generate potent metal-ligand interactions. MOFs have some positive advantages over typical porous materials like extremely high absorptivity, sizable surface areas, controlled pore sizes, surface functions, and superior biocompatibility. Numerous techniques emanated from MOFs have been created for detecting and imaging biomolecules, including surface-enhanced Raman and electrochemiluminescence scattering, photoelectrochemical sensors (59) MRI, and it is very advantageous to create fluorescent nanocomposites for bioimaging in living cells and *in vivo* using MOFs with intriguing binding capacity to fluorescent materials and guest molecules (60) benefits for imaging first off, MOFs make for promising nano vehicles because of their structure and content.

3.3.7.1 Carbon Dot MOFs

Since fluorescent nanoparticles are portable enough to enter cells and infiltrate the body's fluid circulation system, they can be used as building blocks for biosensors that are intended for biomolecule recognition and imaging in living cells, or even *in vivo*. The ZIF-8 is the ideal platform for cancer therapy and fluorescence imaging applications due to its nanoscale size, excellent biocompatibility, and pH-sensitive characteristics (61).

3.3.7.2 Gold Nano-cluster MOFs

Fluorescent gold nanoclusters (Au NCs) are a novel class of emitting materials that have drawn significant interest because of their intriguing characteristics, including high photostability, minimal toxicity, and outstanding biocompatibility. Qu et al. recent study demonstrated that showed that Au NCs (GSH- Au NCs) can have their luminescence altered by modifying their aggregation state according to MOFs (62). Tang and colleagues have found a way to image cells under 980 nm illumination using UCNPs/MBZIF-8. It is important to note that ZIF-8 was crucial in avoiding the leakage of molecules. Additionally, UCNPs offered an in vitro NIR imaging option (63). NUS 2729 NSs ZIF-8 nanocomposites might easily penetrate cancer cells for bioimaging because of the nucleic acid probes' exceptional stability and hydrophilicity, which allow them to be easily endocytosed by cells (64).

3.3.7.3 Near-infrared (NIR) Dye MOFs

Since biological tissues (such as melanin, haemoglobin, etc.) can absorb or scatter visible light, fluorescence imaging is a useful imaging approach for identifying biomolecules in biological systems. Because of its additional advantages, such as less light dispersion, deep tissue penetration, and reduced photodamage to the biosamples, near-infrared fluorescence imaging is an extensively used method in biological research . Fluorescence imaging can now reliably and sensitively detect tumours thanks to ICG-ZIF-8 NPs. However, after a single NIR laser irradiation, ICG-ZIF-8 NPs successfully stimulated photothermal therapy (PTT) (65). More significantly, the active targeting ability of folic acid (FA) may be successfully incorporated into MOFs, allowing for in vivo targeted imaging of MOF-based nanocomposites.

3.3.7.4 Rare Earth-doped UCNPs-MOFs

Inorganic crystal materials tampered with rare earth elements have captivated a lot of recognition because of their exceptional near-infrared stimulated upconversion luminescence (UCL) capabilities, prolonged luminescence life, and good stability. UCNPs convert NIR light into visible light, which is utilized in *in vivo* fluorescence imaging. Binary drug release, UCL imaging, and MRI may be performed with a pH-sensitive responsive nano-system (UCMOFs@D@5) created by Sun et al. (66).

3.3.8 Polydopamine

MRI has both temporal and spatial resolutions, making it a non-invasive diagnostic tool. MRI contrast agents are often utilized to intensify the body's inherently low-sensitive signal intensity by speeding up the proton relaxation of H_2O. Tsai et al. investigated a type of magnetic resonance contrast agent based on PDA coated $Gd_2(CO_3)_3$ for efficient T1-weighted MRI in vivo using calcium/manganese cation-chelated alginate-PDA nanogels (67). Liu et al. employing ferric oxide nanoparticles with a PDA shell (Fe_2O_3-PDA) (68). The technology was next combined with PEG and a peptide that targets tumors (affibody ZIGF1R:4551). The eventual system demonstrated a 68% reduction in tumor-bearing mice's MRI signal, recommending that the Fe_2O_3PDA-affibody platform had a high T2-weighted contrast and was highly effective and selective in tumor identification. Chen et al. proposed a PDA-based coordination complex (PDA-CP3-DOX) for T1/T2 MRI escorted drug delivery in another intriguing work (69).

3.3.9 Metal Nanocluster-based Nanocomposite Application in Imaging

3.3.9.1 In Vitro Luminescence Imaging

As metal NCs have a natural luminescence and are well-suited for biocompatible applications, NC-based composites can be used as reliable optical probes for fluorescence imaging. FR overexpressing cancer cells can now be specifically imaged using folic acid-conjugated NC composites. Cancer cells that overexpress the Tf receptor have also been imaged using CuNCs that have been Tf-functionalized (70). AuNCs-CS or chitosan-AuNC composites functionalized with TPP, use these properties to visualize mitochondria in living cells.

3.3.9.2 In Vivo Multimodal Imaging

Multimodal imaging, which put together two or more imaging modalities that each provides a different type of complementary information, has several advantages. Consequently, there has been a great deal of interests in the evolution of metal NC-based multimodal imaging probes for in-vivo imaging in recent years. In order to make iodinated BSA-AuNC composites for dual-modality fluorescence/CT imaging of thyroid cancer, BSA-AuNCs were oxidised to produce iodide ions (71).

3.4 APPLICATION OF BIO-BASED NANOCOMPOSITES IN DRUG DELIVERY

3.4.1 Nanocomposite of Cellulose in Drug Delivery Applications

In the chemical sector, cellulose has been employed as a tablet coating in conjugation with other pharamaceutical products (72). Serum albumins have been model-carried using biopolymeric bacterial cellulose. Drug loading and release were regulated in the bacterial cellulose. This has led some experts to speculate that this hydrophilic, biocompatible polymer might be used as a cutting-edge medication delivery system (73). In a different study, hydrophobic anticancer medications such as docetaxel, paclitaxel, and etoposide were added to nanocrystalline cellulose (NCCs) that had been surface-modified by cetyl trimethylammonium bromide (CTAB). NCCs demonstrated regulated drug release over two days and cellular absorption by binding to KU-7 (bladder cancer cells), demonstrating their promise as innovative drug delivery systems (74).

3.4.2 Chitosan Nanocomposites in Drug Delivery Applications

Chitosan has emerged as a leading contender for a medicine delivery method. Due to its remarkable biological capabilities, chitosan has become extremely important in the production of biomaterials and has been the subject of in-depth research into drug delivery systems. Chitosan nanocomposites contributed significantly to the biomedical sciences by offering a delivery system that is atoxic, biocompatible, sturdy, target-specific, and biodegradable (75). Other important qualities of chitosan are those that are haemostatic, bacteriostatic, anticholestermic, and anticarcinogenic (76).

3.5 CONCLUSION

Products with main components obtained from living beings are known as bio-based materials. Biomedical research is said to benefit from the use of nanostructured materials since certain tissues and organisms serve as a typical model for nanocomposite materials. Numerous industries, including medical, optical, water treatment, sensors, textiles, energy conversions, cosmetics, and electronics, could benefit from the application of bio nanocomposites. To repair, maintain, or enhance tissue function, tissue engineering helps to comprehend the composition and capabilities of both healthy and diseased mammalian tissues. Bio-based materials such as chitosan, chitin, and gelatin have been explored for application in tissue engineering. Photothermal therapy and photodynamic therapy are newer cancer treatment modalities that use light radiation to generate heat, which leads to thermal ablation and ultimately the death of cancer cells. Considering the harm that both these therapies do to healthy tissue, a therapeutic model with imaging features is ideal. Porphyrins have good photochemical properties, especially the formation of singlet oxygen, which makes them a great choice for photodynamic therapy. Numerous bio-based nanocomposites, including metal-organic frameworks, graphene, carbon dots made from waste paper, graphitic carbon nitride, and chitosan, have demonstrated enormous promise in imaging applications. Nanocomposites based on chitosan, hyaluronic acid, cellulose, and starch have become a top candidate for a drug delivery system.

REFERENCES

1. Kumar, S., Krishnakumar, B., Sobral, A. J., & Koh, J. (2019). Bio-based (chitosan/PVA/ZnO) nanocomposites film: Thermally stable and photoluminescence material for removal of organic dye. *Carbohydrate Polymers, 205,* 559–564.
2. Singla, R., Guliani, A., Kumari, A., & Yadav, S. K. (2016). Nanocellulose and nanocomposites. *Nanoscale Materials in Targeted Drug Delivery, Theragnosis and Tissue Regeneration, 1,* 103–125.
3. Kumar, H., Justa, P., Jaswal, N., Pani, B., & Kumar, P. (2023). Biomimetic and bioinspired composite processing for biomedical applications. *Advanced Materials and Manufacturing Techniques for Biomedical Applications, 1,* 211–239.
4. Kumar, H., Agnihotri, S., Roy, I., Pani, B., & Kumar, P. (2020). Microemulsion mediated multifunction of doxorubicin encapsulated Core–Shell iron oxide/Ormosil nanoparticles as efficient magnetically-guided delivery, bioimaging and In-vitro studies. *Advanced Science, Engineering and Medicine, 12*(9), 1166–1173.
5. Kumar, H., Pani, B., Kumar, J., & Kumar, P. (2023). In vitro and bioimaging studies of mesoporous silica nanocomposites encapsulated iron-oxide and loaded Doxorubicin Drug (DOX/IO@ Silica) as magnetically guided drug delivery system. *Current Pharmaceutical Biotechnology, 24*(10), 1297–1306.
6. Kumar, H., Kumar, A., Gangwar, D. K., Kumar, P., & Singh, G. (2016). Potential application of gold nanostructures in photodynamic therapy. *Journal of Nanomedicine & Nanotechnology, 7*(349), 2.
7. Kumar, S., Umar, M., Saifi, A., Kumar, S., Augustine, S., Srivastava, S., & Malhotra, B. D. (2019). Electrochemical paper based cancer biosensor using iron oxide nanoparticles decorated PEDOT:PSS. *Analytica Chimica Acta, 1056,* 135–145.
8. Kumar, H., Kumar, J., Pani, B., & Kumar, P. (2022). Multifunctional folic acid-coated and doxorubicin encapsulated mesoporous silica nanocomposites (FA/DOX@ Silica) for cancer therapeutics, bioimaging and invitro studies. *ChemistrySelect, 7*(44), e202203113.

9. Zare, E. N., Makvandi, P., Borzacchiello, A., Tay, F. R., Ashtari, B., & Padil, V. V. (2019). Antimicrobial gum bio-based nanocomposites and their industrial and biomedical applications. *Chemical Communications, 55*(99), 14871–14885.

10. Christy, P. N., Basha, S. K., Kumari, V. S., Bashir, A. K. H., Maaza, M., Kaviyarasu, K., ... Ignacimuthu, S. (2020). Biopolymeric nanocomposite scaffolds for bone tissue engineering applications–A review. *Journal of Drug Delivery Science and Technology, 55*, 101452.

11. Bedian, L., Villalba-Rodríguez, A. M., Hernández-Vargas, G., Parra-Saldivar, R., & Iqbal, H. M. (2017). Bio-based materials with novel characteristics for tissue engineering applications–A review. *International Journal of Biological Macromolecules, 98*, 837–846.

12. Kumbar, S. G., James, R., Nukavarapu, S. P., & Laurencin, C. T. (2008). Electrospun nanofiber scaffolds: Engineering soft tissues. *Biomedical Materials, 3*, 15.

13. Jung, H. Y., Le Thi, P., HwangBo, K. H., Bae, J. W., Park & K. D. (2021). Tunable and high tissue adhesive properties of injectable chitosan based hydrogels through polymer architecture modulation. *Carbohydrate Polymers, 261*, 117810.

14. Giannakas, A., Grigoriadi, K., Leontiou, A., Barkoula, N. M., Ladavos, A. (2014). Preparation, characterization, mechanical and barrier properties investigation of chitosan–clay nanocomposites. *Carbohydrate Polymers, 108*, 103–111.

15. Dai, S., Ravi, P., & Tam, K. C. (2008). pH-Responsive polymers: synthesis, properties and applications. *Soft Matter, 4*, 435.

16. Deepthi, S., Venkatesan, J., Kim, S. K., Bumgardner, J. D., & Jayakumar, R. (2016). An overview of chitin or chitosan/nano ceramic composite scaffolds for bone tissue engineering. *International Journal of Biological Macromolecules, 93*, 1338–1353.

17. Wei, G., & Ma, P. X. (2004). Structure and properties of nano-hydroxyapatite/polymer composite scaffolds for bone tissue engineering. *Biomaterials, 25*, 4749–4757.

18. Chang, C., Peng, N., Hea, M., Teramotoc, T., Nishio, Y., & Zhang, L. (2013). Fabrication and properties of chitin/hydroxyapatite hybrid hydrogels as scaffold nano-materials. *Carbohydrate Polymers, 91*, 7–13.

19. Jayakumar, R., Ramachandran, R., Divyarani, V., Chennazhi, K., Tamura, H., & Nair, S. V. (2011). Fabrication of chitin-chitosan/nano TiO2-composite scaffolds for tissue engineering applications. *International Journal of Biological Macromolecules, 48*, 336–344.

20. Millon, L. E., & Wan, W. K. (2006). The polyvinyl alcohol-bacterial cellulose system as a new nanocomposite for biomedical applications. *Journal of Biomedical Materials Research B, 79*, 2.

21. Wang, J., Cao, C., Zhang, Y., & Wan, Y. (2010). Preparation and in vitro characterization of BC/PVA hydrogel composite for its potential use as artificial cornea biomaterials. *Journal of Materials Science: Materials C, 30*, 214–218.

22. Cai, Z., & Kim, J. (2010). Bacterial cellulose/poly(ethylene glycol) composite: characterization and first evaluation of biocompatibility. *Cellulose, 17*, 83–91.

23. Hong, L., Wang, Y. L., Jia, S. R., Huang, Y., Cao, C., & Wan, Y. Z. Hydroxyapatite/bacterial cellulose composite synthesized via a biomimetic route. *Materials Letters*, 60, 1710–1713.
24. Wan, Y. Z., Huang, Y., Yuan, C. D., Raman, S., Zhu, Y., Jiang, H. J., He, F., Gao, C. (2007). Biomimetic synthesis of hydroxyapatite/bacterial cellulose nanocomposites for biomedical applications. *Materials Science and Engineering C*, 27, 855–864.
25. Fang, B., Wan, Y. Z., Tang, T. T., Gao, C., & Dai, K. R. (2009). Proliferation and osteoblastic differentiation of human bone marrow stromal cells on hydroxyapatite/bacterial cellulose nanocomposite scaffolds. *Tissue Engineering A*, 15(5), 1091–1098.
26. Grande, C. J., Torres, F. G., Gomez, C. M., & Bano, M. C. (2009). Nanocomposites of bacterial cellulose/hydroxyapatite for biomedical applications. *Acta Biomaterialia*, 5(5), 1605–1615.
27. Saska, S., Barud, H. S., Caspar, A. M. M., Marchetto, R., Ribeiro, S. J. L., & Messaddeq, Y. (2011). Bacterial cellulose-hydroxyapatite nanocomposites for bone regeneration. *International Journal of Biomaterials*, Article ID: 175362, *2011*, 1–8.
28. Saska, S., Teixeira, L. N., De Oliveira, P. T., Gaspar, A. M. M., Ribeiro, S. J. L., Messaddeq, Y., & Marchetto, R. (2012). Bacterial cellulose-collagen nanocomposite for bone tissue engineering. *Journal of Materials Chemistry*, 22, 22102–22112.
29. Stoica-Guzun, A., Stroescu, M., Jinga, S. I., Jipa, I. M., & Dobre, T. (2013). Microwave assisted synthesis of bacterial cellulose-calcium carbonate composites. *Industrial Crops and Products*, 50, 414–422.
30. Nakayama, A., Kakugo, A., Gong, J. P., Osada, Y., Takai, M., Erata, T., & Kawano, S. (2004). High mechanical strength double-network hydrogel with bacterial cellulose. *Advanced Functional Materials*, 14(11), 1124–1128.
31. Figueiredo, A. G., Figueiredo, A. R., Alonso-Varona, A., Fernandes, S., Palomares, T., RubioAzpeitia, E., et al. (2013). Biocompatible bacterial cellulose-poly (2-hydroxyethyl methacrylate) nanocomposite films. *BioMed Research International*. Article ID 698141, 14 pages. doi:10.1155/2013/698141.
32. Gelatin-Based Nanocomposites: A Review https://doi.org/10.1080/15583724 .2021.1897995.
33. TenHuisen, K. S., & Brown, P. W. (1994). The formation of hydroxyapatite-gelatin composites at 38 degrees C. *Journal of Biomedical Materials Research*, 28, 27–33. doi:10.1002/jbm.820280105.
34. Rajzer, I., Menaszek, E., Kwiatkowski, R., Planell, J. A., & Castano, O. (2014). Electrospun Gelatin/ Poly(e-Caprolactone) fibrous scaffold modified with calcium phosphate for bone tissue engineering. *Materials Science and Engineering: C Materials Biology and Applications*, 44, 183–190. doi:10.1016/j. msec.2014.08.017.
35. Azmana, M., Mahmood, S., Hilles, A. R., Rahman, A., Arifin, M. A. B., & Ahmed, S. (2021). A review on chitosan and chitosan-based bionanocomposites: Promising material for combatting global issues and its applications. *International Journal of Biological Macromolecules*, 185, 832–848.
36. Liu, Y. J., Bhattarai, P., Dai, Z. F., & Chen, X. Y. (2019). Photothermal therapy and photoacoustic imaging via nanotheranostics in fighting cancer. *Chemical Society Reviews*, 48, 2053–2108.

37. Chen, Q., Wen, J., Li, H., Xu, Y., Liu, F., & Sun, S. (2016). Recent advances in different modal imaging-guided photothermal therapy. *Biomaterials, 106,* 144–166.

38. Rabiee, N., Yaraki, M. T., Garakani, S. M., Garakani, S. M., Ahmadi, S., Lajevardi, A., ... Hamblin, M. R. (2020). Recent advances in porphyrin-based nanocomposites for effective targeted imaging and therapy. *Biomaterials, 232,* 119707.

39. Ou, H. L., Li, J., Chen, C., Gao, H. Q., Xue, X., & Ding, D. (2019). Organic/polymer photothermal nanoagents for photoacoustic imaging and photothermal therapy in vivo. *Science China Materials, 62,* 1740–1758.

40. Wang, K., Fan, X., Zhao, L., Zhang, X., Zhang, X., Li, Z., & Wei, Y. (2016). Aggregation induced emission fluorogens based nanotheranostics for targeted and imaging-guided chemo-photothermal combination therapy. *Small, 12*(47), 6568–6575.

41. Ou, H., Dai, S., Liu, R., & Ding, D. (2019). Manipulating the intramolecular motion of AIEgens for boosted biomedical applications. *Science China Chemistry, 62*(8), 929–932.

42. Geng, J., Liao, L. D., Qin, W., Tang, B. Z., Thakor, N., & Liu, B. (2015). Fluorogens with aggregation induced emission: ideal photoacoustic contrast reagents due to intramolecular rotation. *Journal of Nanoscience and Nanotechnology, 15*(2), 1864–1868.

43. Sheng, Z., Guo, B., Hu, D., Xu, S., Wu, W., Liew, W. H., ... Liu, B. (2018). Bright aggregation-induced-emission dots for targeted synergetic NIR-II fluorescence and NIR-I photoacoustic imaging of orthotopic brain tumors. *Advanced Materials, 30*(29), 1800766.

44. Qi, J., Sun, C., Zebibula, A., Zhang, H., Kwok, R. T., Zhao, X., & Tang, B. Z. (2018). Real-time and high-resolution bioimaging with bright aggregation-induced emission dots in short-wave infrared region. *Advanced materials, 30*(12), 1706856.

45. Lee, J. H., Wu, J. H., Lee, J. S., Jeon, K. S., Kim, H. R., Lee, J. H., ... Kim, Y. K. (2008). Synthesis and characterization of ${\rm Fe-FeO} _ {\rm x} $ core-shell nanowires. *IEEE Transactions on Magnetics, 44*(11), 3950–3953.

46. Lim, S. Y., Shen, W., & Gao, Z. (2015). Carbon quantum dots and their applications. *Chemical Society Reviews, 44*(1), 362–381.

47. Yoo, J. M., Kang, J. H., & Hong, B. H. (2015). Graphene-based nanomaterials for versatile imaging studies. *Chemical Society Reviews, 44*(14), 4835–4852.

48. Hemant, K., Pramod, K., Vishal, S., Shashi, P. S., & Balaram, P. (2023). Synthesis and surface modification of biocompatible mesoporous silica nanoparticles (MSNs) and its biomedical applications: A review. *Research Journal of Chemistry and Environment, 27,* 2.

49. Yang, K., Feng, L., Shi, X., & Liu, Z. (2013). Nano-graphene in biomedicine: theranostic applications. *Chemical Society Reviews, 42*(2), 530–547.

50. Wang, J., Mi, P., Lin, G., Wáng, Y. X. J., Liu, G., & Chen, X. (2016). Imaging-guided delivery of RNAi for anticancer treatment. *Advanced drug delivery reviews, 104,* 44–60.

51. Sun, X., Liu, Z., Welsher, K., Robinson, J.T., Goodwin, A., Zaric, S., & Dai, H. (2008). Nanographene oxide for cellular imaging and drug delivery. *Nano Research, 1,* 203–212.

52. Lin, J., Huang, Y., & Huang, P. (2016). Graphene-based nanomaterials in bioimaging. *Biomedical Applications of Functionalized Nanomaterials, 105*(Pt B), 242–254.

53. Liu, Z., Guo, Z., Zhong, H., Qin, X., Wan, M., & Yang, B. (2013). Graphene oxide based surface-enhanced Raman scattering probes for cancer cell imaging. *Physical Chemistry Chemical Physics, 15*(8), 2961–2966.

54. Ma, X., Qu, Q., Zhao, Y., Luo, Z., Zhao, Y., Ng, K.W., & Zhao, Y. (2013). Graphene oxide wrapped gold nanoparticles for intracellular Raman imaging and drug delivery. *Journal of Materials Chemistry B, 1,* 6495–6500.

55. Agnihotri, S., Yadav, K. K., Roy, I., & Kumar, P. (2018). Synthesis of nickel phthalocyanine encapsulated ORMOSIL nanoparticles as efficient phototherapeutic agent. *Advanced Science, Engineering and Medicine, 10*(1), 22–26.

56. Jin, Y., Wang, J., Ke, H., Wang, S., & Dai, Z. (2013). Graphene oxide modified PLA microcapsules containing gold nanoparticles for ultrasonic/CT bimodal imaging guided photothermal tumor therapy. *Biomaterials, 34*(20), 4794–4802.

57. Rong, P., Yang, K., Srivastan, A., Kiesewetter, D. O., Yue, X., Wang, F., Nie, L., Bhirde, A., Wang, Z., Liu, Z., Niu, G., Wang, W., & Chen, X. (2014). Photosensitizer loaded nanographene for multimodality imaging guided tumor photodynamic therapy. *Theranostics, 4,* 229–239.

58. Yan, X., Hu, H., Lin, J., Jin, A. J., Niu, G., Zhang, S., & Chen, X. (2015). Optical and photoacoustic dual-modality imaging guided synergistic photodynamic/photothermal therapies. *Nanoscale, 7*(6), 2520–2526.

59. Wu, C., Wang, S., Luo, X., Yuan, R., & Yang, X. (2020). Adenosine triphosphate responsive metal–organic frameworks equipped with a DNA structure lock for construction of a ratiometric SERS biosensor. *Chemical Communications, 56*(9), 1413–1416.

60. Pan, Y. B., Wang, S., He, X., Tang, W., Wang, J., Shao, A., & Zhang, J. (2019). A combination of glioma in vivo imaging and in vivo drug delivery by metal–organic framework based composite nanoparticles. *Journal of Materials Chemistry B, 7*(48), 7683–7689.

61. Hoop, M., Walde, C. F., Riccò, R., Mushtaq, F., Terzopoulou, A., Chen, X. Z., & Pané, S. (2018). Biocompatibility characteristics of the metal organic framework ZIF-8 for therapeutical applications. *Applied Materials Today, 11,* 13–21.

62. Cao, F. F., Ju, E. G., Liu, C. Q., Li, W., Zhang, Y., Dong, K., Liu, Z., Ren, J. S., & Qu, X. G. (2017). Encapsulation of aggregated gold nanoclusters in a metal-organic framework for real-time monitoring of drug release. *Nanoscale, 9,* 4128–4134.

63. Cai, H. J., Shen, T. T., Zhang, J., Shan, C. F., Jia, J. G., Li, X., & Tang, Y. (2017). A core–shell metal–organic-framework (MOF)-based smart nanocomposite for efficient NIR/H 2 O 2-responsive photodynamic therapy against hypoxic tumor cells. *Journal of Materials Chemistry B, 5*(13), 2390–2394.

64. Meng, H. M., Shi, X., Chen, J., Gao, Y., Qu, L., Zhang, K., & Li, Z. (2020). DNA amplifier-functionalized metal–organic frameworks for multiplexed detection and imaging of intracellular mRNA. *ACS Sensors, 5*(1), 103–109.

65. Cai, W., Gao, H., Chu, C., Wang, X., Wang, J., Zhang, P., & Chen, X. (2017). Engineering phototheranostic nanoscale metal–organic frameworks for multimodal imaging-guided cancer therapy. *ACS Applied Materials & Interfaces, 9*(3), 2040–2051.

66. Ling, D., Li, H., Xi, W., Wang, Z., Bednarkiewicz, A., Dibaba, S. T., & Sun, L. (2020). Heterodimers made of metal–organic frameworks and upconversion nanoparticles for bioimaging and pH-responsive dual-drug delivery. *Journal of Materials Chemistry B*, 8(6), 1316–1325.

67. Xu, H., Liu, X., Su, G., Zhang, B., & Wang, D. (2012). Electrostatic repulsion-controlled formation of polydopamine–gold Janus particles. *Langmuir*, 28(36), 13060–13065.

68. Hong, S., Lee, J. S., Ryu, J., Lee, S. H., Lee, D. Y., Kim, D. P., & Lee, H. (2011). Bio-inspired strategy for on-surface synthesis of silver nanoparticles for metal/organic hybrid nanomaterials and LDI-MS substrates. *Nanotechnology*, 22(49), 494020.

69. Long, Y., Wu, J., Wang, H., Zhang, X., Zhao, N., & Xu, J. (2011). Rapid sintering of silver nanoparticles in an electrolyte solution at room temperature and its application to fabricate conductive silver films using polydopamine as adhesive layers. *Journal of Materials Chemistry*, 21(13), 4875–4881.

70. Zhao, T., He, X. W., Li, W. Y., & Zhang, Y. K. (2015). Transferrin-directed preparation of red-emitting copper nanoclusters for targeted imaging of transferrin receptor over-expressed cancer cells. *Journal of Materials Chemistry B*, 3(11), 2388–2394.

71. Chen, X., Zhu, H., Huang, X., Wang, P., Zhang, F., Li, W., & Chen, B. (2017). Novel iodinated gold nanoclusters for precise diagnosis of thyroid cancer. *Nanoscale*, 9(6), 2219–2231.

72. Jackson, J. K., Letchford, K., & Wasserman, B. Z. (2011) The use of nanocrystalline cellulose for the binding and controlled release of drugs. *International Journal of Nanomedicine*, 6, 321.

73. Müller, A., Ni, Z., Hessler, N., et al (2013) The biopolymer bacterial nanocellulose as drug delivery system: investigation of drug loading and release using the model protein albumin. *Journal of Pharmaceutical Sciences*, 102, 579–592.

74. Jackson, J. K., Letchford, K., Wasserman, B. Z. (2011) The use of nanocrystalline cellulose for the binding and controlled release of drugs. *International Journal of Nanomedicine*, 6, 321.

75. A review on chitosan and its nanocomposites in drug delivery authors: Akbar Ali, Shakeel Ahmed. https://doi.org/10.1016/j.ijbiomac.2017.12.078

76. Saikia, C., Gogoi, P., & Maji, T. K. (2015). Chitosan: A promising biopolymer in drug delivery applications. *Journal of Molecular and Genetic Medicine Science*, 4, 6.

Carbon Nanocomposites

A Good Candidate for Sensing and Detection of Neurotransmitters

*Neeraj Gupta, Vishal Bharati Jaryal,
Sahil, and Abhishek Soni*

4.1 INTRODUCTION

The last century has seen an overwhelming rise in the use of organic polymers as a class of materials. A second step is typically integrated to prepare composite materials in order to further enhance their functionality and extend their applications. Carbon nanocomposites have proven to be most enticing materials for various promising applications. These materials offer special features because to their large abundance, excellent electrical conductivity, structural tunability at the atomic level, high selectivity, good resistance to acidic/alkaline environments, and environmental friendliness.[1] Due to this, these materials can readily be tuned for specific applications. Nanotechnological advancements have made it feasible to shape nanoscale level materials with desired shapes and characteristics. These advancements have permitted the fabrication of carbon nanomaterials into various forms with varying dimensionalities and physico-chemical characteristics. Carbon structures with highly organized zero-, one-, two-, and three-dimensional characteristics have been developed. Fullerene, carbon nanotubes (CNTs), graphene and graphite are some of the examples of carbon nanomaterials.[2,3] Figure 4.1 depicts the structural features of these carbon nanomaterials. Furthermore, amorphous carbon forms including carbon nanofibers, carbon nanofoams and carbon black have also garnered a lot of attention.[4] The complex frameworks and distinctive features of carbon nanomaterials are highly intriguing options for a variety of applications. Carbon nanostructures' diverse architectures and characteristics make them highly engaging materials for a wide range of critical applications. Furthermore, from an economic standpoint, carbon materials with widespread availability, low cost and less toxicity are favourable attributes for carbon-based applications.[5] Carbon nanostructures have amazing features due to their high surface area to volume ratio, in which the bulk of the atoms within the carbon framework are present on the surface and are in close vicinity of surrounding environment.[6] Furthermore, carbon nanomaterials with sp^2 hybridization like graphene and carbon nanotubes provides distinct characteristics including variable electronic properties as well as distinct mechanical, thermal and electrical capabilities.[7]

DOI: 10.1201/9781003470311-4

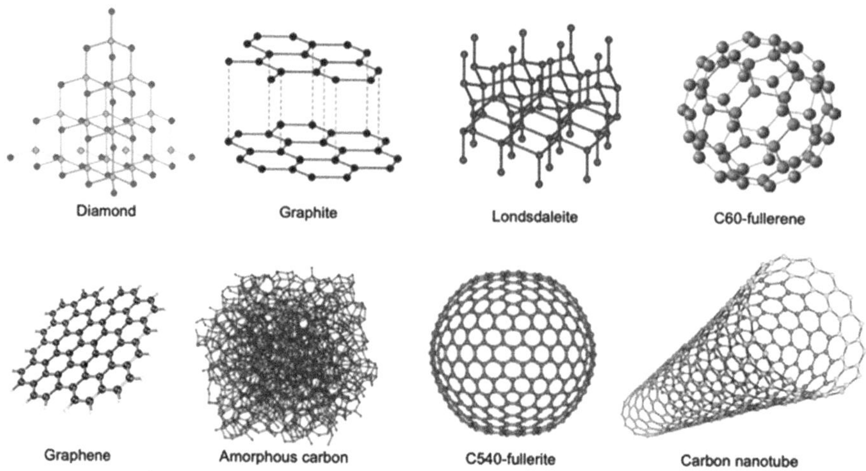

Figure 4.1 Different types of carbon-based nanomaterials. (Reprinted with permission[8]).

Employing carbon nanomaterials as additives in various polymeric materials creates new opportunities for various applications. It combines the excellent characteristics of carbon materials with the advantages of polymeric materials, permitting further enhancement of resulting nanocomposites. The homogenous dispersion of carbon nanofiller and the interaction of the nanofiller with host polymer are crucial components in the production of nanocomposite materials.[9] These parameters have a major influence on the characteristics of nanocomposite materials, which may be modified by regulating the above parameters.[10] Functionalization can improve the dispersion of additives in the nanocomposite. The covalent and non-covalent modification of the nanofillers results in their improved interaction with the host polymer matrix, thereby, increasing their dispersion in the composites. Covalent functionalization, on the other hand, alters the structure of the carbon nanofillers, modifying their hybridization and thereby influencing their thermal, electrical, mechanical and optical properties. To enhance the properties of polymeric nanocomposites, many carbon nanostructures have been used as fillers, from the inexpensive carbon black to the expensive CNTs.[11] Graphene and carbon nanotubes (CNTs) are favourable carbon-based nanofillers for polymeric materials. For more than 20 years, carbon nanotubes (CNTs) have received great attention of researchers because of their exceptional mechanical, electrical, optical, and thermal capabilities, as well as their distinct structure. However, despite many proposals, it is still challenging to produce nano-devices based on carbon nanotubes on an enormous scale.[12] Numerous researchers are becoming interested in investigating carbon nanotubes (CNTs) as bulk materials in an effort to enhance their practical applications.[13] In light of this, the creation of composite materials using polymers provides more insight into the application of CNTs. High mechanical strength, electrical conductivity, and thermal stability have traditionally been offered by CNTs, but low-cost, easily-fabricated polymers with adjustable architectures can be produced via solution or melting processes. As a result, both academic and industrial researchers have made significant efforts to investigate CNT/polymer composite materials. A lot of work has lately been focused on creating graphene/polymer composite materials following the discovery of graphene, a single sheet of graphite.[14] Integrating polymer materials with carbon nanostructures enhance the properties of the resulting nanocomposites, and also opens up a slew of new possibilities such as light-emitting diodes, supercapacitors, solar cells and electronic sensors.[15]

4.1 SYNTHESIS OF CARBON NANOCOMPOSITE MATERIALS

The synthesis of nanomaterials has received great attention, particularly for carbon nanotubes, due to the need to create high-quality CNTs at an affordable price. For decades, carbon fibre impregnated polymer composites have served the scientific community. Other carbon-based allotropic structures such as carbon nanotubes, graphene and buckyballs have joined the club after carbon fibre to improve composite characteristics. However, several carbon compounds incorporating nanoparticles have been explored in recent years with the objective of generating compounds with desirable properties utilizing processes that are less time consuming and use less-toxic reagents. The synthesis of carbon-based nanocomposites is a dynamic and burgeoning field at the intersection of materials science and nanotechnology. These nanocomposites, often composed of carbon nanotubes, graphene, or carbon nanoparticles, combined with various other materials, exhibit extraordinary properties and hold great promise for a plethora of applications. The process typically involves the dispersion of carbon-based materials within a matrix, which can be a polymer, ceramic, or metal, through various techniques such as chemical vapor deposition, solution mixing, or mechanical blending. Carbon-based nanocomposites including nanoparticles can be produced using a variety of approaches. Carbon nanoparticle supports may be constructed using silica matrices,[16,17] as well as by chemical vapour deposition (CVD) on a carbon mould.[18] Impregnation, ball milling, hydrothermal treatment, and sol-gel synthesis are some of the synthetic techniques used to generate nanocomposites.[19,20] More than one approach, such as solvothermal and hydrothermal co-precipitation, can be combined at different phases of the synthesis of nanocomposites, or they can be coupled with metal reduction by the application of a reducing agent[21]. Figure 4.2 depicts the hydrothermal fabrication of

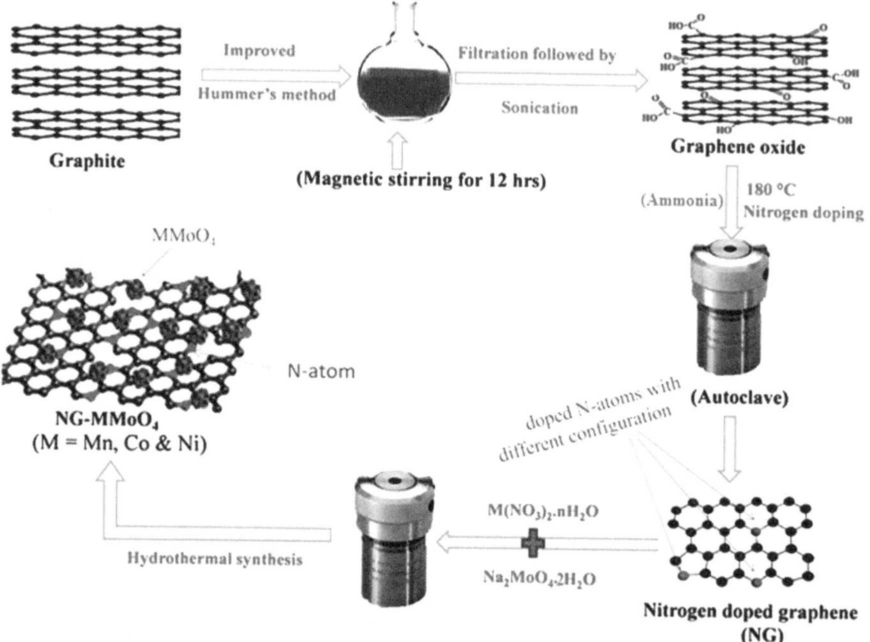

Figure 4.2 Schematic representation of nitrogen-doped graphene nanocomposites with metal molybdates via hydrothermal treatment.[22]

nanocomposites of nitrogen doped graphene and metal molybdates. It has been found that this methods of processing influence the interfaces of a composite and hence its properties.

By tailoring the composition and structure at the nanoscale, researchers can engineer materials with enhanced mechanical, electrical, and thermal properties, making them highly desirable for applications like lightweight structural components, advanced conductive materials, and high-efficiency energy storage devices. The versatility and tunability of carbon-based nanocomposites open doors to innovative solutions for many technological challenges, from aerospace to electronics, and continue to be a subject of intense research and development.

4.2 CARBON NANOCOMPOSITES FOR SENSING OF NEUROTRANSMITTERS

Learning, sleeping, hunger, awareness, memory, muscle contraction and relaxation, and heart rate are all essential to human survival. Neurotransmitters (NTs) are chemical substances inside the neural system that influence these actions and inactions.[23,24] NTs are the chemical substances which transfer signals from axon to dendrites of a neuron resulting in a physiological response. It is worth noting that these chemical messengers are supposed to function optimally in the human system. Epinephrine (EP), norepinephrine (NE), dopamine (DA), acetylcholine (ACh), glycine (Gly), glutamate (Glu), serotonin (SE), and nitric oxide (NO) are a few of the numerous NTs that are frequently studied. Their abnormal concentration in body results in disorders like Parkinson's disease, glaucoma, Alzheimer's disease, schizophrenia, depression, anxiety, myasthenia gravis, and Tourette's syndrome.[25] Determining the concentration of these substances in biological systems is an important scientific endeavor, given the crippling nature of many illnesses. As anticipated, a number of techniques – each with advantages and disadvantages – have been used to identify the concentration of neurotransmitters in human body for diagnosing and treating the illnesses mentioned. A better way of in vivo and in vitro quantification of NTs is desired due to factors like complex sample pretreatment that requires highly skilled instrument handling, expensive instrumentation, and long analysis times. There are several methodologies that have been adopted for the quantification of NTs including mass spectrometry, high-pressure liquid chromatography (HPLC), chemiluminescence, colorimetric technique, capillary electrophoresis, and ion-exchange chromatography. Fortunately, the gap is filled by electrochemical techniques, which are straightforward, sensitive, selective, economical, readily miniaturized, and need nothing in the way of specialized handling expertise. Numerous electrochemical sensors geared towards NT detection have been developed throughout time.[26] Incorporation of carbon nanomaterials such as carbon nanotubes (CNTs), carbon nanofibers and their composites with other materials in bare electrodes (gold, platinum, or glassy carbon electrode) has given birth to electrochemical sensors with high selectivity and sensitivity[27].

4.2.1 Epinephrine (EP)

Carbon nanocomposites have drawn a lot of interest due to their promising uses in electrocatalysis, energy storage, electrochemical sensing and capacitor devices. These materials have been intensively utilized as a promising catalyst for chemical transformations and also as sensing probes for different applications. They have also been used to develop conducting materials for electrochemical sensing of different fluids inside the body with a vision of identifying various acute diseases at the earliest possible stages so that they can be treated in a proper way. One such bodily fluid is the neurotransmitter epinephrine (EP), which is present in human blood serum.[28] Flickering EP levels have been linked to a number of illnesses,[29] including as chronic active hepatitis, hypoglycemia, and adrenal hyperplasia. Additionally, it is utilized as a medication for glaucoma, bronchial infections, emphysema, and several allergic infections.[30] Consequently, EP serves as an emergency pharmaceutical and is crucial for measuring its presence in the human body at the trace level. The literature has documented a number of analytical methods[31] for determining EP, such as capillary electrophoresis, fluorimetry, and HPLC. Their operation at an acidic pH, however, is a noticeable drawback and is very unfavourable, particularly for biological samples.[32] There are several reports in literature on the application of various composites[33,34] coupled with iron, nickel, gold, cobalt, and palladium-based nanomaterials as well as carbon paste electrodes (CPE), glassy carbon electrodes (GCE), and gold electrodes.[29] Nevertheless, because metals are hazardous to biological systems and have limited environmental solidity, they should not be used in the fabrication of biological system sensors. Carbon-based materials and a few modifiers have been utilized to sense EP electrochemically as an alternate to these metal-based analogues. The usage of MWCNTs,[35] graphene,[36] and graphene quantum dots[37] for the electrochemical detection of EP has been reported in a number of publications in the literature. These carbon-based materials are thought to be a great substitute with a wide range of electrochemistry-related applications.

The tailoring of carbon materials for electrochemical sensing can be effectively achieved by modifying their surface, structure and transforming them into various nanocomposites. In this context, the combination of amino groups from electron-rich melamine with graphene oxide has resulted in the formation of a metal-free composite (MGO). This composite exhibits remarkable current response capabilities and provides favourable attachment sites for EP. The analysis through SEM and EDS has unveiled a distinctive surface characterized by wrinkles and granular-shaped aggregates, indicating the inclusion of melamine in between GO sheets.[38] The presence of the highest nitrogen content (31.8%) in MGO confirms the integration of nitrogen rich melamine onto the surface of GO. The CV of MGO-GCE, GO-GCE, bare GCE, and bare GCE without EP were recorded in a 1 mM EP solution. In order to quantify the EP solution including PBS at pH 7.2, the GCE was further modified utilizing GO and MGO.[39] MGO-GCE had a higher Ipa (0.0533 mA) than GCE and GO-GCE. Comparing the MGO-GCE to the unmodified electrode, the current responsiveness was 64.17% greater. The electrocatalytic characteristics of MGO-GCE[39] for EP detection at physiological pH were demonstrated by the CV data. It was suggested that MGO-GCE has more electrocatalytic activity than GO-GCE based on the clear and robust oxidation–reduction peaks of EP. In 2010, Moraes et al.[40] attempted the sensing of epinephrine in a urine sample by employing a paraffin composite electrode and modified MWCNT with cobalt phthalocyanine (CoPc). The analysis of the electrochemical response of SE oxidation via DPV revealed 250 percent increase in peak current as compared to paraffin/MWCNT. The functioning electrode was tagged paraffin/MWCNT/CoPc. This was explained by EP's improved adsorptive capacity in the CoPc layer. During a DPV experiment using the constructed electrode and several doses of EP, a LOD of 15.6 nM was achieved for EP at a linear range of 1.33 to 5.50 µM.

It has been found that nicotine stimulates EP release into the blood stream. In light of this, Goyal and Bishnoi[41] developed a unique electrochemical sensor in 2011 to measure EP in smokers. A fMWCNT was dropped over bare EPPGE to create the working electrode (MWCNT/EPPGE). The sensing of EP at the MWCNT/EPPGE electrode via cyclic voltammetry showed a LOD of 0.15 nM. In contrast to the results of Moraes et al.,[42] our investigation provided a higher LOD. Shahrokhian and Sabre (2011) reported the utilization of an electrochemically deposited oxidized Ppy/MWCNT nanocomposite (pyrrole/MWCNT/GCE) on GCE for the detection of EP[43]. The investigation (using DPV) revealed an EP LOD of 40 nM at the constructed electrode. Using AuNP/MWCNT nanocomposite on ITO support (AuNP/MWCNT/ITO), another 2011 publication[44] reported that the synergy between AuNP and MWCNT, together with the high conductivity of AuNP, resulted in an electrode with a limit of detection of 4.2 nM within an LDR of 5 to 80 nM. The simultaneous measurement of PAR and EP with excellent peak separation demonstrated the adaptability of the AuNP modified electrode. Additionally, compared to non-smokers, smokers' urine had a rise in EP levels by approximately 45 nM, and for every 500 mg PAR consumed, the amount of EP increased five times. The AuNP modified electrode[44] had a rather high LOD, albeit, in contrast to the work done by Goyal and Bishnoi,[41] where a lower limit of detection of 0.15 nM was found. Another novel sensitive electrochemical sensor (GRP-CHIT-Bi_2O_3 or GCB)[45] was synthesized by H. Devnani et al. using precursor bismuth oxide (Bi_2O_3) nanoparticles, graphene (GRP) and chitosan (CHIT). The morphology of nanocomposite was studied with the help of AFM and SEM. The fabricated sensor was used for the EP detection at pH 7.4 using cyclic voltammetry and square wave voltammetry. There was an increase in current response of nanocomposite modified GCE (GCB/GCE) as compared to bare GCE. The sensor detected the neurotransmitter EP with LOD of 3.56 nM and limit of quantification 11.85 nM. Also, the sensor exhibited high sensitivity (1.3 nA/nM) and selectivity for EP. The electrochemical response of EP at nanocomposite modified GCE exhibited dependence on the parameters like scan rate, pH, and concentration. The modified sensor was successfully employed for the detection of EP in both pharmaceutical formulation and human blood serum samples.

4.2.2 Norepinephrine (NE)

Just like dopamine that have been discussed in previous section, this section will cover the efforts made in the last ten years to quantify NE in biological and pharmacological samples. The existence of NE in extracellular fluids with UA and AA is well established. Norepinephrine is acknowledged as a vital catecholamine neurotransmitter within the mammalian central nervous system, originating primarily from the adrenal medulla. Its role holds significance in both health and pathological conditions. Elevated norepinephrine levels are implicated in stress, hypotension, thyroid hormone deficiency, congestive heart failure, and arrhythmias, whereas reduced norepinephrine level is associated with idiopathic postural hypotension. Numerous studies indicate that adherence of leukocytes infected with the HIV-I virus to cardiac endothelial cells and speeds up HIV propagation. Norepinephrine is deemed crucial in the context of mental disorder, DNA damage, diabetes and heart failure.[46] In light of this, Huang et al.'s work[47] on the synchronous measurement of norepinephrine along with UA and AA using an SPCE modified with a composite of MWCNTs and polyacrylic acid (PAA) was made accessible. The MWCNTs dispersion prepared in PAA was drop-casted on the surface of SPCE and was dried at RT in order to create PAA-MWCNT/SPCE as the working electrode. In a CV experiment, anodic peak current was shown to be enhanced for the NE when utilizing PAA-MWCNT/SPCE electrode as opposed to bare SPCE. A limit of detection of 0.131 µM within a linear range of 0 to 10 µM was assessed in the DPV experiment using different amounts of norepinephrine in the presence of constant quantities of AA and UA.

The sulfur nanodots grown on the surface of graphene oxide nanocomposite (nS@GO)[46] was fabricated by N. Jaiswal et al. for the sensing of NE in the absence and presence of tryptophan, acetaminophen and 4-aminophenol. The nanocomposite was fabricated using precursor carbon disulfide as source of sulfur and dimethylformamide as solvent in one-pot method. The fabricated nanocomposite was employed for sensor application through the deposition of nS@GO (dispersed in dimethylformamide) onto a GCE using the drop-casting technique. Differential pulse anodic stripping voltammetry was employed for the sensing of NE in the absence and presence of tryptophan, acetaminophen and 4-aminophenol. Beside this, chronoamperometry and EIS were also used to sense the NE. The nS@GO modified electrochemical sensor exhibited a LOD of 0.26 µM for the sensing of NE in both conditions that is in the absence and presence of other analytes. The electrode modified with the nanocomposite was successfully assessed for its response in real samples, demonstrating effective performance without encountering any cross-reactivity.

D. Queiroz and his workers synthesized a nanocomposite[48] of cobalt ferrite nanoparticles with MWCNTs modified glassy carbon electrode (GC/MWCNT/FCo$_{98}$) for electrocatalytic oxidation and reduction of norepinephrine. The cobalt ferrite underwent characterization through TEM and XRD. The optimized electrode composition involved 10 µL of carbon nanotubes and 4 µL of cobalt ferrite in a 0.1 mol L^{-1} PBS (pH = 7.0). The resultant electrode demonstrated electrochemical response over a broad range of potential (–0.4 to 1.0 V vs. Ag/AgCl), exhibiting excellent durability, stability and conductivity in 0.1 mol L^{-1} PBS. Comparative analysis revealed that the oxidation of NE on the unmodified glassy carbon electrode occurred at +0.60 V vs. Ag/AgCl with a current of 0.17 µA, whereas the modified glassy carbon electrode with carbon nanotubes and cobalt ferrite NPs exhibited catalytic activity at +0.54 V vs. Ag/AgCl with a current of 0.23 mA. The amperometric method for assessing the anodic peak current (Ipa) in relation to norepinephrine concentration at the modified electrode displayed linearity within the concentration range of 0.16–1.91 mmol L^{-1}, with a LOD of 0.76 µmol L^{-1}. Consequently, the nanocomposite modified GCE emerges as a promising tool for neuroscientific applications, particularly in the determination of this neurotransmitter.

Another nanocomposite was prepared using graphene and chitosan which was used too modify the GCE for sensitive and selective quantification of norepinephrine. The morphology of as-prepared nanocomposite was examined through AFM and SEM. EIS and cyclic voltammetry were used for studying the electrochemical behavior of fabricated sensor. The modified sensor exhibited fast electron transfer process and low charge transfer resistance (R_{ct}). The electrochemical response for norepinephrine by nanocomposite-modified sensor was systematically investigated using PBS (pH 7.4) employing square wave and cyclic voltammetry. The modified sensor showed higher in the detection of norepinephrine. Furthermore, the developed method proved effective in determining norepinephrine levels in a pharmaceutical formulation.[49]

4.2.3 Dopamine (DA)

Dopamine (DA) is a neurotransmitter that regulates a variety of bodily behaviors and processes. Abnormal concentrations of DA in the body results in various mental and physical illnesses including Parkinson's disease, attention deficit hyperactivity and obesity.[50] Additionally, it serves as a biomarker for specific cancer types, including heochromocytoma and paraganglioma.[51] Therefore, there is an urgent need for a cheap point-of-care device that can measure dopamine even up to 10^{-12} M in body fluids. Detecting DA in real physiological samples is difficult because the DA concentration in human urine and blood is as low as 274×10^{-9} and 195.8×10^{-12} M respectively. Interfering substances can also complicate the detection process.[51] Early and precise diagnosis of this neurotransmitter is necessary for successful therapy. There are few ways for detecting low levels of DA in laboratories, with few equipment accessible for frontline treatment of afflicted individuals. Diagnostic methods need costly equipment and time-consuming sample preparation, making it difficult to detect DA at the point-of-care. Consequently, a wide range of materials for electrochemical sensing technologies have been developed.

Q. X. Tong et al. had designed a composite of MWCNT and graphene quantum dots[52] for the electrochemical detection of neurotransmitter dopamine. MWCNTs are superior electrode materials, while GQDs, as carbon nanomaterials, have enough surface areas to enhance the conductivity of the modified electrodes. The as synthesized nanocomposite was characterized by TEM, XRD, FT-IR for the identification of various active sites and morphology of the nanomaterial. The sensor exhibits exceptional selectivity for dopamine in comparison to other bio analytes. With a limit of detection of 0.87 nM, the fabricated nanocomposite demonstrated optimal performance for DA measurement under ideal circumstances, displaying strong linearity from 0.005 μM to 100.0 μM. S. C. Peter *et al.* had prepared a $Pt/CeO_2@Cu_2O$ carbon nanocomposite[53] to enhance the electrochemical sensing of the painkiller paracetamol and neurotransmitter dopamine. The nanocomposite was synthesized at low temperature by using Cu_2O as template. The electrochemical behavior of different modified electrodes was recorded using CV and DPV. Out of all, $Pt/CeO_2@Cu_2O$ was observed to be very selective for detection of DA with PA. Sensitive electro-oxidation peak potentials were measured for DA and PA using the DPV approach at 160 mV and 380 mV respectively. The response of both DA and PA is linear within a linear range of 0.5 - 100 μM. For PA and DA, the LOD were found to be 0.079 μM and 0.091 μM, respectively. The $Pt/CeO_2@Cu_2O$-carbon paste electrode (CPE) has practical applications for the detection of DA and PA in pharmaceuticals and in spiked human blood and urine samples. V. Durairaj et al. had developed tetrahedral amorphous carbon electrodes with MWCNTs, nanofibrillar cellulose, and Nafion composite modified for selective Dopamine Detection. The composite membrane is made up of Nafion and sulphated nanofibrillar cellulose (SNFC) dissolved in a matrix of MWCNTs. The SNFC and Nafion ionomers' strong negative charge densities improve the composite's cationic selectivity. FTIR, SEM, TEM and Raman spectroscopy, were used for the characterization the composite. Potential dopamine (DA) electrochemical sensors are being studied using tetrahedral amorphous carbon modified electrodes that have been modified with the developed nanocomposite. The electrodes that were changed with a composite exhibit notable DA selectivity and sensitivity when ascorbic acid and uric acid are present in physiologically appropriate amounts. Using cyclic voltammetry (CV) at 100 mV/s, a linear detection range of 0.05 to 100 μM was achieved for DA with LOD of 65 and 107 nM in PBS and interferent solution respectively.

S. R. Ali et al. have fabricated poly(anilineboronic acid)/carbon nanotube composite[54] for the electrochemical detection of neurotransmitter DA. The transduction mechanism for this nonoxidative DA sensor is the strong affinity between DA and the boronic acid groups inside the polymer, which has a considerable impact on the electrochemical properties of the polyaniline backbone.

SWCNTs functionalized with single-standard DNA had an extraordinary reduction potential and good conductivity, which greatly improved the electrochemical performance of the polymer in a physiological buffer. Additionally, the extensive surface area of CNTs has substantially increased the density of the boronic acid receptors. The carbon nanotubes were used to enhance the electrochemical sensing, whereas PABA was used as the selective DA receptor. The sensor detected DA through CV and DPV technique with limit of detection of 0.6 nM and 16 pM respectively. Q. Huang et al. have synthesized GQDs-MWCNTs composites based electrochemical sensor[55] for the detection of DA in living cells. GQDs were utilized because they have a high surface area, which improves electrode conductivity, and MWCNTs were employed because they serve as ideal electrode materials. Conjugated π-bonds in the nanocomposite facilitate electron transport of DA via the π-π stacking force. Simultaneously, the presence of multiple anionic groups on the graphene quantum dots could effectively attract cations to enhance the selectivity of the sensor. As anticipated, the sensor displayed remarkable selectivity for DA when compared to other interfering bio analytes. The sensor exhibited maximum performance towards DA detection with a LOD of 0.87 nM. D. Sangamithirai et al. have fabricated electrochemical senor based on poly(o-anisidine)/CNTs nanocomposites[56] for the detection of DA. A nanocomposite of carbon nanotubes and poly(o-anisidine) (POA/CNTs) was added to the glassy carbon electrode. POA was used because of its immobilizing matrix, which have π-conjugated backbones to enhance the catalytic activity. Also, POA has excellent biodegradability, biocompatibility, high mechanical strength and susceptibility, and cost effective. The CNTs were used due to their unique properties like electronic structures, high electrical conductivity, chemically active surface, good biocompatibility and favourable chemical stability. Due to the combined effects of the nanocomposite, the modified electrode demonstrated a significant and long-lasting ability to mediate electron transfer, which was influential for the detection of DA. The prepared nanocomposite detected the DA with a limit of detection of 0.12 μM. The sensor showed excellent sensitivity, stability and reproducibility in for DA detection.

4.2.4 Serotonin (SE) or 5-HT

In recent years, the electrochemical sensing of neurotransmitters has emerged as a pivotal area of research, with profound implications for understanding neurobiology and developing diagnostic tools for neurological disorders. Among these neurotransmitters, serotonin, a key player in regulating mood and behavior, has garnered significant attention. This section delves into the realm of electrochemical sensing, focusing on the detection of serotonin utilizing carbon nanocomposites as the sensing platform. The unique properties of carbon nanomaterials, coupled with the electrochemical techniques employed, offer a promising avenue for the selective and sensitive serotonin detection. This section reviews several studies conducted over the last decade on SE sensing employing carbon-based nanocomposites modified electrodes.

M. Raj et al. have designed graphene and poly 4-amino-3-hydroxy-1-naphthalenesulfonic acid based nanocomposites. These nanocomposites were used to fabricate a screen printed carbon sensor for the electrochemical sensing of DA and SE. The electrochemical measurements were done using CV and SWV. EIS and FESEM were utilized to analyze the surface morphology of the modified sensor. The sensor detected DA and SE with a LOD of 2 nM and 3 nM respectively. The designed sensor has exhibited successful detection of SE and DA in pharmacological samples, as well as in human urine and blood samples, demonstrating its efficacy across various matrices. The polymer film containing functional groups and synergistic interaction among graphene and p-AHNSA through π-π stacking, increases the transfer of electrons and displayed a noteworthy catalytic activity towards 5-HT and DA neurotransmitters. Therefore, this technique provided a good methodology for the detection of DA and SE with good sensitivity, selectivity and reproducibility. K. Ghanbari et al. electrochemically synthesized Pt nanoparticles/over-oxidized Polypyrrole nanofibers/reduced graphene oxide (Pt NPs/OPPy/RGO) nanocomposite, and utilized for the electrochemical detection of DA and SE. Initially, graphene oxide was subjected to electrochemical deposition and reduced on GCE surface. Subsequently, OPPy were synthesized through electrodeposition followed by the electrodeposition of Pt NPs on the surface of OPPy to fabricate the nanocomposite Pt NPs/OPPy/RGO/GCE. The PtNPs were used because they exhibit remarkable electrocatalytic activity and heightened sensitivity during electrochemical reactions, signifying improved electron transfer and decreased overpotential. Modifying graphene oxide with Pt NPs not only maximizes the utilization of the electro-active surface area at the nanoscale levels but also enhances the mass transfer rate (movement of reactants to the electro-catalyst). Among the bare GCE, OPPy/RGO/GCE RGO/GCE and Pt NPs/OPPy/RGO/GCE, the modified electrode (Pt NPs/OPPy/RGO/GCE) showed large catalytic activity towards simultaneous detection of DA and SE in the presence of other interferents like ascorbic acid. The sensor's ability to detect DA and SE in human blood serum was assessed using DPV. The sensor simultaneously detected the DA and SE with limit of detection of 42 nM and 106 nM, respectively.

B. Wu et al. have designed a sensitive electrochemical sensor[57] to enhance the detection of SE using nanocomposite, gold nanoparticles on multiwall carbon nanotubes covalently bonded by ferrocene (FeC-AuNPs-MWCNT). The catalytic properties of both high density FeC and AuNPs, along with the excellent electrical conductivity of carbon nanotube networks are responsible to facilitate a sensitive electrochemical response for the oxidation of SE. AuNPs on the surface of MWCT were chemically reduced to create the nanocomposite, and FeC molecules were then covalently functionalized onto the AuNPs. Excellent catalytic activity was demonstrated by the screen-printed carbon electrodes modified with the nanocomposite FeC-AuNPs-MWCNT for the oxidation of SE. The square wave voltammetry was used to confirm the enhanced electrocatalytic activity (61 times higher than the unmodified SPCE) of nanocomposite towards SE detection. The sensor exhibited a limit of detection of 17 nM.

The unique biomaterial for serotonin[58] detection was created by V. V. Becerra et al. using immobilized monoamine oxidase-A on multiwalled carbon nanotubes. The immobilized MAO-A (MWCNT/MAO-A) demonstrated good thermal and pH stability, while maintaining 94.3% of its catalytic activity. Using the bio composite, serotonin was successfully detected by measuring the H_2O_2 generated by enzymes. The modified GCE made of MWCNT/MAO-A was examined using CV and DPV. A linear response of 5.67×10^{-7} M–2.26×10^{-6} M was obtained by electrochemical measurements in simulated body fluid. The quantification limit was 6.73×10^{-7} M (118.7 ng mL^{-1}) and the low detection limit was 2×10^{-7} M (35.6 ng mL^{-1}). These results fall within serotonin levels observed in several neurological diseases. The bio-composite has the potential to be used in the fabrication of biosensors for serotonin detection.

F. Arslan and his co-workers had designed the carbon dot-modified carbon paste electrode[59] for the amperometric detection of ACh. It is found in the central nervous system, lymph nodes of the internal organs' motor systems, and junctions between muscles and nerves. Alzheimer's disease has been linked to a low level of ACh in the brain. It is a significant agent for this illness because of this. To measure the quantity of acetylcholine, a bienzymatic biosensor system containing acetylcholine esterase and choline oxidase was developed using a CPE modified with carbon nanodot (3-aminopropyl)triethoxysilane. Using glutaraldehyde cross-linking, choline oxidase and ACh esterase were immobilized onto a modified CPE. Acetylcholine was measured by oxidizing H_2O_2 that was generated enzymatically at 0.4 V vs. Ag/AgCl. Investigations were conducted into the effects of substrate concentration pH and temperature on the constructed biosensor's cholinergic response. Furthermore, the interference effect, the linear operating range of the biosensor, and the ideal CDs-APTES amount were also examined.

4.2.5 Acetylcholine (ACh)

Compared to previously studied NTs, ACh estimation utilizing modified carbon nanocomposite based electrodes has a limited literature base and may not benefit from the extensive study seen with catecholamines.

Inspired by the fact that exposure to organophosphates (OPs) inhibits the activity of acetylcholinesterase (AChE), Du et al. set out to construct a carbon nanotube (CNT) electrode that can measure AChE.[60] The chitosan-modified GCE surface was covered with MWCNT-Au nanocomposite and applied in a single process, to fabricate an electrode known as AChE-MWCNTs-AuNPs-CHT/GCE. Two nanocomposite modified GCEs (MWCNTs-AuNPs-CHT and AChE-AuNPs-CHT) were prepared for comparison. A limit of detection of 0.10 µM was calculated by the modified electrode in an acetylthiocholine chloride (ATCl) solution. As anticipated, the electrode's current responsiveness to the thiocholine solution decreased significantly after being incubated in malathion. This is due to the pesticide's ability to prevent the enzyme (AChE) from acting, which changes the enzyme's affinity for thiocholine. A LOD of 0.6 ng mL^{-1} was obtained from the current response using CV in the presence of malathion.

Acetylcholinesterase and choline oxidase enzymes were immobilized on iron oxide nanoparticles (Fe_2O_3NPs) and poly(3,4-ethylenedioxythiophene)-rGO nanocomposite modified fluorine doped tin oxide (FTO).[61] They serves as a crucial biological sensor for detection of acetylcholine (ACh). CV, EIS and SEM were employed to test the characteristics of nanocomposites both quantitatively and qualitatively. With a limit of detection of 4.0 nM and a response time of less than 4 seconds, this biological sensor was produced and a linear range from 4.0 nM–800 µM was achieved. Throughout the prolonged storage period, the sensor demonstrated excellent sensitivity, extreme selectivity and stability. The proposed biosensor exhibits a low LOD in addition to its extraordinarily high sensitivity. This was the first reported electrochemical sensor with regards to already developed ACh sensors. The use of Fe_2O_3NPs/rGO/PEDOT modified FTO electrodes to detect ACh levels in serum samples has greatly expanded the biosensor's applicability. This is especially important for individuals with Alzheimer's disease.

Khan and Ghani (2012) developed another AChE-modified MWCNT electrode for concurrently measuring ACh and its metabolite.[58] Poly(o-phenylenediamine) (PoPD) was applied to a carbon fibre electrode (CFE) in order to fabricate this bi-enzyme sensor. This was accomplished by immobilizing AChE and choline oxidase (ChO). Afterwards, electro polymerization of o-phenylenediamine was performed on modified CFE. This structure was subjected to glutaraldehyde for crosslinking before being immersed in a solution containing functionalized CNTs and Nafion. Notably, numerous variants of the electrode were created utilizing varying enzyme ratios and two distinct CFE geometries (elliptical and disc). In the presence of common interferents such as UA, AA amine and alcohols, the NaF-FCNTs/Glu/AChE-ChO/PoPD/CFE modified electrode, was used successfully for the quantification of ACh and Ch. The limit of detection limit of 0.045 µM and a response time of 5 seconds for H_2O_2 was achieved.

4.3 MECHANISM OF DETECTION OF NEUROTRANSMITTERS USING CARBON NANOCOMPOSITES

As previously stated, there are several varieties of NTs with varying chemical structures and their detection methodologies also differs. At the electrode surface, catecholamine such as EP, NE, and DA experiences a distinct redox response than indoleamines NTs. More crucially, the electrochemical setup employed in the literature consists of three electrode system (reference, working and counter electrode). The electrode that undergoes redox reactions is known as the working electrode. In another context, CNTs along with other nanomaterials have been utilized for the surface modification of pristine sensor. The reference electrode, which the potentiostat uses to adjust the potential of the working electrode, usually includes a saturated calomel electrode or an Ag/AgCl electrode. The circuit is completed by the counter electrode, and when current flows between the counter electrode and the working electrode, the current response produced by a redox reaction taking place in the system is recorded.[43]

Apart from acting as a medium in the analyte, supporting electrolyte also aids in circuit completion by lowering solvent resistance. The supporting electrode must always be substantially more concentrated than the analyte to fulfil its intended purpose.[43] Because of the large surface area of carbon nanotubes, ability to facilitate electron transport, and $\pi-\pi$ interaction among carbon nanotubes and DA, the analyte stays near the surface of modified electrode.[62] The analyte (DA) undergoes oxidation at the electrode surface when it loses two electrons and the two H atoms from the OH groups present at the backbone of catechol (Figure 4.3). The flow of current among working and counter electrode is recorded throughout the process.[43] There is a sharp drop in

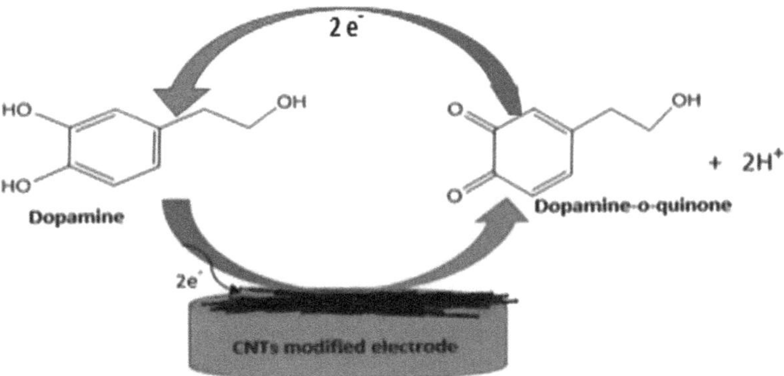

Figure 4.3 Mechanism of electrochemical oxidation of dopamine on the surface of CNTs modified electrode.[43]

the concentration gradient between the diffusion layer and bulk solution as the electrode's reduced form decreases. The analyte's oxidized form is reduced and the initial potential is reversed. Afterwards, the current rate between the working electrode and counter is measured. The anodic and cathodic peak currents represent the highest current under each of the two circumstances.

4.4 CONCLUSION

Over the last decade, there has been an exponential increase in research on carbon nanocomposite based sensors. Researchers are now interested in the emergence of numerous complex carbon nanocomposites, which include porous carbon, graphene-based 2D and 3D carbon composites, graphene quantum dots, carbon nanotubes, carbon nanodiamonds, nanofibers, and conducting polymers. Due to their fascinating characteristics, such as large surface area, tuneable surface functional groups, and superior conductivity, various carbon-based nanocomposites have been investigated for designing electrochemical sensors to detect neurotransmitters in body fluids. Electrochemical sensors based on carbon nanocomposites have emerged as an enticing alternate for various applications due to their high selectivity and fast detection ability. In the near future, constructing skin-like sensors for continuous and real-time sensing of neurotransmitters will be the main objective of electrochemical sensing applications. To accomplish this goal, novel electrochemical approaches for NTs sensing, including fast scan CV are being developed on an ongoing basis. Furthermore, research is also required for developing implantable sensors with fast response time, electrode arrays capable of detecting a panel of NTs at the same time (with effective calibration), smartphone-based and skin-like biomimetic sensors. The creation of high-throughput portable/miniaturized sensor arrays constructed from carbon nanocomposites has been the focus of recent advancements.

This book chapter has collated a large number of published works about the electrochemical detection of neurotransmitters. Furthermore, a detailed discussion of the fundamental idea of employing each carbon-based nanocomposites for surface modification is given. This book chapter will be useful in generating new concepts for the electrochemical methods of selective NTs detection for therapeutic use.

CONFLICT OF INTEREST

The authors declare no competing conflicts of interest.

AUTHOR CONTRIBUTIONS

NG was involved in every stages of this work from planning to execution and internal revision of the chapter. VBJ, S and AS compiled the manuscript in close association with one another.

REFERENCES

1. C. Hu, Y. Xiao, Y. Zou and L. Dai, Carbon-based metal-free electrocatalysis for energy conversion, energy storage, and environmental protection. *Electrochem Energy Rev*, 2018, **1**, 84–112.
2. A. Rabti, N. Raouafi and A. Merkoçi, Bio(sensing) devices based on ferrocene–functionalized graphene and carbon nanotubes. *Carbon N Y*, 2016, **108**, 481–514.
3. D. Jariwala, V. K. Sangwan, L. J. Lauhon, T. J. Marks and M. C. Hersam, Carbon nanomaterials for electronics, optoelectronics, photovoltaics, and sensing. *Chem Soc Rev*, 2013, **42**, 2824–2860.
4. M. J. Beliatis, L. J. Rozanski, K. D. G. I. Jayawardena, R. Rhodes, J. V. Anguita, C. A. Mills and S. R. P. Silva, Hybrid and nano-composite carbon sensing platforms. *Carbon for Sensing Devices*, 2015, 105–132.
5. C. Li, E. T. Thostenson and T. W. Chou, Sensors and actuators based on carbon nanotubes and their composites: A review. *Compos Sci Technol*, 2008, **68**, 1227–1249.
6. E. Llobet, Gas sensors using carbon nanomaterials: A review. *Sens Actuators B Chem*, 2013, **179**, 32–45.
7. M. Pumera, A. Ambrosi, A. Bonanni, E. L. K. Chng and H. L. Poh, Graphene for electrochemical sensing and biosensing. *TrAC Trends in Anal Chem*, 2010, **29**, 954–965.
8. V. Negri, J. Pacheco-Torres, D. Calle and P. López-Larrubia, Carbon nanotubes in biomedicine. *Topics in Curr Chem*, 2020, **378**, 1–41.
9. E. T. Thostenson, Z. Ren and T. W. Chou, Advances in the science and technology of carbon nanotubes and their composites: A review. *Compos Sci Technol*, 2001, **61**, 1899–1912.
10. X. Sun, H. Sun, H. Li, H. Peng, H. Peng, X. Sun, H. Sun and H. Li, Developing polymer composite materials: Carbon nanotubes or graphene? *Adv Mater*, 2013, **25**, 5153–5176.
11. V. Eswaraiah, K. Balasubramaniam and S. Ramaprabhu, Functionalized graphene reinforced thermoplastic nanocomposites as strain sensors in structural health monitoring. *J Mater Chem*, 2011, **21**, 12626–12628.
12. R. H. Baughman, A. A. Zakhidov and W. A. De Heer, Carbon nanotubes--the route toward applications. *Science (1979)*, 2002, **297**, 787–792.
13. X. Gui, J. Wei, K. Wang, A. Cao, H. Zhu, Y. Jia, Q. Shu and D. Wu, Carbon nanotube sponges. *Adv Mater*, 2010, **22**, 617–621.
14. S. Stankovich, D. A. Dikin, G. H. B. Dommett, K. M. Kohlhaas, E. J. Zimney, E. A. Stach, R. D. Piner, S. B. T. Nguyen and R. S. Ruoff, Graphene-based composite materials. *Nature 2006 442:7100*, 2006, **442**, 282–286.

15. G. Mittal, V. Dhand, K. Y. Rhee, S. J. Park and W. R. Lee, A review on carbon nanotubes and graphene as fillers in reinforced polymer nanocomposites. *J Ind Eng Chem*, 2015, **21**, 11–25.

16. C. Vix-Guterl, S. Boulard, J. Parmentier, J. Werckmann and J. Patarin, Formation of ordered mesoporous carbon material from a silica template by a one-step chemical vapour infiltration process. 2002, 1062–1063, https://doi.org/10.1246/cl.2002.1062.

17. F. Ehrburger-Dolle, I. Morfin, E. Geissler, F. Bley, F. Livet, C. Vix-Guterl, S. Saadallah, J. Parmentier, M. Reda, J. Patarin, M. Iliescu and J. Werckmann, Small-angle X-ray scattering and electron microscopy investigation of silica and carbon replicas with ordered porosity. *Langmuir*, 2003, **19**, 4303–4308.

18. C. Zlotea, C. Chevalier-César, E. Léonel, E. Leroy, F. Cuevas, P. Dibandjo, C. Vix-Guterl, T. Martens and M. Latroche, Synthesis of small metallic Mg-based nanoparticles confined in porous carbon materials for hydrogen sorption. *Faraday Discuss*, 2011, **151**, 117–131.

19. A. Rahim, S. B. A. Barros, L. T. Arenas and Y. Gushikem, In situ immobilization of cobalt phthalocyanine on the mesoporous carbon ceramic SiO2/C prepared by the sol–gel process. Evaluation as an electrochemical sensor for oxalic acid. *Electrochim Acta*, 2011, **56**, 1256–1261.

20. A. Tavasoli, K. Sadagiani, F. Khorashe, A. A. Seifkordi, A. A. Rohani and A. Nakhaeipour, Cobalt supported on carbon nanotubes — A promising novel Fischer–Tropsch synthesis catalyst. *Fuel Process Technol*, 2008, **89**, 491–498.

21. V. Sunny, D. S. Kumar, P. Mohanan and M. R. Anantharaman, Nickel/Carbon hybrid nanostructures as microwave absorbers. *Mater Lett*, 2010, **64**, 1130–1132.

22. M. Kumar, R. Singh, H. Khajuria and H. N. Sheikh, Facile hydrothermal synthesis of nanocomposites of nitrogen doped graphene with metal molybdates (NG-MMoO4) (M=Mn, Co, and Ni) for enhanced photodegradation of methylene blue. *J Mater Sci Mater Electron*, 2017, **28**, 9423–9434.

23. Q. Huang, S. Hu, H. Zhang, J. Chen, Y. He, F. Li, W. Weng, J. Ni, X. Bao and Y. Lin, Carbon dots and chitosan composite film based biosensor for the sensitive and selective determination of dopamine. *Analyst*, 2013, **138**, 5417–5423.

24. J. R. Cooper, F. E. Bloom and R. H. Roth, *The Biochemical Basis of Neuropharmacology*, Oxford University Press, New York, 8th edn., 2003.

25. M. Day, Z. Wang, J. Ding, X. An, C. A. Ingham, A. F. Shering, D. Wokosin, E. Ilijic, Z. Sun, A. R. Sampson, E. Mugnaini, A. Y. Deutcch, S. R. Sesack, G. W. Arbuthnott and D. J. Surmeier, Selective elimination of glutamatergic synapses on striatopallidal neurons in parkinson disease models. *Nat Neurosci*, 2006, **9**, 251–259.

26. B. B. Prasad, A. Prasad, M. P. Tiwari and R. Madhuri, Multiwalled carbon nanotubes bearing 'terminal monomeric unit' for the fabrication of epinephrine imprinted polymer-based electrochemical sensor. *Biosens Bioelectron*, 2013, **45**, 114–122.

27. L. C. S. Figueiredo-Filho, T. A. Silva, F. C. Vicentini and O. Fatibello-Filho, Simultaneous voltammetric determination of dopamine and epinephrine in human body fluid samples using a glassy carbon electrode modified with nickel oxide nanoparticles and carbon nanotubes within a dihexadecylphosphate film. *Analyst*, 2014, **139**, 2842–2849.

28. K. Bala, D. Sharma and N. Gupta, Carbon-nanotube-based materials for electrochemical sensing of the neurotransmitter dopamine. *Chem Electro Chem*, 2019, **6**, 274–288.

29. D. M. Fouad and W. A. El-Said, Selective electrochemical detection of epinephrine using gold nanoporous film. *J Nanomater*, doi:10.1155/2016/6194230.

30. L. I. N. Tomé and C. M. A. Brett, Polymer/Iron oxide nanoparticle modified glassy carbon electrodes for the enhanced detection of epinephrine. *Electroanalysis*, 2019, **31**, 704–710.

31. H. N. Luk, T. Y. Chou, B. H. Huang, Y. S. Lin, H. Li and R. J. Wu, Promotion effect of palladium on BiVO4 sensing material for epinephrine detection. *Catalysts*, 2021, **11**, 1083.

32. H. Beitollahi, M. Safaei and S. Tajik, Voltammetric and amperometric sensors for determination of epinephrine: A short review (2013–2017): Original scientific paper. *J Electrochem Sci Eng*, 2019, **9**, 27–43.

33. N. G. Mphuthi, A. S. Adekunle and E. E. Ebenso, Electrocatalytic Oxidation of Epinephrine and Norepinephrine at Metal Oxide Doped Phthalocyanine/ MWCNT Composite Sensor. *Sci Rep*, 2016, **6**, 1–20.

34. M. Mazloum-Ardakani, F. Farbod and L. Hosseinzadeh, An electrochemical sensor based on nickel oxides nanoparticle/ graphene composites for electrochemical detection of epinephrine. *J Nanostruct*, 2016, **6**, 293–300.

35. S. D. Sukanya, B. E. K. Swamy, J. K. Shashikumara, S. C. Sharma and S. A. Hariprasad, A novel, extreme low-cost poly (erythrosine) modified pencil graphite electrode for determination of adrenaline. *Sci Rep*, 2023, **13**, 1–9.

36. H. Beitollahi, M. Safaei and S. Tajik, Voltammetric and amperometric sensors for determination of epinephrine: A short review (2013–2017): Original scientific paper. *J Electrochem Sci Eng*, 2019, **9**, 27–43.

37. X. Ma, M. Chao and Z. Wang, Electrochemical detection of dopamine in the presence of epinephrine, uric acid and ascorbic acid using a graphene-modified electrode. *Anal Methods*, 2012, **4**, 1687–1692.

38. S. Sun, X. Gou, S. Tao, J. Cui, J. Li, Q. Yang, S. Liang and Z. Yang, Mesoporous graphitic carbon nitride (g-C3N4) nanosheets synthesized from carbonated beverage-reformed commercial melamine for enhanced photocatalytic hydrogen evolution. *Mater Chem Front*, 2019, **3**, 597–605.

39. K. Sen, S. Ali, D. Singh, K. Singh and N. Gupta, Development of metal free melamine modified graphene oxide for electrochemical sensing of epinephrine. *Flat Chem*, 2021, **30**, 100288.

40. F. C. Moraes, D. L. C. Golinelli, L. H. Mascaro and S. A. S. MacHado, Determination of epinephrine in urine using multi-walled carbon nanotube modified with cobalt phthalocyanine in a paraffin composite electrode. *Sens Actuators B Chem*, 2010, **148**, 492–497.

41. R. N. Goyal and S. Bishnoi, A novel multi-walled carbon nanotube modified sensor for the selective determination of epinephrine in smokers. *Electrochim Acta*, 2011, **56**, 2717–2724.

42. F. C. Moraes, D. L. C. Golinelli, L. H. Mascaro and S. A. S. MacHado, Determination of epinephrine in urine using multi-walled carbon nanotube modified with cobalt phthalocyanine in a paraffin composite electrode. *Sens Actuators B Chem*, 2010, **148**, 492–497.

43. S. E. Elugoke, A. S. Adekunle, O. E. Fayemi, B. B. Mamba, T. T. I. Nkambule, E.-S. M. Sherif and E. E. Ebenso, Progress in electrochemical detection of neurotransmitters using carbon nanotubes/nanocomposite based materials: A chronological review. *Nano Select*, 2020, 1, 561–611.

44. R. N. Goyal and S. Bishnoi, Simultaneous determination of epinephrine and norepinephrine in human blood plasma and urine samples using nanotubes modified edge plane pyrolytic graphite electrode. *Talanta*, 2011, 84, 78–83.

45. H. Devnani, S. P. Satsangee and R. Jain, A novel graphene-chitosan-Bi2O3 nanocomposite modified sensor for sensitive and selective electrochemical determination of a monoamine neurotransmitter epinephrine. *Ionics (Kiel)*, 2016, 22, 943–956.

46. N. Jaiswal and I. Tiwari, Sulphur nanodots decorated graphene oxide nanocomposite for electrochemical determination of norepinephrine in presence and absence of 4-aminophenol, acetaminophen and tryptophan. *J Electroanal Chem*, 2021, 881, 114956.

47. S. H. Huang, H. H. Liao and D. H. Chen, Simultaneous determination of norepinephrine, uric acid, and ascorbic acid at a screen printed carbon electrode modified with polyacrylic acid-coated multi-wall carbon nanotubes. *Biosens Bioelectron*, 2010, 25, 2351–2355.

48. D. F. de Queiroz, T. R. de L. Dadamos, S. A. S. Machado and M. A. U. Martines, Electrochemical determination of norepinephrine by means of modified glassy carbon electrodes with carbon nanotubes and magnetic nanoparticles of cobalt ferrite. *Sensors*, 2018, 18, 1223.

49. H. Devnani, S. P. Satsangee and R. Jain, Nanocomposite modified electrochemical sensor for sensitive and selective determination of noradrenaline. *Mater Today Proc*, 2016, 3, 1854–1863.

50. M. Michaelides, P. K. Thanos, N. D. Volkow and G. J. Wang, Dopamine-related frontostriatal abnormalities in obesity and binge-eating disorder: Emerging evidence for developmental psychopathology. *Int Rev Psychiatry*, 2012, 24, 211–218.

51. T. E. Osinga, T. P. Links, R. P. F. Dullaart, K. Pacak, A. N. A. Van Der Horst-Schrivers, M. N. Kerstens and I. P. Kema, Emerging role of dopamine in neovascularization of pheochromocytoma and paraganglioma. *The FASEB J*, 2017, 31, 2226–2240.

52. Q. Huang, X. Lin, L. Tong and Q. X. Tong, Graphene quantum dots/multi-walled carbon nanotubes composite-based electrochemical sensor for detecting dopamine release from living cells. *ACS Sustain Chem Eng*, 2020, 8, 1644–1650.

53. A. R. Rajamani and S. C. Peter, Novel nanostructured Pt/CeO2@Cu2O carbon-based electrode to magnify the electrochemical detection of the neurotransmitter dopamine and analgesic paracetamol. *ACS Appl Nano Mater*, 2018, 1, 5148–5157.

54. S. R. Ali, R. R. Parajuli, Y. Balogun, Y. Ma and H. He, A nonoxidative electrochemical sensor based on a self-doped polyaniline/carbon nanotube composite for sensitive and selective detection of the neurotransmitter dopamine: A Review. *Sensors*, 2008, 8, 8423–8452.

55. Q. Huang, X. Lin, L. Tong and Q. X. Tong, Graphene quantum dots/multi-walled carbon nanotubes composite-based electrochemical sensor for detecting dopamine release from living cells. *ACS Sustain Chem Eng*, 2020, 8, 1644–1650.

56. D. Sangamithirai, S. Munusamy, V. Narayanan and A. Stephen, Fabrication of neurotransmitter dopamine electrochemical sensor based on poly(o-Anisidine)/CNTs nanocomposite. *Surf Interfaces*, 2016, **4**, 27–34.
57. B. Wu, S. Yeasmin, Y. Liu and L. J. Cheng, Sensitive and selective electrochemical sensor for serotonin detection based on ferrocene-gold nanoparticles decorated multiwall carbon nanotubes. *Sens Actuators B Chem*, 2022, **354**, 131216.
58. A. Khan and S. A. Ghani, Multienzyme microbiosensor based on electropolymerized O-phenylenediamine for simultaneous in vitro determination of acetylcholine and choline. *Biosens Bioelectron*, 2012, **31**, 433–438.
59. O. C. Bodur, S. Dinç, M. Özmen and F. Arslan, A sensitive amperometric detection of neurotransmitter acetylcholine using carbon dot-modified carbon paste electrode. *Biotechnol Appl Biochem*, 2021, **68**, 20–29.
60. D. Du, M. Wang, J. Cai, Y. Qin and A. Zhang, One-step synthesis of multiwalled carbon nanotubes-gold nanocomposites for fabricating amperometric acetylcholinesterase biosensor. *Sens Actuators B Chem*, 2010, **143**, 524–529.
61. N. Chauhan, S. Chawla, C. S. Pundir and U. Jain, An electrochemical sensor for detection of neurotransmitter-acetylcholine using metal nanoparticles, 2D material and conducting polymer modified electrode. *Biosens Bioelectron*, 2017, **89**, 377–383.
62. H. Cheng, H. Qiu, Z. Zhu, M. Li and Z. Shi, Investigation of the electrochemical behavior of dopamine at electrodes modified with ferrocene-filled double-walled carbon nanotubes. *Electrochim Acta*, 2012, **63**, 83–88.

Chapter 5

Bioinspired Nanocomposites
Multifunctional Materials towards Sustainable Alternatives

Nipun Jain, Yusuf Olatunji Waidi, Ranjit Barua, Samir Das, Vilay Vannaladsaysy, Arbind Prasad, and Sudipto Datta

5.1 INTRODUCTION

Nature has developed the ability to create hierarchical, multifunctional materials that greatly outperform manufactured materials in many aspects.[1] It uses a wide variety of simple molecular reactions amongst a small number of building components in ambient circumstances. This has allowed for some astounding results in the field of nanocomposites. Recent material technology is greatly inspired, in particular, by the progressive growth of multilayered layered structures that possess paradoxical qualities, including simultaneous superior strength and toughness. Damage-resistant structures can be created by modeling the microstructures. Some biologically inspired substances have previously been used in a variety of applications.[2] Creating multipurpose, ecologically friendly, and dynamical composites is essential for the field's advancement. However, numerous obstacles exist, such as the need for rapid large-scale production, fundamental coupling, the ability to create molecular-scale preciseness, and the ability to maintain structural integrity without losing functional characteristics.[3]

The widespread use of synthetic polymers in everyday applications has brought significant benefits to industry and consumers, offering desirable properties like durability, affordability, and diverse functionalities. However, their extensive use, particularly in packaging, has dramatically risen in recent decades.[4] This reliance on non-biodegradable, petrochemical-based plastics poses a major threat to environmental sustainability. The ever-growing accumulation of plastic waste highlights the urgent need for alternative materials and responsible management practices to ensure a sustainable future.[5] The reliance on fossil means can be significantly decreased by developing bio-based materials derived from renewable sources. This is evident in the expanding bioplastics market, which is currently experiencing a growth rate that is 30% higher than the synthetic plastic market. Researchers are actively exploring the production of novel bio-based compounds through various methods, including chemical modifications and industrial biotechnological processes.[6] This includes utilizing microorganisms and plants to create biopolymers or their building

DOI: 10.1201/9781003470311-5

blocks, such as exopolysaccharides and polyesters. Researchers are also exploring blending different polymers to enhance material properties, resulting in composite materials.[7–12] Furthermore, incorporating nanoscale reinforcements into these composites creates what are known as nanocomposite materials, offering even more advanced functionalities.

While waste-based biomass utilization drives a sustainable, bio-based economy, and it is crucial to differentiate between bio-based and biodegradable plastics.[13]. Although often used interchangeably, these terms hold distinct meanings. Bio-based plastics can be derived from renewable resources like biopolymers but may not necessarily be biodegradable. Conversely, some plastics made from non-renewable resources like petroleum can be engineered to be biodegradable. Understanding these distinctions is essential when traversing the diverse range of plastics available (Figure 5.1).

Achieving control over various aspects like composition, gradients, interfaces, microstructures, morphology, and dynamic responses remains a significant obstacle in developing bioinspired composites.[14] While synthetic composites, often employed in temperature-critical fields like automotive and aerospace, may surpass bioinspired options in specific areas, the latter offer distinct advantages. These components can be manufactured eco-friendly by merging conventional approaches with newly developed programs, producing materials with remarkable properties and reduced

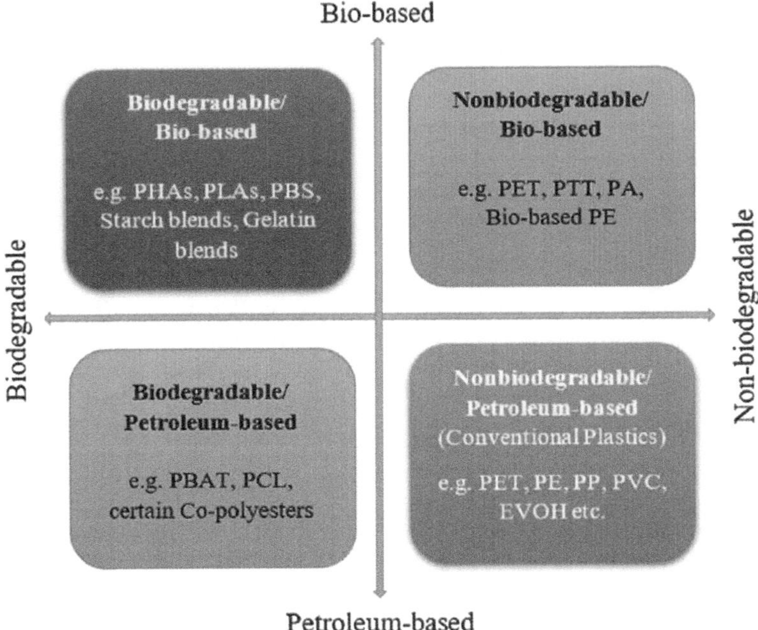

Figure 5.1 Numerous kinds of polymers are available. (Reproduced from[5].)

environmental impact.[15] Extensive research on nature's most resilient materials has unveiled fundamental design principles, particularly emphasizing the crucial role of molecular interactions and hierarchical structures. This remarkable ability of organisms to engineer mineral-based materials into anisotropic architectures allows them to create load-bearing elements spanning vast size scales.[16] This unique unification of stiffness and high durability has proved advantageous in developing bioinspired synthetic analogs, as current synthetic composites often exhibit trade-offs between strength and toughness (Figure 5.2).

Establishing new nanohybrid materials for tailoring polymer matrices is an emerging field at the intersection of nanotechnology, material sciences, and life sciences. The term "nanobiotechnology" emerged in the last decade to describe nanohybrid materials that combine natural or bio-based polymers with non-organic components.[17] Scientists have been drawn to the exceptional properties of nanocomposites for functional and structural applications, including applications in electrochemical devices and heterogeneous catalysts.[18] The creation of bio-nanocomposites, which exhibit exceptional qualities akin to synthetic materials (such as enhanced tensile and barrier properties), is currently the focus of future experiments.[19] Apart

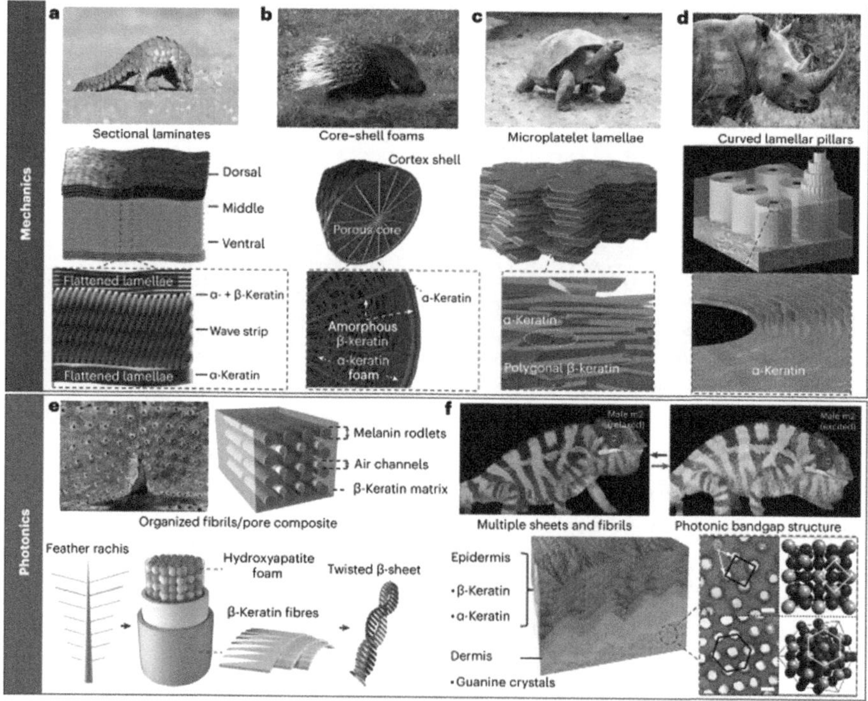

Figure 5.2 Illustration of keratin-based structure with different hierarchy composites that yield various functional applications. (Reproduced from [8].)

from these attributes, these exhibit notable benefits such as biodegradability, biocompatibility, and, occasionally, bioactive functional features.[20–29]

5.2 SCALE-SPANNING HIERARCHICAL INTERACTIONS

Natural materials exhibit a special combination of mechanical and functional qualities linked to systematic association at different length scales. This hierarchical organization can also evolve, ranging from molecular ordering to macro-scale congregation (Figure 5.3). Hard/soft interfaces that are widely present and highly structured act as a mediator for this kind of synergistic self-organization.[30] Depending on the volume limitations and end-goal functionality, hierarchical structures can have spatial dimensions ranging from 0-D to N-D that differ significantly. Additional proportions, for instance, time or previously approachable material alterations, may also be incorporated into ND structures. The property interfaces also influence the physical characteristics, which control numerous layers of macroscale structure[31] (Figure 5.3 a–e).

The strength, toughness, stiffness, and adhesive and shear capabilities of a substance are ultimately determined by the mix of its strong and weak surfaces. Nature can modify shape and qualities that respond to stimuli thanks to the reversible remodeling of barriers by molecular and formed phase changes. Realizing morphing and responsive behavior involves several chemical processes, such as rebounding or adjusting molecules, nanoparticles, and groups with properties. The reaction, attachment, moderation, and distribution of structural essentials occur on timeframes ranging from picoseconds to milliseconds. Additional procedures that generate materials over similar time spans include accumulation, crystallization, dissolution, leisure, controlled deformation and morphing, phase separation, emergence, and auto-healing of structural materials. As a result, creating artificial structural arrangements with the mechanical robustness and functionality seen in nature is difficult.[32] The intricacy of various parts and interfaces is still challenging to replicate and program into artificial processes. Creating composition gradients, combining multiple material phases, and accomplishing among the issues are reusable energy loss and exceptional influence on global and local mechanics.

5.3 NANOCOMPOSITES MADE OF RENEWABLE MATERIALS

One issue that is becoming more and more of a worry for academics and industrialists is using ecologically friendly materials to replace non-biodegradable ones. The goal of this change is to lessen the buildup of plastic garbage. The development of bio-degradable components that can be used in the food, healthcare, and agricultural sectors is the main goal of many research investigations. Natural, organic, and biodegradable substitutes

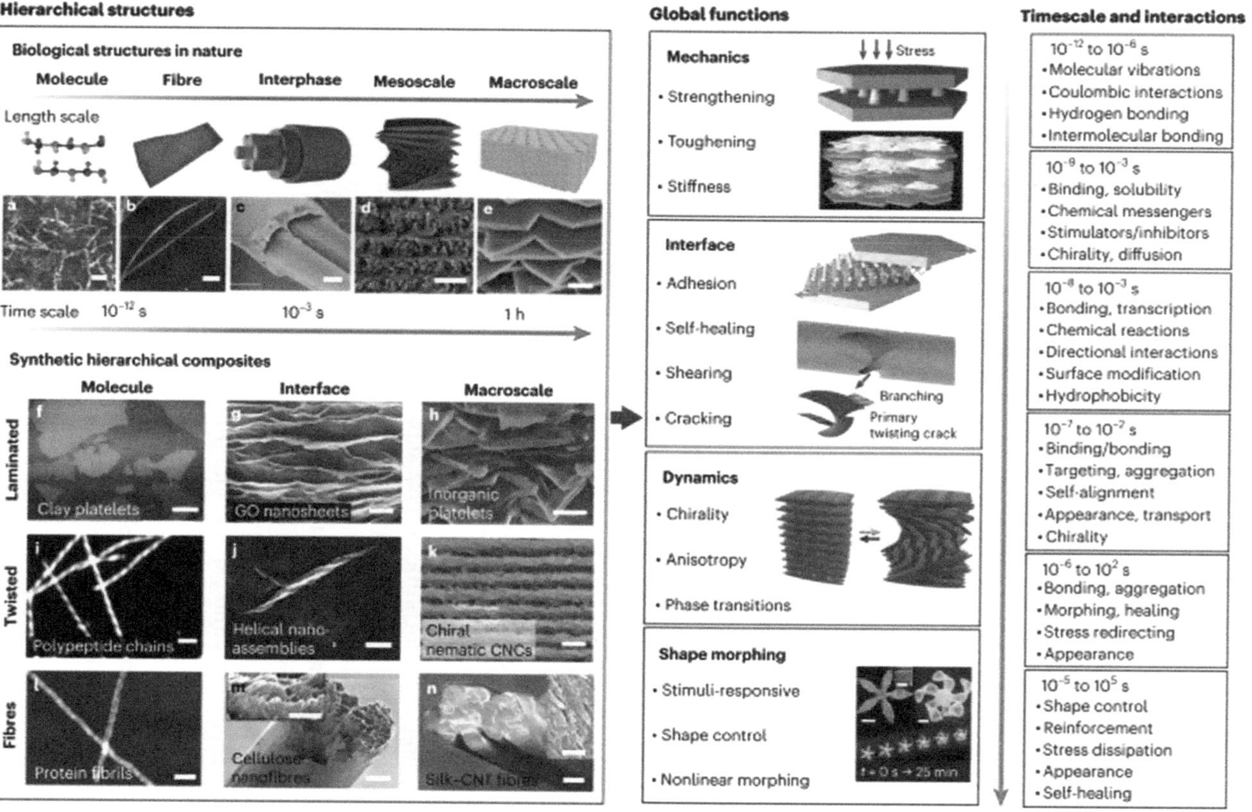

Figure 5.3 Schematic representation of different structures based on different levels of natural hierarchy. (Reproduced from [8].)

for petroleum-based products are progressively taking their place as they are renewable in the environment. For example, the production of biodegradable packaging materials uses components including cellulose, starch, polycaprolactone, and PLA.[33] These renewable resources are made up of non-toxic substances that can be broken down biologically by different types of soil microbes. This new way of thinking has the potential to drastically lessen the harm that petrochemical reliance does to the environment.

Numerous scientific investigations are devoted to producing increased-quality bio-based materials because of the major advantages of renewable materials with ecologically sustainable features and their wide variety of industrial and healthcare uses.[34] As a result, biodegradable nanocomposites that have better qualities than bioplastics without reinforcement have been produced. Nanocomposites are frequently made using natural polymers such as cellulose, starch, and their derivatives, or biomacromolecules.[35] These materials contain either natural or manufactured clay minerals or modified clay minerals, such as nanofillers, which offer compounds for intercalation or exfoliation. In these investigations, silicates such as montmorillonite and cloisite are commonly used as nanofillers to strengthen the biopolymer material and increase the mechanical strength of the resulting biopolymeric films.

Plasticizers are chemicals used with synthetic resins to increase their fluidity and flexibility, reducing the final product's brittleness. Plasticizers such as glycerol, vegetable oil, and triethyl citrate are typically added to avoid deterioration and produce high-quality thermoplastic polymers. Additionally, plasticizers improve how nanofillers are distributed throughout the matrix, enhancing the material's exceptional mechanical qualities. The most popular biopolymer for creating bioplastics mixed with organically modified silicates is thermoplastic PLA, which is produced by the fermentation of cornstarch.[36] Better biodegradation, similar to $TiO2$, is achieved when titanate is added as a nanofiller to PLA bioplastics.[37]

The development of nano-based biocomposites is still in its early stages. Creating innovative biopolymers to improve the materials' compatibility with inorganic components is essential for future improvement. Incorporating natural macromolecules (such as polysaccharides) with other nanofillers would improve the mechanical qualities. Clay films show enhanced heat stability, gas barrier, and increased mechanical characteristics.[38] Synthetic polymer nanocomposites display a "tortuous" pathway phenomenon, in which its dispersion in the matrix causes changes in the gas diffusion characteristics. Other inorganic minerals have also been used as reinforcements in biopolymer composites. For example, sepiolite dispersion improves natural rubber's mechanical characteristics.[39] SiC nanoparticles and single-walled carbon nanotubes (SWCNTs) increase the natural rubber's mechanical strength, outperforming those derived from SWCNTs alone. Comparable results are obtained when multi-walled carbon nanotubes (MWCNTs) are dispersed, thus improving the biopolymer's mechanical, chemical, and physical characteristics[40] (Figure 5.4).

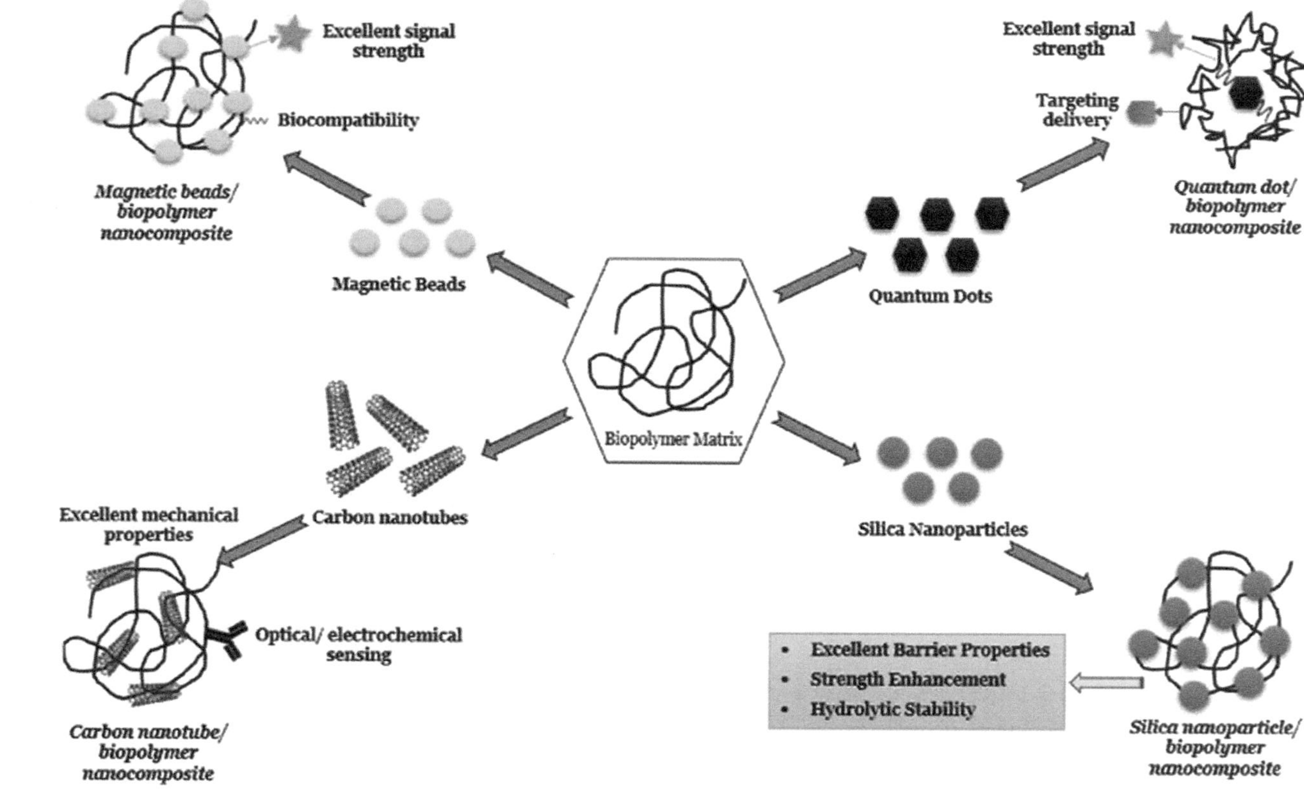

Figure 5.4 Various forms of nanostructured components within the matrix to achieve the intended properties. (Reproduced from [5].)

5.4 FORMATION OF MATERIALS FOR NANOCOMPOSITES

Creating new orientations and arrangements, dissolving intermolecular bonds with lower energy requirements, and creating novel interactions and bonds all work together to form a new 3D network of polymeric substances in developing nanohybrid materials. The polymer's shape (length/diameter ratio) and the surrounding environment are among the variables that affect the creation of new intermolecular forces. Different kinds of bonding, such as covalent, hydrogen, hydrophobic, and electrostatic, stabilize the resultant material. Biopolymer-based nanocomposites are often synthesized using wet and dry processing techniques.[41]

In dry processing, disulfide/sulfhydryl exchange reactions are induced by mechanical and heat treatments, which are based on the thermoplastic qualities of the polymer. However, wet processing (continuous spreading) is widely used to create bio and nanocomposites from organic materials such as lipids, proteins, and carbohydrates (Figure. 5.5A). In wet processing, the polymer is mixed with an appropriate solvent to make a solution that forms films. The solution contains various chemicals, including plasticizers, fillers, antioxidants, antibacterial substances, nano- and microparticles, and cross-linking agents. The process then entails spreading the film and letting the solvent evaporate. It is advantageous to include plasticizers because they provide flexibility and ease of handling by reducing stiffness and intermolecular attractions. This process improves the mechanical qualities of the final product and is very helpful for the creation of packing materials.[42]

As previously mentioned, thermoplastic characteristics of plastics play a crucial part in the development of composite materials, which is the basis

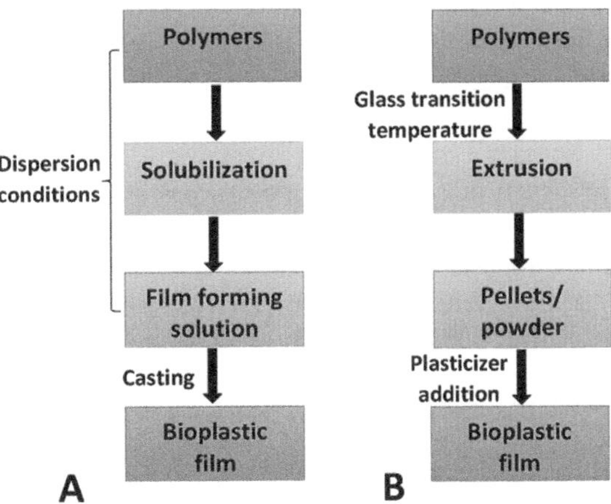

Figure 5.5 Techniques for developing bio/nanocomposites: (A) wet processing; (B) dry processing. (Reproduced from [5].)

for this method. It correlates with the glass transition principle, which states that the glassy materials transform into a viscosity condition with a particular temperature. Transitional states generally cause disorder, movement, and free volume by altering the material's biomechanical and physical characteristics.[43] Typically, adding plasticizer at high temperatures and applying a shear force will form polymers into an ideal substance. When proteins are heated to higher temperatures, the molecules' bonds dissolve, and novel bonds form, changing the characteristics of the substance.[44] There are many approaches to developing materials based on the polymeric dry process, including heating and extrusion (Figure 5.5B). The methods, notably employing extrusion as a mixture and restricted modifications and the heating process to produce the final item, may be applied separately or simultaneously.

5.5 HYDROMECHANICAL PROPERTIES AND STABILIZATION OF NANOCOMPOSITES USING STRONG BONDS

Water greatly impacts the characteristics of the above-mentioned bioinspired nanocomposites. The water impact can be useful by understanding the basics of the polymeric phase's dynamization. Conversely, it is critical to identify barriers against water-induced mechanical deterioration in a scientific setting.[45] The impact of moisture on several bioinspired nanocomposites has been studied using nanoclays. Poly(vinyl alcohol) (PVA) has varying aspects and behaves as nano clay in the study. Beyond 60% relative humidity, every compound shows a substantial water uptake.[46] The nanoclays display extended inelastic deformations caused by friction slides. Nanocomposites use the finest possible particles of nano clays (LAP, MTM) that exhibit a rigid/strong-to-ductile change to increase the moisture content further. However, the biggest nano clay (NTS) hardly shows any inelastic deformations and can only be exhibited when PVA/NTS is submerged under water.[47] Dynamic mechanical investigation showed that the glass-transition temperature of the nanoscale-confined plastics decreases as the percentage RH increases. This pattern makes sense when considering a shear-lag concept and the plasticizing matrices. These studies highlight the significance of comprehending the proportions of polymeric dynamics in rigid deformation and demonstrate how dampness regulates mechanical achievements. Cross-linking is necessary for moisture stability and helps prevent the hydrophilic–hydrophobic structures. Various cross-linking techniques were investigated, including ionic bonding, covalent cross-linking produced by photochemical and thermal processes, and mineralization.[48] Sodium carboxymethylcellulose with montmorillonite nacre-mimetics ((Na+) CMC/MTM) was employed for ionic cross-linking and following film production. As a result, there was a macroscopic strengthening due

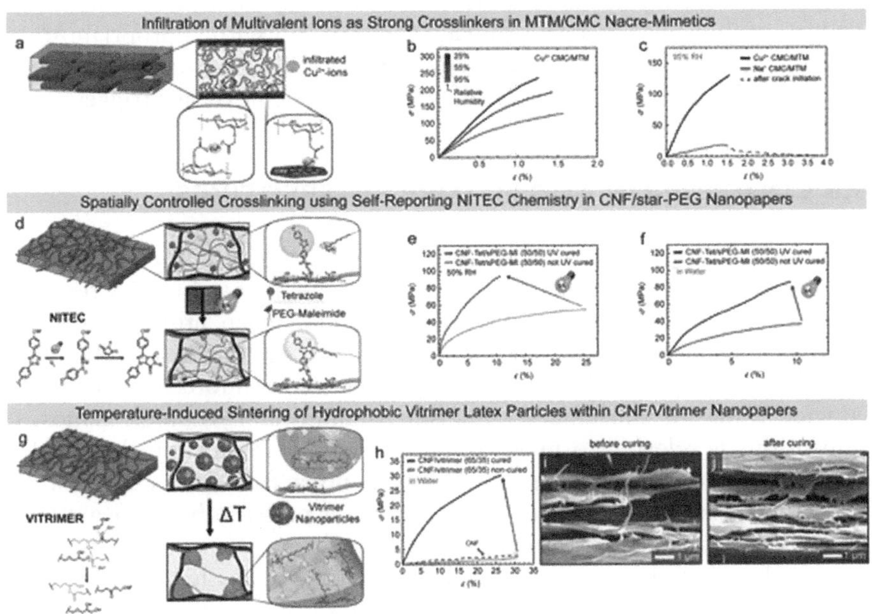

Figure 5.6 Stabilization processes during cross-linking. (Reproduced from [30].)

to an ionic interaction between the negative-charged MTM surfaces and the acid groups of the CMC. A slight decrease was seen in tensile testing at high relative humidity percentages (Figure 5.6 a-c).[49] As an outcome, the post-infiltration of diverse ions stabilizes their mechanical characteristics in higher percentages of relative humidity. The components gain water from the photo-cross-linking at 50% RH, as evidenced by the self-reporting strong fluorescence. Following UV light, there is a noticeable stiffness and strengthening [50] (Figure 5.6 d-f). Without cross-linking, films become softer and lose their cohesiveness when submerged in water, while a photo-cured film keeps its high mechanical properties. Covalent bonding between a polymer and CNF causes this transformation.

Studies are also done by combining CNFs with latex particles, which employ β-hydroxy ester linkages attached to poly(dimethylsiloxane) (PDMS) and can undergo transesterification. Sintering occurs between the vitrimer and CNF as a result of heating [51] (Figure 5.6g). Significantly, during film casting, these nanoparticles seamlessly integrate into the continuous matrix phase, which is further strengthened after curing. The water uptake at the interface is inhibited by the creation of covalent bonds at the vitrimer/CNF junction, which also promotes interfacial adhesion. Improved interfacial strength is confirmed by cross-sectional SEMs that show meso-scale layer transitions upon curing [50] (Figure 5.6 i,j). Studies of various nanocomposites show that bonding during cross-linking is highly effective in stabilization. Hydrophobic materials and strong interfacial bonding are important, but the latter must always be balanced with appropriate structure creation specific to aqueous environments. Even spatial control over mechanical patterns can arise from well-maintained exterior triggers.[52–57]

5.6 CONCLUSION AND FUTURE PERSPECTIVES

Utilizing bioinspired nanocomposites as an alternative source of research has caught the interest of material researchers and nanotechnology researchers. For instance, there are some disadvantages when utilizing neat biopolymers, including their deteriorating physical characteristics, that may be solved successfully by using nanoparticles as reinforcement elements. A wide range of substances possessing a minimum of single nanoscale dimensions is referred to under the term "nanomaterials," including dendrimers that are nanocrystals, nanotubes, nanoparticles, and multiple other inorganic substances. Due to their environment friendly, biodegradable, and biocompatible characteristics, "green" chemical methods offer substantial benefits above conventional material processes for creating nano/biocomposite materials. A key characteristic of applying such nanohybrid substances in the food industry, biological engineering, and therapeutic fields within health care is its biological compatibility. The development of non-viral DNA vectors for personalized medicine and customized administration of drugs represent two additional important uses of nanohybrid substances. Furthermore, several kinds of important nanohybrid substances in electronics and devices are currently being developed. The development of organic nanohybrid products that include organic polymers such as chitosan, which have strong ion-exchange abilities and effective sensors for electricity, is interesting. Employing an array of inorganic compounds for trapping enzymes has generated functional nano bio-composites, which are ideal for application in biosensors and bioreactors. Another growing field of research is the development of creative nanocomposites with improved characteristics and multipurpose use. The building elements of tomorrow will be composite which are durable, flexible, and adaptable, including morphing, adapting, sensing, and healing abilities. This overview highlights the individualization of the material's confinement, interphases, and architecture to generate flexible and combinatorial reactions. It additionally covers modern developments and ideas in bioinspired nanocomposites. We show key situations of organic substances having unique mixtures of mechanical characteristics derived from fairly straightforward elements produced in natural conditions in aqueous conditions. Particular importance is given to architectural topologies, which cover multiple length scales to achieve resiliency and multipurpose use. We additionally cover present advances, trends, and possibilities for merging artificial and organic components, in addition to innovative modeling and characterization methods to assess the physics underlying nature-inspired architecture and mechanical behaviors over an array of scales of length. Future work will include enhancing prediction and normative construction for the next generation of building materials at multilength levels across various uses. These multidisciplinary methods additionally encourage a collaborative improvement of specific material qualities.

REFERENCES

1. Liu, Z.; Meyers, M. A.; Zhang, Z.; Ritchie, R. O. Functional Gradients and Heterogeneities in Biological Materials: Design Principles, Functions, and Bioinspired Applications. *Prog Mater Sci*, **2017**, *88*, 467–498. https://doi.org/10.1016/j.pmatsci.2017.04.013.
2. Clancy, A. J.; Anthony, D. B.; De Luca, F. Metal Mimics: Lightweight, Strong, and Tough Nanocomposites and Nanomaterial Assemblies. *ACS Appl Mater Interfaces*, **2020**, *12* (14), 15955–15975. https://doi.org/10.1021/acsami.0c01304.
3. Jain, N.; Singh, S. Glycans in Scaffold Design in Tissue Reconstruction. *J Bioact Compat Polym*, **2021**, *36* (3), 185–196. https://doi.org/10.1177/0883911521997847.
4. Sommerhuber, P. F.; Welling, J.; Krause, A. Substitution Potentials of Recycled HDPE and Wood Particles from Post-Consumer Packaging Waste in Wood–Plastic Composites. *Waste Manag*, **2015**, *46*, 76–85. https://doi.org/10.1016/j.wasman.2015.09.011.
5. Ahmad Qamar, S.; Asgher, M.; Khalid, N. Bioinspired Nanocomposites: Functional Materials for Sustainable Greener Technologies. In *Renewable Energy - Resources, Challenges and Applications*. IntechOpen, **2020**. https://doi.org/10.5772/intechopen.92876.
6. Asgher, M.; Urooj, Y.; Qamar, S. A.; Khalid, N. Improved Exopolysaccharide Production from Bacillus Licheniformis MS3: Optimization and Structural/Functional Characterization. *Int J Biol Macromol*, **2020**, *151*, 984–992. https://doi.org/10.1016/j.ijbiomac.2019.11.094.
7. Prasad, A. Biomaterial-based Nanofibers Scaffolds in Tissue Engineering Application. In Sougata Jana, Subrata Jana (Eds.), Functional Biomaterials: Drug Delivery and Biomedical Applications (pp. 245–264). Singapore: Springer Singapore, 2022.
8. Katiyar, V.; Prasad, A.; Sankar, M. R. Process for the Preparation of Resorbable Polymeric Composite Bone Stable, 2022. (Indian Patent No. 393675).
9. Datta, S.; Waidi, Y. O.; Prasad, A. Metal 3D Printing for Emerging Healthcare Applications. *Advanced Materials and Manufacturing Techniques for Biomedical Applications*, **2023**, 383–409. https://doi.org/10.1002/9781394166985.ch15.
10. Prasad, A.; Shaikh, A.; De, S.; Kumar, R.; Srivastava, M. K. Aspects of Bioabsorbable Polymeric Composites in Biomedical Applications. In R. Kumar, A. Prasad, and A. Kumar (Eds.), *Sustainable Smart Manufacturing Processes in Industry 4.0* (pp. 73–87). CRC Press, **2023**.

11. Katiyar, V.; Prasad, A.; Sankar, M. R. Resorbable Composite Bone Plate, 2024. (Indian Patent No. 500905).
12. De, S.; Das, D.; Prasad, A.; Kumar, A.; Chattopadhyay, D. Insights into Multifunctional Smart Hydrogels in Wound Healing Applications. In A. Prasad, A. Kumar and M. Gupta (Eds.), *Advanced Materials and Manufacturing Techniques for Biomedical Applications*, 2023. https://doi.org/10.1002/9781394166985.ch3.
13. Dietrich, K.; Dumont, M.-J.; Del Rio, L. F.; Orsat, V. Sustainable PHA Production in Integrated Lignocellulose Biorefineries. *N Biotechnol*, 2019, *49*, 161–168. https://doi.org/10.1016/j.nbt.2018.11.004.
14. Nepal, D.; Kang, S.; Adstedt, K. M.; Kanhaiya, K.; Bockstaller, M. R.; Brinson, L. C.; Buehler, M. J.; Coveney, P. V.; Dayal, K.; El-Awady, J. A.; et al. Hierarchically Structured Bioinspired Nanocomposites. *Nat Mater*, 2023, *22* (1), 18–35. https://doi.org/10.1038/s41563-022-01384-1.
15. Huang, W.; Restrepo, D.; Jung, J.; Su, F. Y.; Liu, Z.; Ritchie, R. O.; McKittrick, J.; Zavattieri, P.; Kisailus, D. Multiscale Toughening Mechanisms in Biological Materials and Bioinspired Designs. *Advanced Materials*, 2019, *31* (43). https://doi.org/10.1002/adma.201901561.
16. Wang, B.; Yang, W.; McKittrick, J.; Meyers, M. A. Keratin: Structure, Mechanical Properties, Occurrence in Biological Organisms, and Efforts at Bioinspiration. *Prog Mater Sci*, 2016, *76*, 229–318. https://doi.org/10.1016/j.pmatsci.2015.06.001.
17. Qamar, S. A.; Asgher, M.; Khalid, N.; Sadaf, M. Nanobiotechnology in Health Sciences: Current Applications and Future Perspectives. *Biocatal Agric Biotechnol*, 2019, *22*, 101388. https://doi.org/10.1016/j.bcab.2019.101388.
18. Zhang, W.-D.; Xu, B.; Jiang, L.-C. Functional Hybrid Materials Based on Carbon Nanotubes and Metal Oxides. *J Mater Chem*, 2010, *20* (31), 6383. https://doi.org/10.1039/b926341a.
19. Sanchez-Garcia, M. D.; Lopez-Rubio, A.; Lagaron, J. M. Natural Micro and Nanobiocomposites with Enhanced Barrier Properties and Novel Functionalities for Food Biopackaging Applications. *Trends Food Sci Technol*, 2010, *21* (11), 528–536. https://doi.org/10.1016/j.tifs.2010.07.008.
20. Prasad, A. State of Art Review on Bioabsorbable Polymeric Scaffolds for Bone Tissue Engineering. *Mater Today: Proc*, 2021, *44*, 1391–1400.
21. Prasad, A.; Bhasney, S.; Katiyar, V.; Sankar, M. R. Biowastes Processed Hydroxyapatite Filled Poly (Lactic Acid) Bio-composite for Open Reduction Internal Fixation of Small Bones. *Mater Today: Proc*, 2017, *4* (9), 10153–10157.
22. Prasad, A.; Devendar, B.; Ravi Sankar, M.; Robi, P. S. Micro-Scratch Based Tribological Characterization of Hydroxyapatite (HAp) Fabricated through Fish Scales. *Mater Today: Proc*, 2015, *2* (4–5), 1216–1224.
23. Prasad, A.; Ravi Sankar, M.; Katiyar, V. State of Art on Solvent Casting Particulate Leaching Method for Orthopedic Scaffolds Fabrication. *Mate Today: Proc*, 2017, *4* (2), 898–907.
24. Sarkar, K.; Dutta, K.; Chatterjee, A.; Sarkar, J.; Das, D.; Prasad, A.; Chattopadhyay, D.; Acharya, K.; Das, M.; Verma, S. K.; De, S. Nanotherapeutic Potential of Antibacterial Folic Acid-Functionalized Nanoceria for Wound-Healing Applications. *Nanomedicine*, 2023, *18* (2), 109–123.

25. Bhoi, S.; Prasad, A.; Kumar, A.; Sarkar, R. B.; Mahto, B.; Meena, C. S.; Pandey, C. Experimental Study to Evaluate the Wear Performance of UHMWPE and XLPE Material for Orthopedics Application. *Bioengineering*, **2022**, *9* (11), 676.

26. Katiyar, V.; Prasad, A.; Sankar, M. R. Process for the Preparation of Polymer Composite Based Cortical Screw, **2023**. (Indian Patent No. 449153).

27. Katiyar, V.; Prasad, A.; Sankar, M. R; Bhasney, S. M. Process for the Preparation of Polymer Composite Based Cancellous Screw and Pins, **2022**. (Indian Patent No. 401811).

28. Prasad, A.; Datta, S.; Kumar, A.; Gupta, M. Introduction to Next-Generation Materials for Biomedical Applications. In *Advanced Materials and Manufacturing Techniques for Biomedical Applications* (pp. 1–24). Scrivener Publishing, **2023**. https://doi.org/10.1002/9781394166985.

29. Datta, S.; Barua, R.; Prasad, A. Additive Manufacturing for the Development of Artificial Organs. In *Advanced Materials and Manufacturing Techniques for Biomedical Applications* (pp. 411–427). Wiley, **2023**. https://doi.org/10.4018/979-8-3693-1306-0.ch001.

30. Ren, J.; Wang, Y.; Yao, Y.; Wang, Y.; Fei, X.; Qi, P.; Lin, S.; Kaplan, D. L.; Buehler, M. J.; Ling, S. Biological Material Interfaces as Inspiration for Mechanical and Optical Material Designs. *Chem Rev*, **2019**, *119* (24), 12279–12336. https://doi.org/10.1021/acs.chemrev.9b00416.

31. Gao, H.-L.; Chen, S.-M.; Mao, L.-B.; Song, Z.-Q.; Yao, H.-B.; Cölfen, H.; Luo, X.-S.; Zhang, F.; Pan, Z.; Meng, Y.-F.; et al. Mass Production of Bulk Artificial Nacre with Excellent Mechanical Properties. *Nat Commun*, **2017**, *8* (1), 287. https://doi.org/10.1038/s41467-017-00392-z.

32. Natarajan, B.; Gilman, J. W. Bioinspired Bouligand Cellulose Nanocrystal Composites: A Review of Mechanical Properties. *Philos Transac Royal Soc: Math Phy Eng Sci*, **2018**, *376* (2112), 20170050. https://doi.org/10.1098/rsta.2017.0050.

33. Mangaraj, S.; Yadav, A.; Bal, L. M.; Dash, S. K.; Mahanti, N. K. Application of Biodegradable Polymers in Food Packaging Industry: A Comprehensive Review. *J Packag Technol Res*, **2019**, *3* (1), 77–96. https://doi.org/10.1007/s41783-018-0049-y.

34. Meite, N.; Konan, L. K.; Bamba, D.; Goure-Doubi, B. I. H.; Oyetola, S. Structural and Thermomechanical Study of Plastic Films Made from Cassava-Starch Reinforced with Kaolin and Metakaolin. *Materials Sciences and Applications*, **2018**, *9* (1), 41–54. https://doi.org/10.4236/msa.2018.91003.

35. Syafri, E.; Kasim, A.; Abral, H.; Sudirman; Sulungbudi, G. T.; Sanjay, M. R.; Sari, N. H. Synthesis and Characterization of Cellulose Nanofibers (CNF) Ramie Reinforced Cassava Starch Hybrid Composites. *Int J Biol Macromol*, **2018**, *120*, 578–586. https://doi.org/10.1016/j.ijbiomac.2018.08.134.

36. Tabasum, S.; Younas, M.; Zaeem, M. A.; Majeed, I.; Majeed, M.; Noreen, A.; Iqbal, M. N.; Zia, K. M. A Review on Blending of Corn Starch with Natural and Synthetic Polymers, and Inorganic Nanoparticles with Mathematical Modeling. *Int J Biol Macromol*, **2019**, *122*, 969–996. https://doi.org/10.1016/j.ijbiomac.2018.10.092.

37. Sun, J.; Shen, J.; Chen, S.; Cooper, M.; Fu, H.; Wu, D.; Yang, Z. Nanofiller Reinforced Biodegradable PLA/PHA Composites: Current Status and Future Trends. *Polymers (Basel)*, **2018**, *10* (5), 505. https://doi.org/10.3390/polym10050505.

38. Tang, M. C.; Agarwal, S.; Alsewailem, F. D.; Choi, H. J.; Gupta, R. K. A Model for Water Vapor Permeability Reduction in Poly(Lactic Acid) and Nanoclay Nanocomposites. *J Appl Polym Sci*, **2018**, *135* (30). https://doi.org /10.1002/app.46506.

39. Zaini, N. A. M.; Ismail, H.; Rusli, A. Tensile, Thermal, Flammability and Morphological Properties of Sepiolite Filled Ethylene Propylene Diene Monomer (EDPM) Rubber Composites. *Iran Polym J*, **2018**, *27* (5), 287–296. https://doi.org/10.1007/s13726-018-0609-6.

40. Wang, X.; Yang, C.; Jin, J.; Li, X.; Cheng, Q.; Wang, G. High-Performance Stretchable Supercapacitors Based on Intrinsically Stretchable Acrylate Rubber/MWCNTs@conductive Polymer Composite Electrodes. *J Mater Chem A Mater*, **2018**, *6* (10), 4432–4442. https://doi.org/10.1039/C7TA11173H.

41. Oksman, K.; Aitomäki, Y.; Mathew, A. P.; Siqueira, G.; Zhou, Q.; Butylina, S.; Tanpichai, S.; Zhou, X.; Hooshmand, S. Review of the Recent Developments in Cellulose Nanocomposite Processing. *Compos Part A Appl Sci Manuf*, **2016**, *83*, 2–18. https://doi.org/10.1016/j.compositesa.2015.10.041.

42. Farris, S.; Introzzi, L.; Piergiovanni, L. Evaluation of a Bio-coating as a Solution to Improve Barrier, Friction and Optical Properties of Plastic Films. *Packag Technol Sci*, **2009**, *22* (2), 69–83. https://doi.org/10.1002/pts.826.

43. Wang, Y.; Wang, W.; Zhang, Z.; Xu, L.; Li, P. Study of the Glass Transition Temperature and the Mechanical Properties of PET/Modified Silica Nanocomposite by Molecular Dynamics Simulation. *Eur Polym J*, **2016**, *75*, 36–45. https://doi.org/10.1016/j.eurpolymj.2015.11.038.

44. Miaudet, P.; Derré, A.; Maugey, M.; Zakri, C.; Piccione, P. M.; Inoubli, R.; Poulin, P. Shape and Temperature Memory of Nanocomposites with Broadened Glass Transition. *Science (1979)*, **2007**, *318* (5854), 1294–1296. https://doi.org/10.1126/science.1145593.

45. Das, P.; Malho, J.-M.; Rahimi, K.; Schacher, F. H.; Wang, B.; Demco, D. E.; Walther, A. Nacre-Mimetics with Synthetic Nanoclays up to Ultrahigh Aspect Ratios. *Nat Commun*, **2015**, *6* (1), 5967. https://doi.org/10.1038/ ncomms6967.

46. Lossada, F.; Hoenders, D.; Guo, J.; Jiao, D.; Walther, A. Self-Assembled Bioinspired Nanocomposites. *Acc Chem Res*, **2020**, *53* (11), 2622–2635. https://doi.org/10.1021/acs.accounts.0c00448.

47. Walther, A.; Lossada, F.; Benselfelt, T.; Kriechbaum, K.; Berglund, L.; Ikkala, O.; Saito, T.; Wågberg, L.; Bergström, L. Best Practice for Reporting Wet Mechanical Properties of Nanocellulose-Based Materials. *Biomacromolecules*, **2020**, *21* (6), 2536–2540. https://doi.org/10.1021/acs .biomac.0c00330.

48. Yao, J.; Fang, W.; Guo, J.; Jiao, D.; Chen, S.; Ifuku, S.; Wang, H.; Walther, A. Highly Mineralized Biomimetic Polysaccharide Nanofiber Materials Using Enzymatic Mineralization. *Biomacromolecules*, **2020**, *21* (6), 2176–2186. https://doi.org/10.1021/acs.biomac.0c00160.

49. Das, P.; Walther, A. Ionic Supramolecular Bonds Preserve Mechanical Properties and Enable Synergetic Performance at High Humidity in Water-Borne, Self-Assembled Nacre-Mimetics. *Nanoscale*, **2013**, *5* (19), 9348. https://doi.org/10.1039/c3nr02983b.

50. Hoenders, D.; Guo, J.; Goldmann, A. S.; Barner-Kowollik, C.; Walther, A. Photochemical Ligation Meets Nanocellulose: A Versatile Platform for Self-Reporting Functional Materials. *Mater Horiz*, **2018**, *5* (3), 560–568. https://doi.org/10.1039/C8MH00241J.

51. Lossada, F.; Guo, J.; Jiao, D.; Groeer, S.; Bourgeat-Lami, E.; Montarnal, D.; Walther, A. Vitrimer Chemistry Meets Cellulose Nanofibrils: Bioinspired Nanopapers with High Water Resistance and Strong Adhesion. *Biomacromolecules*, **2019**, *20* (2), 1045–1055. https://doi.org/10.1021/acs.biomac.8b01659.

52. Prasad, A.; Bhasney, S. M.; Prasannavenkadesan, V.; Sankar, M. R.; Katiyar, V. Polylactic Acid Reinforced with Nano-Hydroxyapatite Bioabsorbable Cortical Screws for Bone Fracture Treatment. *J Polym Res*, **2023**, *30* (5), 177.

53. Prasad, A.; Bhasney, S. M.; Prasannavenkadesan, V.; Sankar, M. R.; Katiyar, V. Nano-Hydroxyapatite Reinforced Polylactic Acid Bioabsorbable Cancellous Screws for Bone Fracture Fixations. *J Appl Polym Sci*, **2023**, *140* (43), e54577.

54. Chakraborty, G.; Padmashree, R.; Prasad, A. Recent Advancement of Surface Modification Techniques of 2-D Nanomaterials. *Mater Sci Eng B*, **2023**, *297*, 116817.

55. Prasad, A.; Bhasney, S. M.; Sankar, M. R.; Katiyar, V. Fish Scale Derived Hydroxyapatite Reinforced Poly (Lactic Acid) Polymeric Bio-films: Possibilities for Sealing/Locking the Internal Fixation Devices. *Mater Today: Proc*, **2017**, *4* (2), 1340–1349.

56. Gupta, A.; Prasad, A.; Mulchandani, N.; Shah, M.; Ravi Sankar, M.; Kumar, S.; Katiyar, V. Multifunctional Nanohydroxyapatite-Promoted Toughened High-Molecular-Weight Stereocomplex Poly (Lactic Acid)-Based Bionanocomposite for both 3D-Printed Orthopedic Implants and High-Temperature Engineering Applications. *ACS Omega*, **2017**, *2* (7), 4039–4052.

57. Prasad, A. Bioabsorbable Polymeric Materials for Biofilms and Other Biomedical Applications: Recent and Future Trends. *Mater Today: Proc*, **2021**, *44*, 2447–2453.

Bio-based Starch Blends in Active Food Packaging Applications

Shazia Hussain, Priya, and Shiwani Berry

6.1 INTRODUCTION

Food packaging material made from petroleum-derived plastics used for the protection and increasing lifespan of all types of foods. It has become increasingly common for packaging materials based on petrochemicals, such as polystyrene (PS), polyethylene (PE), polypropylene (PP), and polyamide (PA) etc., due to their better mechanical properties, tear and tensile strength, barrier properties against gases (CO_2, O_2), anhydride and aromatic compounds, and heat salability, along with their availability at relatively low prices (Rahman, 2019). The performance and ease of production of plastics has led to its widespread use in packaging materials over the past 50 years. For food applications, petroleum-based packaging materials are increasingly in demand because of the advent of the food processing industry. Tremendous elevation in the use of plastics, however, their non-biodegradability has created serious environmental problems (Mangaraj et al., 2019a). The various issues with regular plastic food packaging and food wastage that affect the environment and human health compelled researchers to develop some biodegradable materials for food packaging. The usage of such non-biodegradable materials not only poses a harm to the environment but also harmful for human health. Bio based products are more preferable due to its many benefits, such as biodegradability, biocompatibility, non-toxicity. There are so many bio-based plastic materials are available for food packaging like starch blends, bio-PE, and PLA. Due to consumer trends towards greener packaging and reducing waste, the use of bio-based materials in sustainable packaging is growing rapidly (Reichert et al., 2020). In recent years, renewable resources, such as chitin, lignin, cellulose, plant-based fatty acids, and caseinates, have been used to develop sustainable polymers. By chemically modifying and/or physically blending these biopolymers, defined properties can be achieved (Pavon et al., 2021). In nature, starch typically appears as granules, a polysaccharide made by the combination of numbers of glucose molecules that are plentiful and low cost. As a natural biodegradable material, starch is suitable for biofilm formation and biocompatibility due to its hydroxyl structure. Starch is being used

DOI: 10.1201/9781003470311-6

by some researchers as a packaging substrate in food packaging industry (Song et al., 2022). Starch's availability, accessibility, and cost-effectiveness make it a desirable material for packaging applications. One method to create packaging material by combining biopolymers with starch for creating novel polymer blends which are sustainable and biodegradable, the resulted combined components are with high biodegradation (Falua et al., 2022). Starch-based materials can be produced using a blend of starches and other biodegradable materials, such as chitosan, cellulose, or glycerol, to improve their mechanical and barrier properties. These blends can be used to produce various types of packaging, such as films, bags, trays, and containers. Starch-based packaging materials have several advantages over traditional plastics. They are biodegradable and compostable, meaning they can break down into natural compounds and do not accumulate in the environment. They also have low toxicity and do not release harmful chemicals during decomposition. Additionally, starch-based materials can be produced from cassava, corn, potatoes, making them a more sustainable option. Overall, starch blends have the potential to offer a more sustainable and environmentally friendly solution for food packaging, while also providing the necessary functional properties required for packaging materials.

6.2 STARCH

When numbers of monomers unit combine together to form a structure unit then it is called polysaccharides. Polysaccharides are complex structure of starch, cellulose, glycogen. The structure of starch is shown in Figure 6.1 (Arfin & Sonawane, 2018). Plants create starch through their photosynthesis process. A plant produces glucose through photosynthesis, which is necessary for its growth and development. To produce glucose, the plant uses atmospheric carbon to convert it into glucose molecules. Glucose is the basic molecule used in the synthesis of starch polymers. Amylose and amylopectin are the two components of starch. Amylose is composed of helical α-D-glucose units and in amylopectin linear addition of glucose units will occur in the highly branched manner. With every 22–30 glucose repeating units, there is a branching at the α-(1-6) bonds (Niranjana Prabhu

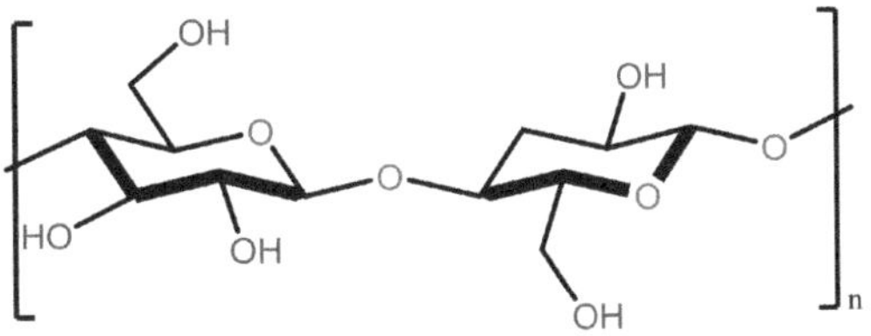

Figure 6.1 Structure of starch.

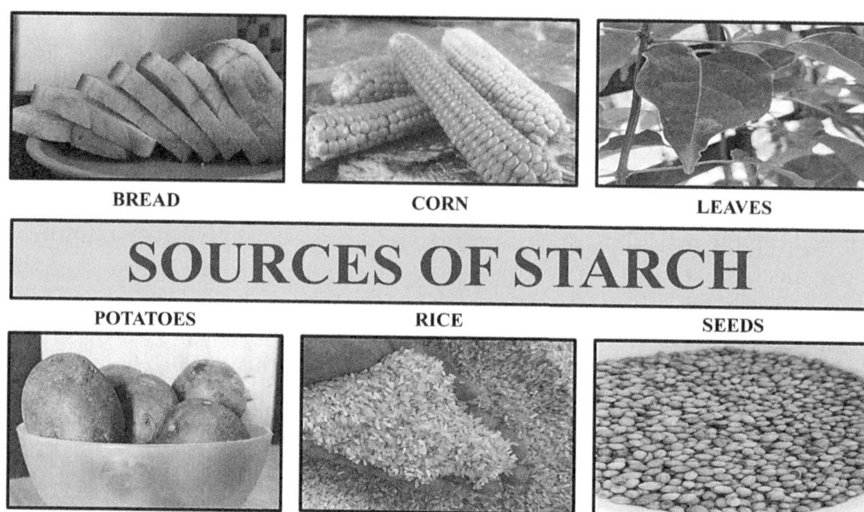

Figure 6.2 Sources of starch.

& Prashantha, 2018). Depending on the source, starch contains 80–90% amylopectin and 10–20% amylose, respectively (Mangaraj et al., 2019b).

Starch makes up the majority of natural polymers, followed by cellulose as the most abundant polymer in nature. Among the benefits of starch are that it is a low cost, sustainable, plentiful, renewable, consumable and biodegradable polymer. There are several types of roots, stalks, and seeds that are used to extract it, including rice, potatoes, tapioca, wheat, and corn as shown in Figure 6.2 (Sanyang et al., 2018a).

6.2.1 Starch Blends

Blends of polymers create new materials with different physical properties by blending two or more polymers together. Developing polymeric materials with versatility for commercial applications has been made easier and more cost-effective by blending polymers (Parameswaranpillai et al., 2014). The global presence of polymer blends in consumer products proves their potential technological significance (Muthuraj et al., 2018). It is possible to categorize polymer blends into two types based on their miscibility or immiscibility. A miscible blend has a single phase and a single glass transition temperature. An unmixable polymer blend, on the other hand, is characterized by separate phases, each component exhibiting a different glass transition and melting temperature (Gunawardene et al., 2021).

As a substitute to synthetic polymers, starch blending with another biopolymer is a promising approach as it will help sustain starch's biodegradability and renewable quality (Sanyang et al., 2018a).

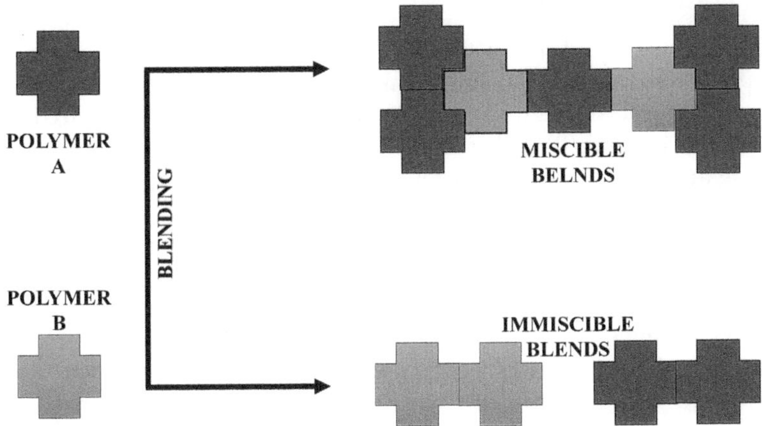

Figure 6.3 Types of polymer blends.

6.2.2 Starch Blends Preparation

Researchers have used a variety of techniques to manufacture starch-based blends, including solution casting, compression moulding, hot pressing, extrusion and injection moulding.

6.2.2.1 Starch/PCL Blends

Singh et al. prepared four types of PCL/Starch blends by mechanical kneading and hydrophobic coating was applied to granular starch to investigate its compatibility with PCL grafted dextran copolymer and used as a compatibilizer in corn starch/PCL blends. In this study, the rate of biodegradation of blend compounds was faster than pure PCL due to the incorporation of starch. According to the authors, compatibilized starch/PCL blends compatible with PGD display a lower degradation rate than pure PCL/starch blends. Furthermore, biodegradation of PCL/starch blends result due to the consumption of starch and continues as natural filler content increases, regardless of the compatibilizing agent (Singh et al., 2003).

Kim et al. prepared poly (acrylic acid)-g-polycaprolactone and compatibilized with starch/PCL blended films. According to the authors, the tensile strength and modulus of the compatible blends decreased with the increasing graft degree of PAA-g-PCL, as a result of a decrease in crystallinity of the PCL matrix with increase in graft degree of PAA-g-PCL. A blend containing PAA-g-PCL showed the most elongation and tensile strength at break. It was also found that reducing graft length by 11 mol% resulted an elevation in elongation and tensile strength. Thus, PAA-g-PCL showed superior compatibility in PCL/starch blends (Kim et al., 2001).

6.2.2.2 Starch/PVA Blends

Jose et al. synthesized starch/PVA and carbon nanotubes solution by mixing to find out the effect of carbon nanotubes as a compatibilizer. Plasticizer glycerol added to the starch dispersion as a plasticizer. When compared to PVA thin film with starch/PVA there are reduction in tensile properties. Hydrogen bonding among polymer –OH groups and O-containing groups on the CNT surface resulted in a tortuous path that decreased water uptake due to strong physical bonds. Moreover, the results indicate the depression in water uptake by 60-43% alongwith the addition of carbon nanotubes (Jose et al., 2015).

Cano et al. synthesized starch/PVA films with Ag nanoparticles to acquire biological activity such as antimicrobial properties. In starch/PVA films embedded with silver nanoparticles, its antibacterial activity against *E. coli* and *Listeria innocua* was remarkable. It also had an antifungal activity against *Peniccilium expansum* and *Aspergillus niger*. Furthermore, silver nanoparticle content has a significant role to play in both antifungal and antibacterial activity (Cano et al., 2016).

6.2.2.3 Starch/PBAT Blends

Fourati et al. Synthesized a blend of TPS and PBAT sheets was prepared to study the compatibilization effects of citric acid (CA), maleic anhydride (MA) and PBAT-grafted MA (PBAT-g-MA). TPS initially had a low strain at break (7%) but increased to 185% when blended with PBAT without compatibilizers. The strain at break decreased, though, with the addition of 2% of MA or 2% of CA. The evolution did not appear to change significantly with an additional 6% addition of MA or CA. According to the authors, PBAT-g-MA enhanced interfacial adhesion via ester-linking of starch and MA grafted onto MA (Fourati et al., 2018).

Ren et al. synthesized the TPS/PBAT/PLA starch blends by the methods of one step extrusion process for exploring the effects of MA as a compatibilizer. The study's findings showed that adding a small quantity of compatibilizer to the blends enhanced the tensile strength and elongation of the blend at break point across the board. From SEM images it is find that the starch granules generally melted and with synthetic polymer matrix result a continuous phase, when compared to compatibilized blends, non-compatibilized blends had inferior mechanical properties. Also, it was noted that as the PBAT level grew from 0% to 50%, the water content elevated from 16% to 20%. Even though, the compatibilized blends' equilibrium water uptake was significantly less than that of the non-compatibilized blends (Ren et al., 2009).

6.2.2.4 Starch/PLA Blends

Wang et al. prepared the corn starch/ PLA blends for studied the compatibilizing impact of low-toxicity maleic anhydride. According to the authors, TPS and PLA were more evenly dispersed while PLA and MA significantly reduced the size of starch granules compared to control mixes. Also, it was shown that when the starch amounts in the blends increased, the mechanical characteristics significantly degraded (Wang et al., 2007).

Akrami et al. prepared the starch/PLA blend for analyzed the impact of grafted maleic anhydride on polyethylene glycol. This research showed that spherical particles developed in compatibilized mixes and that a superior dispersion was attained. In addition, the authors' research found that the compatibilizer had no discernible impact on degradation. This behavior is a result of the TPS's consistent presence in all samples, which is essential for the start and progression of degradation (Akrami et al., 2016).

6.2.2.5 Starch/PBS Blends

Fahrngruber et al. synthesized the properties of thin TPS/poly (butylene succinate) films, and assessed the potential positive changes achieved by the use of hydrophilic/hydrophobic compatibilizer systems. In terms of morphology, TPS dispersion was excellent (under optimized processing conditions), with an average particle size of 1.5 m. The preparation of the compatibilizers used two different raw material approaches: (a) destructurized TPS and (b) native corn starch. Compounding was conducted with 0.5 and 1.0 weight percent of the compatibilizer systems (a) and (b). Comparatively, the introduction of the TPS-based compatibilizer led to increase TPS incorporation, in addition, the material was stronger and more resistant to tears. A biodegradable film with a good bio-based content is the result of this work, and it has a lot of potential for usage in single-use packaging (Fahrngruber et al., 2020).

Yin et al. synthesized the starch/PBS blends by a two-step extrusion method. An efficient interfacial compatibilizer was created by grafting maleic anhydride onto PBS (rPBS). Investigations were done on the TPS/PBS blend's miscibility, morphology, thermal behavior, and mechanical characteristics. It was discovered that compatibilized TPS/PBS blends had a enhanced strength, high-water resistance and good biodegradability. It was anticipated that the TPS/PBS blend would make an effective packing substance (Yin et al., 2015).

6.3 COMMERCIAL PRODUCTION OF STARCH-BASED ACTIVE PACKAGING MATERIALS

Starch is a biopolymer consist of glucose units linked together via glycosidic linkage, and exist as linear and branched units amylose and amylopectin units respectively, it extracted from the various sources like plants, fruits, vegetables, seeds, cassava, corn etc. (Ortega et al., 2022; Diyana et al., 2021) but due to its water and oxygen permeability not suitable for the packaging industry and need to be modified (Pausescu et al., 2022; Alhanish & Abu Ghalia, 2021). Starch/PLA blends with improved properties studied to increase its application area (Alhanish & Abu Ghalia, 2021). Starch/PLA blends with improved properties studied to increase its application area (Molina-Ramírez et al., 2020). Starch modified to thermoplastic starch-based polymers which can be used as an substitute to the conventional non-biodegradable plastics such material result by the various compositions of starch with plasticizers result as biofilms (Ortega et al., 2022), plasticizers used to increase the strength and flexibility of the films prepared to avoid cracking. Plasticizers are non-volatile compounds some of them are glycol, glycerol, sucrose, sorbitol, urea, fructose and amino acids (Diyana et al., 2021). Bioplasticizers such as succinic acid, isosorbide with starch also studied. Starch/PLA blends with citrate species extract as plasticizer with enhanced mechanical properties, flexibility and processibility to result flexible biofilms (Alhanish & Abu Ghalia, 2021). Along with this even sunflower oil also used in thermoplastic composites. Thermoplastic composites fabricated by the combination of starch with biopolymeric units from the citric fruits, bamboo, sugar palm, sugarcane, sunflower oil, PLA etc. Commercial production of thermoplastic starch-based bioplastic films helps to substitute non-biodegradable plastic from packaging industry. Starch based material is modified by various techniques such as blending, derivatization, plasticization and copolymerization which help to enhance its various properties which are must needed to widen its application, biodegradability, biocompatibility, flexibility, and elasticity are the main properties which is considered mainly to its use in biofilm formation, electronic devices, food packaging, cutlery etc. (Diyana et al., 2021). TPS is plastarch material from corn starch used in the packaging as bags, foams, compostable films, pens etc. (Patel et al., 2020). According to a study the market of modified starch can reach at USD 10,700 million till 2023, and predicted to grow at CAGR of 4.2% from 2017–2023 (Falua et al., 2022). Chitosan and starch blend prepared with glycerol plasticizer and little amount of dye to result as an intelligent biodegradable biofilm (Pausescu et al., 2022), other blends such as starch-gelatine, starch-polyvinyl alcohol also studied widely to use as starch based material with better mechanical and barrier (gas, water) in food packaging industry (Falua et al., 2022) With improved water resistivity by adding kaolin, caffeine etc. and with good gas permeability, use of starch blends as a good material for packaging to increase the self-life of food. Similarly Starch-PLA blend is also used to replace the conventional plastic used as cups, food containers, plates etc. (Markevičiūtė & Varžinskas, 2022). Recent studies shows that the modified starch result bio-nanocomposities, carbon dots (fluorescent films), pH sensitive films, film for food packaging, aerogels, medicines, textiles, biofoams, nanofillers. Ezati et al. studied that the pH sensitive intelligent packaging used for food packaging to maintain the food freshness. Colorimetric films of cassava starch-bayberry extract (anthocyanin rich) are with good tensile strength and antioxidant properties, introduction of *Lycium ruthenicum anthocyanins* in cassava starch improve the properties such as antioxidant and water permeability with minimum UV barrier. Anthocyanin rich extract from red cabbage, purple sweet potato and ginger with starch also studied for improved mechanical, moisture content, and water solubility properties result as pH sensitive intelligent films (Falua et al., 2022).

Starch and other biopolymers such as polysaccharides, lipids and proteins used to synthesize bio-based and biodegradable packaging material edible films. Starch and starch derivatives such as amylose, hydroxypropylated amylose considered as easily available and excellent material to develop packaging films, edible coatings with good transparency, elasticity, and mechanical properties (Amin et al., 2021). Starch based-PLA foams investigated recently as a substitute to synthetic polystyrene food trays, rice starch biofoams with good tensile strength, flexibility and good density (Falua et al., 2022). Pavon et al. investigated different properties of five TPS blends with varies concentration of resin derivatives (10 wt%): i) disproportionate gum rosin, ii) pentaerythritol ester of gum rosin, iii) gum rosin, iv) glycerol ester of gum rosin and v) modified gum rosin-maleic anhydride, different properties such as surface wettability, water absorptivity, thermo-mechanical properties, color patterns, X-ray diffraction on the basis of composting conditions, resulted blends are find good for biodegradable food packaging (Pavon et al., 2021). In another study thermoplastic yam starch and epoxidized sesamum oil blends are prepared for semi-rigid food packaging material (Ortega-Toro et al., 2021). Bio-based plastic material prepared from starch used in cutlery, coffee machine capsules, tableware and bottles (Mendes & Pedersen, 2021). In food packaging starch nanocomposites are used which are combination of nanofillers and polymer matrix, i.e., Clay ZnO/PEA starch, Starch nanocrystal/Potato starch, Cellulose whiskers/PEA starch, Chitin whiskers/starch etc. show various applications like as biodegradable edible packaging films, drug release, and other medical application. Starch from potato, wheat and corn used to fabricate biodegradable and encapsulation packaging material, in another investigation, MMT clay used to produce nanocomposites, with different polymers, i.e., starch, PVS, nylon, PE and different nanomaterial's such as Ag, SO_2, halloysite, cellulose nanofiber (Basavegowda & Baek, 2021). Numerous applications of starch base bioplastic with different compositions are reported recently with different brands: BIOPLAST®300, BIOPLAST®400, and BIOPLAST®500 (With different composition of potato starch + Biopolymer) used as waste bags, vegetable and fruit bags, Terratek®SC50 and Terratek®SC65 (With different percentage of wheat starch + polypropylene) used as injection molding material, PaperFoam® (potato + bio-based material) used as egg cartoons, etc. (Jayarathna et al., 2022).

Table 6.1 Starch-based packaging material market products, sources, additional ingredients/material and possible applications

Starch source	Ingredients added	Market brands/products	Possible applications	References
Potato starch	Biopolymers	BIOPLAST®GF 106/02 Bioplast®300, BIOPLAST®400, BIOPLAST® 500	Blown film extrusion uses. Blown film extrusion uses as fruit and vegetable packaging and mailing film.	(*Advanced Biopolymers for Building a Better Tomorrow*, n.d.),
Potato starch	Bio-based material Seed or root flour-based material	PaperFoam® Solanyl	Injection molding uses Sheet, film casting, profile extrusion, injection and thermoforming molding uses.	(*Sustainable Packaging: PaperFoam® - Environment-Friendly*, n.d.), (*PRODUCTS - Rodenburg Biopolymers*, n.d.)
Wheat Starch	Polypropylene (50% and 65%)	Terratek®SC50, Terratek®SC65	Injection molding uses.	(*Starch Composites*, n.d.)
Starch	Polyethylene	Terratek®SC200012, Terratek®SC200041	Injection molding uses	(*Starch Composites*, n.d.)
Starch	Polyester + additives	Mater-Bi® types (Mater-Bi® NF803 (grade N))	Injection, extrusion, filming and thermoforming.	(Jayarathna et al., 2022)

6.4 ENVIRONMENTAL IMPACT OF ACTIVE PACKAGING MATERIALS

Packaging industry is major source of pollution and it is a great matter of concern. Annual growth in use of plastic as food packaging material is about 5% (Sadeghizadeh-Yazdi et al., 2019). Important part of food industry is food packaging, so food industry sector has more attention on the use of biodegradable packaging material in order to reduce waste, transportation cost and use of waste material. Use of plastic material for food packaging is important to increase shelf life by preventing the growth of microorganisms. But plastic degrade very slowly and have negative impact on environment and some plastics are non- renewable which become burden on environment. During photodecomposition it has bad impact on marine life and land animals, and cause bad effect on the balance of ecosystem and food chain, extreme effect of this problem can cause extinction of species (Onyeaka et al., 2022). So new strategies for food packaging based on green material derived from renewable resources is required (Sanyang et al., 2018b). There is increased interest to conduct new researches in food packaging areas because of awareness about limited natural resources and impact of package waste on environment. There is also increased demand of consumers for food with safe, high quality and long shelf life. So bio-based renewable material that are environment friendly can be used for green packaging (Pelissari et al., 2019). Green packaging is defined as plant-based packaging material, don't have bad impact on environment, livestock and human health, can be easily degraded and recycled (Singh & Pandey, 2018). Use of biodegradable polymers for packaging is still limited because, they are difficult to process and also show some poor properties. Blending of biodegradable polymer with synthetic plastic can be ideal solution to overcome these limitations. This will reduce packaging price with retained quality of packaging material. It is crucial from ecological stand point that formed bio-based material must contain major part as biopolymer in the blend so that microorganisms present in the nature can decompose and consume this bio-polymer along with synthetic plastic due to oxidation chain reactions (Turković et al., 2019). Out of many bio-polymers, starch used as green packaging material because of its ability to form various coatings and films. It is made up of amylose and amylopectin and their composition depends on the type of starch. It is essential component of human diet and also a good source of energy, present in many plant sources, e.g., maize, bean, rice and wheat. Because of its properties such as renewable, affordable, safe to consume, biodegradable in nature and also show compatibility with other bio-polymers, starch is considered as an ideal raw material to use for green packaging (Sanyang et al., 2018b). So to solve the harmful impact of synthetic plastic waste, starch is an alternative to it because of low production cost and easy availability. Films made from starch have low carbon footprints as compared to conventional plastic (Żołek-Tryznowska & Holica, 2020). There is a growing need for starch due to its many uses in the food packaging industry, particularly as water retaining agent (e.g., swelling properties and thickening agent to change viscosity or texture (Bangar, Purewal et al., 2021a). Property of gelatinization of starch is very unique. It is only bio- polymer that can undergo gelatinization. Mechanical properties and different barrier properties of starch-based packaging films can be improvised by the introduction of other polymers. Introduction of essential oils will improve antibacterial properties of material (Żołek-Tryznowska & Holica, 2020). It undergo thermoplastic processing with the addition of water and plasticizer such as glycerol, urea glycerine sorbitol (Bangar, Whiteside et al., 2021b) which can also obtained from different biowastes.

Double derived starches are produced by crosslinking and combining chemically modified derivatization for example: Aerogels formed from ionic crosslinking of biopolymers by sol-gel technique, can be used in advanced packaging applications in food industry. In order to make the corresponding aerogels, starch suspensions are first cross-linked to increase their hardness then formation of gel and freeze drying. Food products with starch add functional and physicochemical properties (crystallinity, gelatinization, composition). The starches from millets, cereals and pulses have all been researched for use in food packaging. To create environmentally friendly packing materials, starch can be used as the base blending material (Bangar, Purewal et al., 2021a). In order to form starch based green nanocomposites crosslinking films which are in accordance with ecological and economic needs. Owi et al. studies that, with the development of nanotechnology, tapioca starch green composites were reinforced with nanocellulose that was chemically extracted from oil palm empty fruit bunches (EFB). In order to crosslink the molecules of tapioca starch in the films, a cross-linking agent called citric acid was added and plasticizer such as glycerol was also used to enhance film processing (Owi et al., 2017). Francisco et al. studied the use of biodegradable hydroxyethyl cellulose (HEC) and acetylated cassava starch (ACS) based coatings to elevate the shelf life of guavas and decreased impact of conventional plastic packaging material on environment thickness, water vapor transport, opacity and solubility were used to describe films and also examine the texture, titratable acidity, fruits weight loss, skin color, soluble solids, vitamin C content of biodegradable films. They reported that hygroscopic and transparency character increased with high HEC concentration and by using 75% HEC and 25% ACS leads to reduced ripening (Lasting for 13 days), retained green skin color and increased firmness (Francisco et al., 2020). Gunkaya et al. compared the impact of LDPE (low density polyethylene) films with that of biodegradable films of pectin jelly-corn starch derived from orange peel on environment and their life cycle assessment and biodegradability. They reported that in contrast, the bio-composite film's maximum level of biodegradation is 78.4%, compared to the LDPE film's maximum level of 40.4% (Günkaya

& Banar, 2016). In order to evaluate the environmental impact and energy efficiency of manufacturing cassava starch-based film based on casting in Brazil, Lies et al. used LCA (life cycle assessment). Results show that the production of films, cassava crops, ethanol additives, and the use of fossil glycerine are the main causes of impacts. To minimise the product's impact on the environment and energy use, resource efficiency and cleaner production techniques were developed (de Léis et al., 2017). Development of cheaper and enviro-friendly material needs multidisciplinary approach for successful commercialization and implementation of biopolymer-based eco-friendly packaging materials (Bangar et al., 2021b).

6.5 FUTURE SCOPE AND CONCLUSION

Starch-based packaging material has been used widely in past few years, it produced continuously and expected that it shows tremendous growth in future because of the recent researches and possible future scope as increase its market production. As the literature give information about starch and its properties such as gas and water resistibility, flexibility, mechanical strength, tensile strength etc. concluded that starch-based material can used in market as smart, intelligent material in active packaging industry. Starch blends and composites with other biopolymers or natural material which are less toxic, emerged as safe and smart packaging raw material. But because we still dealing with negative impact of synthesized non-biodegradable packaging material, in future we need to completely substitute the conventional non-biodegradable packaging material with non-toxic, active-biodegradable packaging material and use of starch-based material can help in this matter very deeply. By using starch from different types of biomass and its combination with other biopolymers (which are also extracted from other biomass) help to decrease load of biowaste generated by natural process such as agricultural process, and industrial process such as industrial biowaste, effluents from oil refinery, food waste, etc. Industries like packaging, textile, electronic industry, etc. are focusing on creating bio-based and biodegradable material to replace petroleum-based synthetic material. Creating such smart and intelligent material came with new opportunities for ongoing and incoming researches, and help to create a collaborative environment with various industries to produce biodegradable plastic material. Recent researches on starch-based material as a smart packaging material in food and other packaging industries, and due to the biodegradability along with antioxidant and antimicrobial properties, water and gas permeability etc. it can concluded that in future this area of research attract many researchers, and help to find that this area of research can help to create a future with active, biodegradable starch-based plastic industry, so that future will be without or atleast with less amount of non-biodegradable plastic.

REFERENCES

Advanced biopolymers for building a better tomorrow. (n.d.). Retrieved May 10, 2023, from https://www.biotec.de/

Akrami, M., Ghasemi, I., Azizi, H., Karrabi, M., & Seyedabadi, M. (2016). A new approach in compatibilization of the Poly(Lactic Acid)/Thermoplastic Starch (PLA/TPS) blends. *Carbohydrate Polymers, 144,* 254–262. https://doi.org/10.1016/j.carbpol.2016.02.035

Alhanish, A., & Abu Ghalia, M. (2021). Developments of biobased plasticizers for compostable polymers in the green packaging applications: A review. *Biotechnology Progress, 37*(6). https://doi.org/10.1002/btpr.3210

Amin, U., Khan, M. U., Majeed, Y., Rebezov, M., Khayrullin, M., Bobkova, E., Shariati, M. A., Chung, I. M., & Thiruvengadam, M. (2021). Potentials of polysaccharides, lipids and proteins in biodegradable food packaging applications. *International Journal of Biological Macromolecules, 183,* 2184–2198. https://doi.org/10.1016/j.ijbiomac.2021.05.182

Arfin, T., & Sonawane, K. (2018). Bio-based materials: Past to future. In S. Ahmed (Ed.), *Bio-based materials for food packaging* (pp. 1–32). Springer Singapore. https://doi.org/10.1007/978-981-13-1909-9_1

Bangar, S. P., Purewal, S. S., Trif, M., Maqsood, S., Kumar, M., Manjunatha, V., & Rusu, A. V. (2021). Functionality and applicability of starch-based films: An eco-friendly approach. *Foods, 10*(9), 2181. https://doi.org/10.3390/foods10092181

Bangar, S. P., Whiteside, W. S., Ashogbon, A. O., & Kumar, M. (2021). Recent advances in thermoplastic starches for food packaging: A review. *Food Packaging and Shelf Life, 30,* 100743. https://doi.org/10.1016/j.fpsl.2021.100743

Basavegowda, N., & Baek, K.-H. (2021). Advances in functional biopolymer-based nanocomposites for active food packaging applications. *Polymers, 13*(23), 4198. https://doi.org/10.3390/polym13234198

Cano, A., Cháfer, M., Chiralt, A., & González-Martínez, C. (2016). Development and characterization of active films based on starch-PVA, containing silver nanoparticles. *Food Packaging and Shelf Life, 10,* 16–24. https://doi.org/10.1016/j.fpsl.2016.07.002

de Léis, C. M., Nogueira, A. R., Kulay, L., & Tadini, C. C. (2017). Environmental and energy analysis of biopolymer film based on cassava starch in Brazil. *Journal of Cleaner Production, 143,* 76–89. https://doi.org/10.1016/j.jclepro.2016.12.147

Diyana, Z. N., Jumaidin, R., Selamat, M. Z., Ghazali, I., Julmohammad, N., Huda, N., & Ilyas, R. A. (2021). Physical properties of thermoplastic starch derived from natural resources and its blends: A review. *Polymers, 13*(9), 1396. https://doi.org/10.3390/polym13091396

Fahrngruber, B., Fortea-Verdejo, M., Wimmer, R., & Mundigler, N. (2020). Starch/Poly(butylene succinate) compatibilizers: Effect of different reaction-approaches on the properties of thermoplastic starch-based compostable films. *Journal of Polymers and the Environment, 28*(1), 257–270. https://doi.org/10.1007/s10924-019-01601-0

Falua, K. J., Pokharel, A., Babaei-Ghazvini, A., Ai, Y., & Acharya, B. (2022). Valorization of starch to biobased materials: A review. *Polymers*, *14*(11), 2215. https://doi.org/10.3390/polym14112215

Fourati, Y., Tarrés, Q., Mutjé, P., & Boufi, S. (2018). PBAT/thermoplastic starch blends: Effect of compatibilizers on the rheological, mechanical and morphological properties. *Carbohydrate Polymers*, *199*, 51–57. https://doi.org/10.1016/j.carbpol.2018.07.008

Francisco, C. B., Pellá, M. G., Silva, O. A., Raimundo, K. F., Caetano, J., Linde, G. A., Colauto, N. B., & Dragunski, D. C. (2020). Shelf-life of guavas coated with biodegradable starch and cellulose-based films. *International Journal of Biological Macromolecules*, *152*, 272–279. https://doi.org/10.1016/j.ijbiomac.2020.02.249

Gunawardene, O. H. P., Gunathilake, C., Amaraweera, S. M., Fernando, N. M. L., Wanninayaka, D. B., Manamperi, A., Kulatunga, A. K., Rajapaksha, S. M., Dassanayake, R. S., Fernando, C. A. N., & Manipura, A. (2021). Compatibilization of starch/synthetic biodegradable polymer blends for packaging applications: A review. *Journal of Composites Science*, *5*(11), 300. https://doi.org/10.3390/jcs5110300

Günkaya, Z., & Banar, M. (2016). An environmental comparison of biocomposite film based on orange peel-derived pectin jelly-corn starch and LDPE film: LCA and biodegradability. *The International Journal of Life Cycle Assessment*, *21*(4), 465–475. https://doi.org/10.1007/s11367-016-1042-8

Jayarathna, S., Andersson, M., & Andersson, R. (2022). Recent advances in starch-based blends and composites for bioplastics applications. *Polymers*, *14*(21), 4557. https://doi.org/10.3390/polym14214557

Jose, J., De, S. K., AlMa'adeed, M. A.-A., Dakua, J. B., Sreekumar, P. A., Sougrat, R., & Al-Harthi, M. A. (2015). Compatibilizing role of carbon nanotubes in poly(vinyl alcohol)/starch blend. *Starch - Stärke*, *67*(1–2), 147–153. https://doi.org/10.1002/star.201400074

Kim, C.-H., Cho, K. Y., & Park, J.-K. (2001). Effect of poly(acrylic acid)-g-PCL microstructure on the mechanical properties of starch/PCL blend compatibilized with poly(acrylic acid)-g-PCL. *Polymer Engineering & Science*, *41*(3), 542–553. https://doi.org/10.1002/pen.10751

Mangaraj, S., Yadav, A., Bal, L. M., Dash, S. K., & Mahanti, N. K. (2019a). Application of biodegradable polymers in food packaging industry: A comprehensive review. *Journal of Packaging Technology and Research*, *3*(1), 77–96. https://doi.org/10.1007/s41783-018-0049-y

Mangaraj, S., Yadav, A., Bal, L. M., Dash, S. K., & Mahanti, N. K. (2019b). Application of biodegradable polymers in food packaging industry: A comprehensive review. *Journal of Packaging Technology and Research*, *3*(1), 77–96. https://doi.org/10.1007/s41783-018-0049-y

Markevičiūtė, Z., & Varžinskas, V. (2022). Smart material choice: The importance of circular design strategy applications for bio-based food packaging preproduction and end-of-life life cycle stages. *Sustainability*, *14*(10), 6366. https://doi.org/10.3390/su14106366

Mendes, A. C., & Pedersen, G. A. (2021). Perspectives on sustainable food packaging: Is bio-based plastics a solution? *Trends in Food Science & Technology*, *112*, 839–846. https://doi.org/10.1016/j.tifs.2021.03.049

Molina-Ramírez, C., Cañas-Gutiérrez, A., Castro, C., Zuluaga, R., & Gañán, P. (2020). Effect of production process scale-up on the characteristics and properties of bacterial nanocellulose obtained from overripe Banana culture medium. *Carbohydrate Polymers*, *240*, 116341. https://doi.org/10.1016/j.carbpol.2020.116341

Muthuraj, R., Misra, M., & Mohanty, A. K. (2018). Biodegradable compatibilized polymer blends for packaging applications: A literature review. *Journal of Applied Polymer Science*, *135*(24), 45726. https://doi.org/10.1002/app.45726

Niranjana Prabhu, T., & Prashantha, K. (2018). A review on present status and future challenges of starch based polymer films and their composites in food packaging applications. *Polymer Composites*, *39*(7), 2499–2522. https://doi.org/10.1002/pc.24236

Onyeaka, H., Obileke, K., Makaka, G., & Nwokolo, N. (2022). Current research and applications of starch-based biodegradable films for food packaging. *Polymers*, *14*(6), 1126. https://doi.org/10.3390/polym14061126

Ortega, F., Versino, F., López, O. V., & García, M. A. (2022). Biobased composites from agro-industrial wastes and by-products. *Emergent Materials*, *5*(3), 873–921. https://doi.org/10.1007/s42247-021-00319-x

Ortega-Toro, R., López-Córdoba, A., & Avalos-Belmontes, F. (2021). Epoxidised sesame oil as a biobased coupling agent and plasticiser in polylactic acid/thermoplastic yam starch blends. *Heliyon*, *7*(2), e06176. https://doi.org/10.1016/j.heliyon.2021.e06176

Owi, W. T., Lin, O. H., Sam, S. T., Villagracia, A. R., & Santos, G. N. C. (2017). Tapioca starch based green nanocomposites with environmental friendly cross-linker. *Chemical Engineering Transactions*, *56*, 463–468. https://doi.org/10.3303/CET1756078

Parameswaranpillai, J., Thomas, S., & Grohens, Y. (2014). Polymer blends: State of the art, new challenges, and opportunities. In S. Thomas, Y. Grohens, & P. Jyotishkumar (Eds.), *Characterization of polymer blends* (pp. 1–6). Wiley-VCH Verlag GmbH & Co. KGaA. https://doi.org/10.1002/9783527645602.ch01

Pavon, C., Aldas, M., López-Martínez, J., Hernández-Fernández, J., & Arrieta, M. P. (2021). Films based on thermoplastic starch blended with pine resin derivatives for food packaging. *Foods*, *10*(6), 1171. https://doi.org/10.3390/foods10061171

Pelissari, F. M., Ferreira, D. C., Louzada, L. B., dos Santos, F., Corrêa, A. C., Moreira, F. K. V., & Mattoso, L. H. (2019). Starch-based edible films and coatings. In *Starches for food application* (pp. 359–420). Elsevier. https://doi.org/10.1016/B978-0-12-809440-2.00010-1

PRODUCTS - Rodenburg Biopolymers. (n.d.). Retrieved May 10, 2023, from https://biopolymers.nl/biopolymer/

Rahman, R. (2019). Bioplastics for food packaging: A review. *International Journal of Current Microbiology and Applied Sciences*, *8*(3), 2311–2321. https://doi.org/10.20546/ijcmas.2019.803.274

Reichert, C. L., Bugnicourt, E., Coltelli, M.-B., Cinelli, P., Lazzeri, A., Canesi, I., Braca, F., Martínez, B. M., Alonso, R., Agostinis, L., Verstichel, S., Six, L., Mets, S. D., Gómez, E. C., Ißbrücker, C., Geerinck, R., Nettleton, D. F., Campos, I., Sauter, E., … Schmid, M. (2020). Bio-based packaging: Materials, modifications, industrial applications and sustainability. *Polymers*, *12*(7), 1558. https://doi.org/10.3390/polym12071558

Ren, J., Fu, H., Ren, T., & Yuan, W. (2009). Preparation, characterization and properties of binary and ternary blends with thermoplastic starch, poly(lactic acid) and poly(butylene adipate-co-terephthalate). *Carbohydrate Polymers*, 77(3), 576–582. https://doi.org/10.1016/j.carbpol.2009.01.024

Sadeghizadeh-Yazdi, J., Habibi, M., Kamali, A. A., & Banaei, M. (2019). Application of edible and biodegradable starch-based films in food packaging: A systematic review and meta-analysis. *Current Research in Nutrition and Food Science Journal*, 7(3), 624–637. https://doi.org/10.12944/CRNFSJ .7.3.03

Sanyang, M. L., Ilyas, R. A., Sapuan, S. M., & Jumaidin, R. (2018a). Sugar palm starch-based composites for packaging applications. In M. Jawaid & S. K. Swain (Eds.), *Bionanocomposites for packaging applications* (pp. 125–147). Springer International Publishing. https://doi.org/10.1007/978-3-319-67319 -6_7

Sanyang, M. L., Ilyas, R. A., Sapuan, S. M., & Jumaidin, R. (2018b). Sugar palm starch-based composites for packaging applications. In M. Jawaid & S. K. Swain (Eds.), *Bionanocomposites for packaging applications* (pp. 125–147). Springer International Publishing. https://doi.org/10.1007/978-3-319-67319 -6_7

Singh, G., & Pandey, N. (2018). The determinants of green packaging that influence Buyers' Willingness to pay a price premium. *Australasian Marketing Journal*, 26(3), 221–230. https://doi.org/10.1016/j.ausmj.2018.06.001

Singh, R. P., Pandey, J. K., Rutot, D., Degée, P., & Dubois, P. (2003). Biodegradation of poly(ε-caprolactone)/starch blends and composites in composting and culture environments: The effect of compatibilization on the inherent biodegradability of the host polymer. *Carbohydrate Research*, 338(17), 1759–1769. https://doi.org/10.1016/S0008-6215(03)00236-2

Song, T., Qian, S., Lan, T., Wu, Y., Liu, J., & Zhang, H. (2022). Recent advances in bio-based smart active packaging materials. *Foods*, 11(15), 2228. https:// doi.org/10.3390/foods11152228

Starch Composites. (n.d.). Green dot bioplastics. Retrieved May 10, 2023, from https://www.greendotbioplastics.com/materials/starch-composites/

Sustainable packaging: PaperFoam®—Environment-friendly. (n.d.). Retrieved May 10, 2023, from https://paperfoam.com/sustainable-packaging/

Turković, A., Govorčin Bajsić, E., Zovko, R., Jozinović, A., Kučić Grgić, D., Mandić, L., & Ocelić Bulatović, V. (2019). Environmentally friendly packaging materials based on thermoplastic starch. *Chemical & Biochemical Engineering Quarterly*, 33(3), 347–361. https://doi.org/10.15255/CABEQ .2018.1548

Wang, N., Yu, J., & Ma, X. (2007). Preparation and characterization of thermoplastic starch/PLA blends by one-step reactive extrusion. *Polymer International*, 56(11), 1440–1447. https://doi.org/10.1002/pi.2302

Yin, Q., Chen, F., Zhang, H., & Liu, C. (2015). Fabrication and characterisation of thermoplastic starch/poly(butylene succinate) blends with maleated poly(butylene succinate) as compatibiliser. *Plastics, Rubber and Composites*, 44(9), 362–367. https://doi.org/10.1179/1743289815Y.0000000031

Żołek-Tryznowska, Z., & Holica, J. (2020). Starch films as an environmentally friendly packaging material: Printing performance. *Journal of Cleaner Production*, 276, 124265. https://doi.org/10.1016/j.jclepro.2020.124265

Chapter 7

Smart and Self-healing Hydrogels for Biomedical Applications

Yusuf Olatunji Waidi, Nipun Jain, Ranjit Barua, Vilay Vannaladsaysy, Samir Das, Arbind Prasad, and Sudipto Datta

7.1 INTRODUCTION

Hydrogels, with their crosslinked networks of polymer and huge water holding capability, have arose as talented materials for biomedical uses due to their biocompatibility, elasticity, and likeness to the extracellular matrix [1]. Inspired by the inherent curative capability of living creatures, researchers have developed self-healing hydrogels that can autonomously repair damage and restore their original properties. Early attempts incorporated microcapsules, releasing healing molecules at the defect site [2, 3]. Nevertheless, these approaches often involve permanent healing processes and prospective complications from fillers, limiting their applicability [4, 5]. Additionally, several dynamic hydrogels rely on external stimuli like heat, low pH, or light to trigger self-healing, which could pose risks to surrounding cells and tissues [6, 7]. This chapter of the book focuses on a new generation of self-healing hydrogels designed for automatic and reversible repair, offering significant advantages for various biomedical needs. Self-healing hydrogels offer a unique combination of self-repairing properties and diverse functionalities, making them highly promising for various applications. These materials are formed through dynamic covalent bonds or non-covalent interactions, enabling them to heal damage and reform their structure [8]. The type of interaction influences the healing process, with covalent bonds providing slower but more stable healing, while non-covalent interactions offer faster but potentially weaker self-repair. This versatility allows for tailoring the mechanical properties of the hydrogels, ranging from robust to cell-adaptable or shear-thinning, making them suitable for diverse applications like soft robotics, drug/cell delivery, and 3D printing.

7.2 SELF-HEALING MECHANISM OVERVIEW

The remarkable hydrogels self-healing property stems from the reversible nature of their crosslinked structures. These crosslinks can be designed

DOI: 10.1201/9781003470311-7

by the covalent bonds that are dynamic like Schiff base, borate ester, Diels–Alder, and disulfide bonds [9–13] or through dynamic non-covalent connections like hydrophobic interactions, hydrogen bonding, host-guest interactions and metal coordination [14–19]. The interplay between these bonds' number, strength, and type directly influences the hydrogel's stability, self-healing capability, and mechanical properties. Understanding these underlying mechanisms empowers researchers to develop hydrogels with tailored self-healing capabilities for diverse applications. Traditionally synthesized hydrogels with covalently crosslinked polymer networks suffer from irreversible damage and fatigue during use due to their permanent bonds. In contrast, dynamic covalent bonds, with their reversible "fracture-formation" process in mild environments, offer self-healing capabilities in hydrogels. Additionally, dynamic non-covalent interactions, characterized by natural reversibility and stable fracture recombination, present another promising avenue for designing self-healing hydrogels due to their inherent physical interactions. These dynamic bond approaches offer advantages over traditional methods in creating robust and self-repairing hydrogels.

7.2.1 Dynamic Covalent Bond Base Approach

The hydrogels prepared using conventional covalent interactions are fragile, making them highly vulnerable to wear and tear. Self-healing hydrogels have been designed using the dynamic covalent link (which can be reversible) in a mild environment. The basic approaches for creating hydrogels that can mend themselves using reversible covalent connections are as follows.

7.2.1.1 Imine Bond/Schiff Bond

The reversible combination of a primary amine and a carbonyl functional group creates this chemical link. It is commonly utilized in hydrogel networks, such as chitosan and polyethylene imine, because of its dynamic nature. Figure 7.1 demonstrates the self-healing approach [20]. The basic interface (–CH=N–) amongst the amino group the PEG aldehyde and PEI allows the hydrogel to self-heal. Zhao et al. [21] produced a hydrogel that is self-healing by utilizing the communication between three polymers (sodium alginate, adipic dihydrazide and N-carboxyethyl chitosan). This hydrogel system demonstrates exceptional capability of self-healing along with high effectiveness (equal to 95%) under biological settings.

7.2.1.2 Diels–Alder Reactions

This is regarded as the best covalent connection in crosslinked hydrogels owing to its greater selectivity, efficiency, speed, absence of side products, reversibility, and capability to self-heal. Shao et al. [23] created a straightforward and efficient technique for creating a nanocomposite

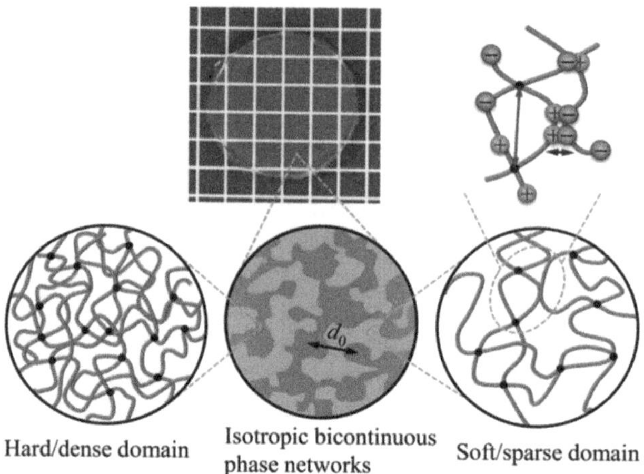

Figure 7.1 The structural hierarchy of PA gel. Ionic crosslinking stabilized the polymer network of hard and soft phases (reprinted with permission of *PNAS*, from [22]).

hydrogel by using a reversible DA reaction to crosslink furan-based modified with poly(ethylene glycol) PEGalong with cellulose nanocrystals (CNC). The hydrogel exhibited excellent mechanical characteristics and fatigue resistance. At 90°C, the hydrogel's self-healing was enhanced, and 78% of its mechanical qualities were restored. The hydrogels had exceptional physical characteristics, exhibiting a high elongation of up to 690%. The CNC-PEG hydrogels' strong self-healing capabilities offer a novel concept for creating efficient, biocompatible hydrogels. Zhao and his colleagues [24] disclosed the production of a DA reaction using dextran in biological circumstances (pH = 7.4, 37°). Under physiological settings, the hydrogels demonstrated outstanding self-healing capabilities. This work expands the potential uses of self-healing in biological domains like cell encapsulation and offers a straightforward technique for creating polysaccharide hydrogels that mend themselves.

7.2.1.3 Disulfide Bonds

Disulfide bonds are found in all living things. They are crucial for preserving cellular redox reactions and the tertiary arrangement of molecules [25, 26]. This particular covalent link can be quickly altered with mercaptan (oxidation-reducing agent) because of the changes in pH and is commonly utilized in creating self-healing networks [27–29]. Barcan and co-authors [30] used ring-opening polymerization to reveal a crosslinked water-soluble triblock (ABA) hydrogel using dithiol. The synthetic hydrogel demonstrated significant self-healing properties in the dynamical stepwise strain study. The energy storage modulus G dropped to 65 Pa as the strain grew to 800%, and it swiftly returned to its initial value when the strain was recovered. A similar hydrogel based on acyl hydrazone and disulfide linkages was created by Deng et al. [31]. The hydrogel demonstrated self-healing settings by the mercaptan transformation process. The technique could be initiated at 37°C, and the stress-strain curve for 2 days presented that the strain and fracture stress might surpass 50% of the initial strength. Additionally, acyl hydrazone allows the gel to self-heal in acidic and neutral environments.

7.2.2 Covalent Bond Base Strategy (Non-dynamic)

7.2.2.1 Ionic Interaction

One typical tactic to draw polymer chains together and generate a hydrogel is ionic contact between oppositely charged groups. This tactic depends on the dispersion of groups with opposing charges. It can sometimes be as simple as mixing oppositely charged components to create an ionic cross-linked hydrogel. For instance, adding calcium can produce a Ca-alginate-based hydrogel; the Ca2+ ions act as CRAM cationic donors. This hydrogel works well as a superficial wound dressing and is a classic example of an auto-healing hydrogel based on ionic interaction. However, hydrogels that depend on ionic contact still have a problem since an inhomogeneous material will emerge if the components in charge interact too strongly. As a result, creating and gelling strategies is essential [32].

Dynamic designs allow for a wide range of products since many mechanical attributes, like strength, auto-healing capability, and stiffness, depend on the hydrogel's ionization level and particle size. Ionic bond-based hydrogels have a lot of promise, as demonstrated by subsequent research that tuned various interactions and hierarchical topologies. A hydrogel with adjustable toughness and viscoelasticity was presented by Sun et al. [33]. Within the hydrogel, weak and strong ionic connections either maintain its shape or improve its resistance and auto-healing properties. The hydrogel demonstrated favorable mechanical qualities and biocompatibility by maintaining a significant bond of ionization density and equilibrium of various interfaces, allowing its use as a structural biomaterial. Resistance to fatigue fracture was shown by an additional polyampholyte gel featuring exact structured configurations [22]. In this study, mechanical examination showed the three-tier structure of polyampholyte hydrogels (Figure 7.1). The local aggregation of the crosslinked polymers caused by creating an ionic connection also led to larger-scale hard/soft phase systems and a milder advancement of weariness cracks.

7.2.2.2 The Hydrogen Bonding

Like oxygen, a hydrogen atom and an electronegative atom combine to form a hydrogen bond. While a solution of water including organic compounds offers amides and hydroxyl groups as intermediates, it is typical of biological processes. As a result, hydrogels that rely on hydrogen bonds typically have strong histocompatibility. Since the hydrogen bonds are far feebler than ionic and covalent interactions, their straightforward application is less attractive for applications needing significant mechanical strength [34]. Nonetheless, there are still methods to enhance the hydrogen bond act. Hard tissue, including bone and cartilage, can be treated with the improved methods [34–37].

For instance, Wang et al. [38] created a robust self-healing hydrogel. The numerous hydrogen relationships generated by the pair of NH2 and 2′-F compounds in addition to the water molecules themselves provided plenty of durability and backing to the multi-hydrogen binding system they created, which had its foundation on the monomeric gelator 2-FA). The hydrogel's injectability, mechanical durability, and capacity to control inflammation made it a practical and efficient tooth-extraction socket healing cause.

In addition to the intended supramolecule, hydrogen bonding can be found in various common and biodegradable biopolymers. It is possible to alter these materials to enhance their mechanical qualities. A biobased hydrogel including PVA starch and glycerol [34] was presented, which spontaneously provided the hydrogen bond formation conditions. Additionally, the hydrogel demonstrated excellent conductivity and resilience to freezing, which raised the prospect of employing organic hydrogels in flexible technology.

7.2.2.3 Hydrophobic Interaction

The repulsive forces of hydrophobic groups with water are how hydrophobic bonding functions. In polar solutions, the hydrophobic components of molecules spontaneously collect closer by folding and forming clusters since water hinders them. Appel and colleagues [39] reported that a hydrogel created using NPs having an altered hydrophobic polymer and hydrophobic contact helped a hydrogel repair itself. Because the hydrogel is biocompatible and discharges drugs with cells through erosion, it is a minimally invasive drug delivery device. Because the hydrogel is biocompatible and releases drugs with cells through erosion, it is a minimally invasive drug delivery device. Additional research found that the mechanical characteristics might be even better by combining hydrogen bonding with the hydrophobic cage shape. Following the construction of sizable hydrophobic chains copolymerized by hydrophiles like acrylamide or UPy motifs, the hardness of self-healing hydrogels was improved [40, 41].

Once detergents were added to this kind of hydrophobic spherical, micelle and hydrogel chains encircled through molecules accomplish the purpose of crosslinking cores to encourage better self-healing. Tuncaboylu [42] described a straightforward method for integrating hydrophobic sequences through the membrane polymeric reaction to produce a hydrogel modeling using hydrophobic bonds (Figure 7.2). Furthermore, they selected an

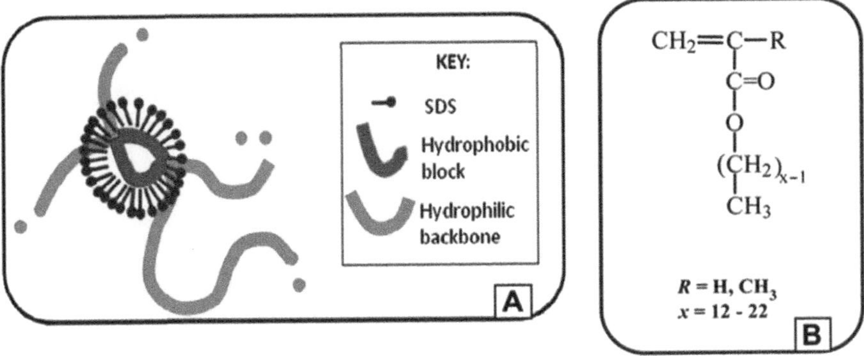

Figure 7.2 (A) Gels showing self-healing properties (B) shows the molecules that are hydrophobic (reprinted with the permission of Elsevier from [42]).

alkyl side chain length optimization for 18 carbon atoms. The effectiveness of the self-healing hydrogel using the big hydrophobic molecule known as stearyl methacrylate (C18) together with its detergent SDS was evaluated by Gulyuz and Okay [43]. They discovered that surfactant significantly improves their strength and quickens the self-healing process. Comparing the SDS-infused gel to a virgin hydrogel, the former demonstrated far better self-healing capabilities and excellent stability.

7.2.2.4 Coordinating Interaction in Metals

Metal cations function like electron receivers, cooperating with ligands to transfer electrons by coordinating metals. The adhesive nature of mussels serves as an inspiration among the most popular metal coordinating approaches for self-healing hydrogel [44–46]. Fe and catechol formed a coordination bond. The interaction may generate the sacrifice connection, offering appropriate mechanical strength and breaks in stress before inflicting harm within the hydrogel's centre. A pH-sensitive, Fe-catechol coordinating bonded in a dual-dynamic-bond hydrogel had been developed by Liang et al. [47]. Due to its antibacterial abilities, this works well as a covering for wound incisions that may be taken off as needed when paired with QCS [48].

Other hydrogels made from metal coordination exhibit numerous appealing properties caused by various metallic ions. Shi et al. [49] created the hydrogel by combining the HA solutions and BP pairs (HA-BP) with silver (Ag+) ions. The hydrogel can be molded and self-healed, making it appropriate for filling various wound beds. Synchronization with the polymerization phase makes this possible. More specifically, the hydrogel's slow breakdown of Ag+ ions – a wide-ranging antibacterial element – makes avoiding infections possible. Because of these characteristics, the hydrogel

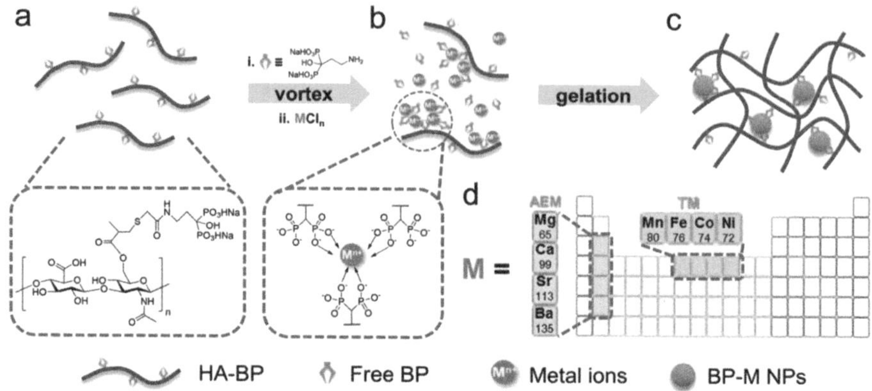

Figure 7.3 The hydrogels of HA-BP-M nanocomposites self-assembling structures (a–c), typical components (d). (Reprinted with permission of John Wiley and Sons from [50]).

is a ready-to-use option for wound healing materials. A popular technique that suggests adding various basic metallic ions, such as Fe2+, Mg2+, and Ca2+, to form a restorable hydrogel was recommended due to the coordinating ability of HA-BP [50] (Figure 7.3).

7.3 SELF-HEALED HYDROGELS USED IN BIOMEDICINE

SHH exhibits remarkable potential as a biological material due to its close resemblance to normal tissues [51–53]. Normal tissues can repair themselves, increasing their longevity, mechanical strength, and resilience [54]. Self-healed hydrogels' practical uses include synthetic tissue engineering, medication delivery, soft robots, carrying platforms for transferring different guest molecules inside cells, catalyst science, and electrochemical uses like sensing technological advances. These are all made possible by the hydrogels' remarkably comparable characteristics to those of natural tissues.

7.3.1 Tissue Engineering

Normal tissue has an incredible capacity to mend itself, which increases its resilience and strength [54]. Hydrogels are among the components with high promise for healthcare engineering due to their self-healed characteristics, which are motivated by biological processes [55]. Hydrogels are nearly identical in real tissue regarding their strength and water concentration [56]. Quick adhesion, stimulus reactivity, and excellent conductivity are characteristics of hydrogels that have broad applications, particularly in tissue engineering [57]. Figure 7.4 shows some examples of the different possible uses for SSH.

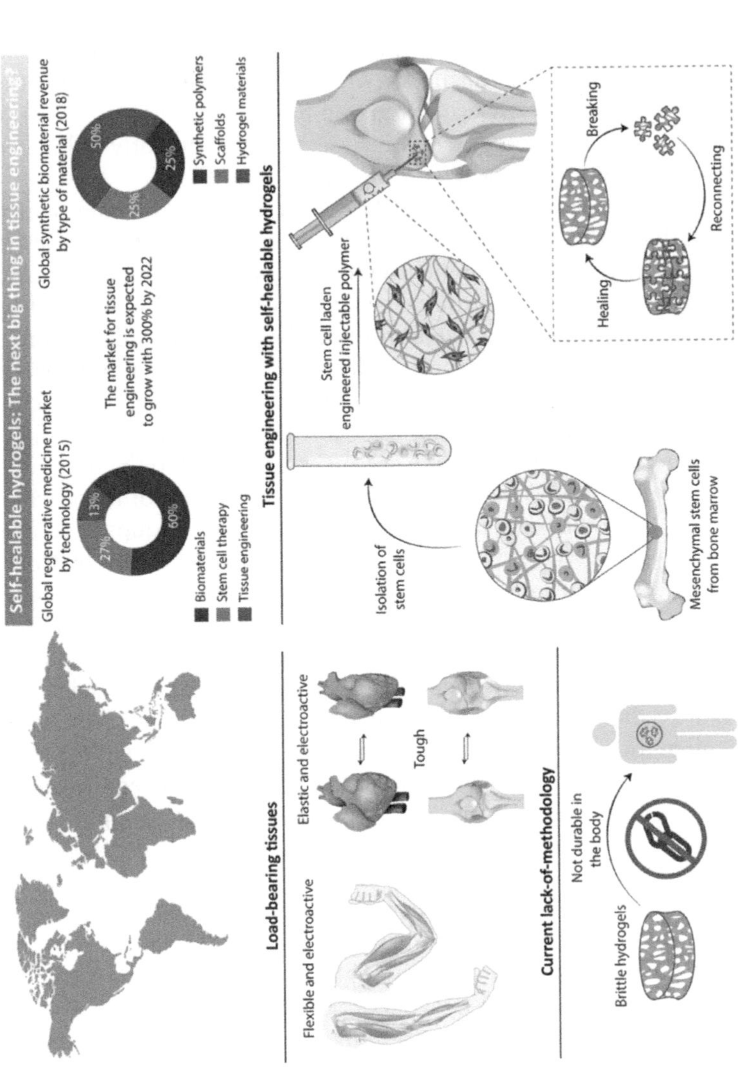

Figure 7.4 Numerous uses of hydrogels that are self-healing in different tissue engineering circumstances. Talebian et al. [58] helped the inspiration for this figure. The study can be used, shared, adapted, distributed, and reproduced in any manner or media according to the Creative Commons Attribution 4.0 International License. Nonetheless, a link to the Creative Commons license and due attribution to the original author(s) and source must be included. (http://creativecommons.org/licenses/by/4.0/, accessed on 19 October 2022).

Myocardial infarction, sometimes called a heart attack, is the result of inadequate oxygen delivery to specific areas of the heart muscle. Self-healing hydrogels (SHH) of the host-guest type are widely used to treat myocardial infarction. By adding pathogenic endothelial cells (PECs) to the hydrogel and implanting them into cardiac tissues[59], Agrawal et al. [60] created a host-guest-based SHH system. The hydrogel was made of β-cyclodextrin (β-CD) and adamantine-modified hyaluronic acid (HA). Interestingly, in this system, β-CDs-HA were the hosts while adamantine-HA were the guests. The hydrogel with PECs was evaluated for effectiveness in a mouse model of myocardial infarction. Vasculogenesis was significantly enhanced when the HA-based hydrogel and PECs were used separately.

To prevent left ventricular remodeling, Loebel et al. [61] created a hydrogel that is injectable and having shear-thinning properties what was uses to Michael addition and host-guest interaction to administer minimally invasive treatment to the infarcted myocardium. Hyaluronic acid (HA) modified by adamantane/thiol and CD/methacrylate formed the hydrogel; adamantane/thiol was the guest, and CD/methacrylate was the host. Through a reversible host-guest connection and stable Michael addition, this method offered excellent retention and shear slimming injection [62, 63]. Epicardial injection of the hydrogel produced noteworthy changes compared to the untreated group and hydrogel without Michael's inclusion in rat models of myocardial infarction [61, 62]. Furthermore, ureidopyrimidinone (UPy) groups functionalized by poly(ethylene glycol) (PEG) were present in a self-healing hydrogel that was recently created as a growth factor delivery method [64]. A pocket placed under the kidney capsule of rats included the PEG hydrogel modified by UPy, which incorporated an antifibrotic growth factor. After injecting hydrogels containing growth factors, the quantity of myofibroblasts in the healthy kidney did not change; nevertheless, it grew dramatically when hydrogel or saline alone was injected [65, 66]. In a different investigation, growth factors were delivered to the infarcted myocardium for repair using a PEG hydrogel that had been changed via UPy [66]. A catheter mapping system with a long, narrow lumen might be used to administer this pH-switchable hydrogel, which quickly transforms into a hydrogel when it comes into contact with tissue in a myocardial infarction model in pigs [67].

Tseng et al. [68] developed self-healing hydrogels (SHH) related on the difunctionalized poly(ethylene glycol) (GC-DP) and glycol chitosan to address CNS repair. Injection of GC-DP hydrogel containing neurospheres expedited the process of functional regeneration in zebrafish with CNS damage. Within the hydrogel, neurosphere-like progenitors demonstrated increased proliferation and differentiation. Optogenetic techniques and GC-DP hydrogel were used in a different strategy to treat neurodegenerative illnesses utilizing a temporal-spatial approach [69]. When CNS-impaired zebrafish were injected with a hydrogel containing neural stem cells and the bacteriorhodopsin plasmid, their neural tissue recovered, particularly when came in contact to green light. The GC-DP hydrogel was also employed to promote blood capillary development [69]. Besides the fibrin gel, a mixed hydrogel structure has been developed with a fibrin polymer network and interpenetrating GC-DP [69]. Vascular endothelial cells were induced to produce capillary-like patterns alone in this hydrogel, and hydrogel injections by themselves promoted angiogenesis in zebrafish and repaired circulation to mice whose hindlimbs suffered ischemic.

7.3.2 Management of Wounds

The process of replacing lost or injured cellular structures and tissue layers is known as wound healing, and it is dynamic and complicated [70, 71]. SHH could reduce the need to change dressings, sparing patients from needless suffering [72, 73]. Furthermore, causing network disintegrations can dissolve certain stimuli-responsive SHH [74]. Moreover, SHH can reduce burn patients' suffering during dressing changes and satisfy the need for surgical debridement [71, 73]. Figure 7.5 [75] demonstrated that the hydrogel MF-Lip@PEG exhibited anti-necrotic, anti-inflammation, anti-infection, pro-neovascularization properties. Wang et al. [76] developed FHE@exo, an oxidative hyaluronic acid-based stem cell hybrid that releases exosomes made from adipose-derived mesenchymal stem cells, and Poly-ε-L-lysine, an antimicrobial peptide, for treating wounds that persist. Multifunctional

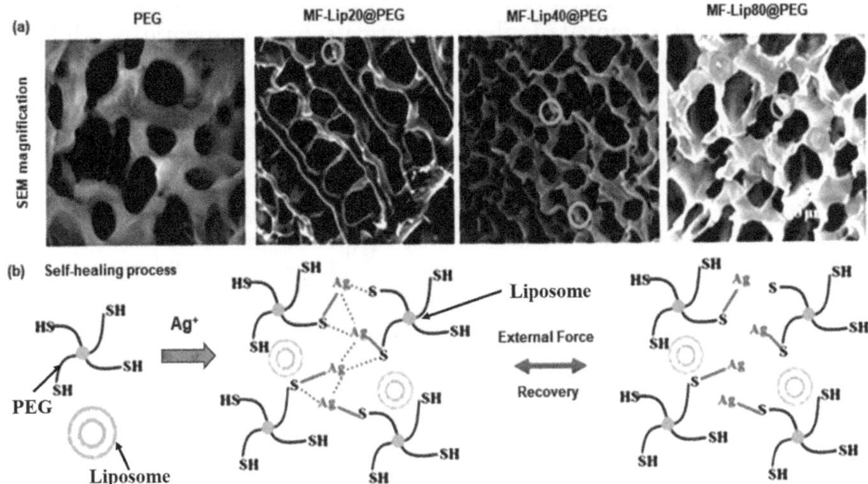

Figure 7.5 MF-Lip@PEG hydrogels: microscopic analysis and unique characteristics. (A) SEM pictures: yellow circles show liposomes. (a) Drug release kinetics in vitro: the self-healing process. The source of this figure is Mao et al. [75]. PEG is indicated by a green marked line connecting to a solid yellow circle, whereas a yellow bilayer circle represents a liposome. The study can be used, shared, adapted, distributed, and reproduced in any format as long as the original author(s) and source are properly credited, and a link to the Creative Commons license (http://creativecommons.org/licenses/by/4.0/, accessed on October 19, 2022) is provided. The study is licensed under the Creative Commons Attribution 4.0 International License. Mangiferin liposomes (MF-Lip) with polyethylene glycol (PEG).

features of hydrogel FHE@exo included injectability, stimuli-responsive exosome release, self-healing, and antibacterial activity. In HUVEC cells, this SHH that are bioactive markedly enhanced angiogenesis, proliferation, and migration. Furthermore, it accelerated the development of granulation tissue, reepithelialization, collagen remodeling, and neovascularization in a diabetic mouse model [76]. Chouhan et al. [77] used gellan gum and sodium chloride solution to create decorin-releasing SHH eye drops to treat retinal scarring. Decorin, a leucine-rich glycoprotein, is a molecule of anti-scarring that prevents TGF-β1 and TGF-β2 to reduce fibrotic damaging. Human corneal cells were not incompatible with the decorin-loaded SHH. Additionally, decorin was released at a progressive rate (45%) for three hours in an injury model of corneal of a rat ex vivo, which promoted reepithelialization [77].

7.3.3 Delivery of Drugs

Lipophilicity is an important factors influencing the cytotoxicity and cellular absorption of pharmaceuticals or therapeutic candidates. It has a connection to the pharmacokinetics of substances as well. Drug-like molecules must have the proper ratio of lipophilicity to hydrophobicity to be optimal [78]. Regarding drug delivery, SHH or polymers have several advantages over traditional hydrogels or polymers [79, 80]. SHH provides homogenous encapsulation of conjugated pharmaceuticals or therapeutic candidates, thereby mitigating side effects, enhancing potency and selectivity, and preventing drug diffusion. Most importantly, the continuous release effect ensures long-term therapeutic effectiveness, and the medicines' release can be regulated by external stimulation (Figure 7.6) [81–83].

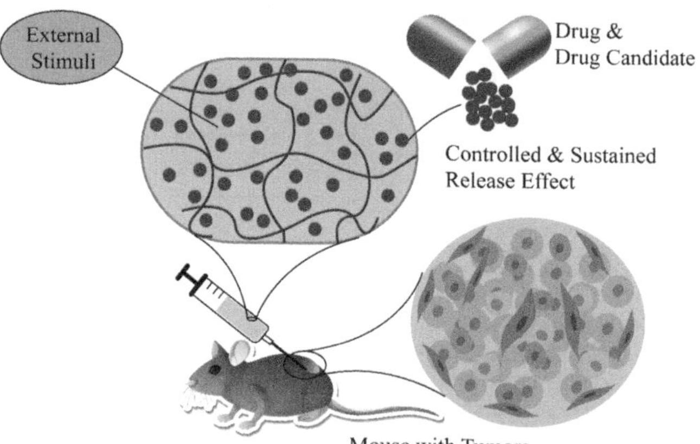

Figure 7.6 Delivering medicinal drugs through SHH. Therapeutic medicines are efficiently delivered to the target tissue by SHH. Furthermore, extrinsic stimuli (magnetic field, pressure, and temperature) can control the drug release. Hydrogels that self-heal.

A water-soluble anticancer medication licensed by the FDA, doxorubicin (DOX) is used to treat a variety of cancers, counting haematological, lung, breast and, thyroid malignancies [78, 84]. In order to transport DOX inside the hepatocellular cancer cells, i.e., HepG2, Using dibenzaldehyde-terminated poly(ethylene glycol) and N-carboxyethyl chitosan, Qu et al. [85] developed a polysaccharide-based SHH. Hydrogels with a vibrant covalent Schiff-base assembly established rapid self-healing capabilities deprived of an outside response [85]. Furthermore, in the in vitro system, the pH-controlled hydrogels showed gels which are pH-dependent that breakdown and releases DOX [85, 86]. The cytotoxicity assays validated the concentration and time-dependent cytotoxic effects of the DOX-loaded hydrogel toward HepG2 cells [87–89]. More significantly, in mouse L929, fibroblast cells, the hydrogel that are loaded with DOX exhibits outstanding biocompatibility and superior or similar cytotoxic efficacy to free DOX, suggesting the hydrogel's potential for use in cancer therapy [85, 90]. The promising results suggested that the SHH might be applied to stop tumor reappearance. Likewise, isoguanosine, borate, and guanosine were used to create supramolecular hydrogel (isoGBG), which demonstrated self-healing qualities, anticancer activity, and biocompatibility. Through apoptosis, hydrogel isoGBG reduced the cancer cells viability and inhibited tumor recurrence [91–94].

Biomolecules, Drug Candidates and Drugs can have their sustained release effect(s) enhanced through SHH [69, 95]. The hydrophilic and hydrophobic natures of beneficial drugs could be adjusted using SSH [96, 97]. As an illustration, the SHH made by HA, Fe3+, and EDTA (ethylene-diaminetetraacetic acid) showed outstanding antibiotic properties against organisms such as S. aureus and E. coli. Fe3+ complexation with EDTA and HA guaranteed Fe3+ release over time, showing antibacterial properties. More importantly, compared to the control, the Fe3+ trapped EDTA-HA-based hydrogel significantly accelerated the healing of female damages in C57BL/6 mice and demonstrated remarkable biocompatibility towards L-929 mouse fibroblast cells. In addition, hydrogel used topically for 10 days improved cutaneous regeneration, produced inflammation, and prevented S. aureus from growing (Figure 7.7) [98]. SHH could additionally be employed for monitoring the ejection of chemotherapy drugs. In the study by Pandit et al. [99], injectable SHH based on N, O-carboxymethyl chitosan with CGC (metaldehyde guar gum) demonstrated outstanding mechanical assets (having high modulus of approximately 1625 Pa) and biocompatibility against red blood cells (HEK-293) and human embryonic kidney. Astonishingly, its pH could be altered to manage the CGG hydrogels' ability to swell. Whenever the pH altered, the drug release kinetics of the DOX-loaded CGG hydrogel differed. For example, at functional pH which is at around 7.4, the hydrogel of CGG freed DOX 32.13% while 67.06% DOX at the tumoral microenvironment of the tumoral, i.e., pH of about 5.5. Furthermore, MCF-7 breast cancer cells demonstrated significant cytotoxicity (~72.13%) when subjected to DOX-CGG hydrogel [99].

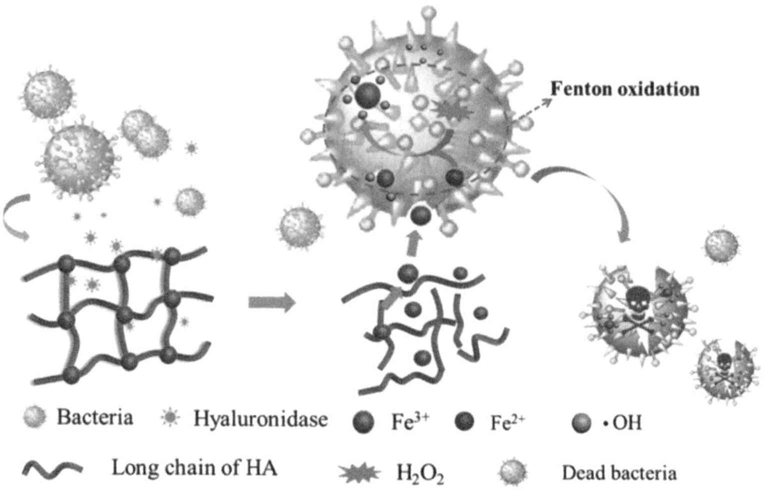

Figure 7.7 Properties of Fe3+- SHH loaded upon prolonged release. SHH: Bacteria rapidly adsorbed the Fe^{3+}-HA composite, altering Fe^{3+} to Fe^{2+} in this manner. Fe^{2+} and H_2O_2 recombine to create radicals with hydroxyl groups, i.e., ·OH, that damage the nuclear acids or bacterial proteins. Tian et al. [98] is from where the image is taken. The reading may be employed, shared, adapted, given away, and copied in any format as long as the original author(s) and source are correctly acknowledged and a link to the CCC (http://creativecommons.org/licenses/by/4.0/, accessed on September 26, 2022) is provided. The study has been licensed under the CCC 4.0 International License. SHH: Self-healing hydrogel; ·OH: Hydroxyl radical, HA: Hyaluronic acid.

7.4 CONCLUSION AND POSSIBILITIES FOR FUTURE GENERATIONS

Because SHH is biocompatible with natural tissues, they are presented as appealing drug delivery choices and tissue engineering choices. Achieving an appropriate mix of elastic and viscous features is unique to the main problem in SHH development. Recently, noteworthy advancements have been attained in refining the mechanical features and additional aspects of the SHH for multifaceted purposes in biomedical engineering, like prescribing medications and tissue engineering [100]. Still, numerous problems have been addressed to guarantee hydrogels' real-world approval for their intended biomedical purpose. Achieving an appropriate mix of viscous and elastic assets is one of the main encounters in SHH development. SHH's primary issue regarding hydrogels that are utilized for delivering drugs is their lipophilicity. A hydrophilic polymer with many gaps and hydrophilic domains is called hydrogel [101]. If there is hydrophobic, there may be limitations on the quantity and how consistently the drug can be incorporated into the gel matrix [102]. In addition, hydrophilic drugs might possess rapid-release kinetics because of their high water content and porous structure [103]. Patients might suffer serious side effects from that. SHH's stability in the real world is a further significant factor. Most SHH, particularly the physically crosslinked hydrogels, become unstable during the swelling phase and degrade quickly in water [104, 105]. Most naturally crosslinked SHH can't act out the self-healing system, even in a water medium [106]. Yet, a self-healing hydrogel is required to expand and retain water for longer to replace internal tissue or organs [107]. The chemically crosslinked hydrogels provide small self-healing percentage terms that are insufficient for biomedical technological use. They need actual time recovery, even if they are durable and persistent in water [108]. The exchange among physical durability, biocompatibility, and self-healing is a further obstacle that severely restricts biological uses for hydrogel. Covering the dynamic discharge profiles attained using hydrogels in the system of drug delivery continues to bring problems [102]. If the time required for release could be widened, this might be favorable, and the gels might serve the place of hydrophilic tiny particle systems in overdue release uses [109]. Since hydrogels possess a greater degree of biological compatibility, that could be beneficial. Hydrogels with various degradation rates and segments responsive to their surrounding environment might be capable of assisting with these kinetic difficulties [110, 111]. In addition, SHH needs a boost in mechanical characteristics [101]. The mechanically unstable gel could probably have adverse impacts on the human body. Gels that are self-healing and mechanically strong reduce the discomfort and suffering while maintaining the injury's state of being and increasing the lifespan of the covering substance [112]. For utilizing in biomedical fields like systems for tissue engineering and drug delivery& healing wounds, the mechanical characteristics of the SHH must be modified. Lastly, it is essential to consider the medicinal possibilities, overtime security, and possible SSH risks before starting future clinical trials(s).

REFERENCES

1. Wang, H.; Heilshorn, S.C. Adaptable hydrogel networks with reversible linkages for tissue engineering. *Adv. Mater.* 2015, 27(25), 3717–3736.
2. White, S.R.; Sottos, N.R.; Geubelle, P.H.; Moore, J.S.; Kessler, M.R.; Sriram, S.R.; Brown, E.N.; Viswanathan, S. Autonomic healing of polymer composites. *Nature.* 2001, 409(6822), 794–797.
3. Toohey, K.S.; Sottos, N.R.; Lewis, J.A.; Moore, J.S.; White, S.R. Self-healing materials with microvascular networks. *Nat. Mater.* 2007, 6(8), 581–585.
4. Bergman, S.D.; Wudl, F. Mendable polymers. *J. Mater. Chem.* 2008, 18(1), 41–62.
5. Syrett, J.A.; Becer, C.R.; Haddleton, D.M. Self-healing and self-mendable polymers. *Polym. Chem.* 2010, 1(7), 978–987.
6. Murphy, E.B., Wudl, F. The world of smart healable materials. *Prog. Polym. Sci.* 2010, 35(1–2), 223–251.
7. Harada, A.; Takashima, Y.; Nakahata, M. Supramolecular polymeric materials via cyclodextrin–guest interactions. *Acc. Chem. Res.* 2014, 47(7), 2128–2140.

8. Zou, W.; Dong, J.; Luo, Y.; Zhao, Q.; Xie, T. Dynamic covalent polymer networks: From old chemistry to modern day innovations. *Adv. Mater.* 2017, 29(14), 1606100.

9. Zhang, Q.; Niu, S.; Wang, L.; Lopez, J.; Chen, S.; Cai, Y.; Du, R.; Liu, Y.; Lai, J.-C.; Liu, L.; et al. An elastic autonomous self-healing capacitive sensor based on a dynamic dual crosslinked chemical system. *Adv. Mater.* 2018, 30, 1801435.

10. Imato, K.; Nishihara, M.; Kanehara, T.; Amamoto, Y.; Takahara, A.; Otsuka, H. Self-healing of chemical gels crosslinked by diarylbibenzofuranone-based trigger-free dynamic covalent bonds at room temperature. *Angew. Chem. Int. Ed.* 2012, 51, 1138–1142.

11. Deng, C.; Brooks, W.; Abboud, K.; Sumerlin, B. Boronic acid-based hydrogels undergo self-healing at neutral and acidic pH. *ACS Macro Lett.* 2015, 4, 220–224.

12. Pratama, P.A.; Sharifi, M.; Peterson, A.M.; Palmese, G.R. Room temperature self-healing thermoset based on the Diels-Alder reaction. *ACS Appl. Mater. Interfaces.* 2013, 5, 12425–12431.

13. Zhang, L.; Qiu, T.; Zhu, Z.; Guo, L.; Li, X. Self-healing polycaprolactone networks through thermo-induced reversible disulfide bond formation. *Macromol. Rapid Commun.* 2018, 39, e1800121.

14. Guadagno, L.; Vertuccio, L.; Naddeo, C.; Calabrese, E.; Barra, G.; Raimondo, M.; Sorrentino, A.; Binder, W.H.; Michael, P.; Rana, S. Self-healing epoxy nanocomposites via reversible hydrogen bonding. *Compos. Part B Eng.* 2019, 157, 1–13.

15. Andersen, A.; Krogsgaard, M.; Birkedal, H. Mussel-inspired self-healing double-cross-linked hydrogels by controlled combination of metal coordination and covalent crosslinking. *Biomacromolecules* 2018, 19, 1402–1409.

16. Wang, X.-H.; Song, F.; Xue, J.; Qian, D.; Wang, X.-L.; Wang, Y.-Z. Mechanically strong and tough hydrogels with excellent anti-fatigue, self-healing and reprocessing performance enabled by dynamic metal-coordination chemistry. *Polymer* 2018, 153, 637–642.

17. Miyamae, K.; Nakahata, M.; Takashima, Y.; Harada, A. Self-Healing, Expansion-contraction, and shape-memory properties of a preorganized supramolecular hydrogel through host-guest interactions. *Angew. Chem. Int. Ed. Engl.* 2015, 54, 8984–8987.

18. Takashima, Y.; Yonekura, K.; Koyanagi, K.; Iwaso, K.; Nakahata, M.; Yamaguchi, H.; Harada, A. Multifunctional stimuli-responsive supramolecular materials with stretching, coloring, and self-healing properties functionalized via host–guest interactions. *Macromolecules* 2017, 50, 11.

19. Xia, N.N.; Xiong, X.M.; Rong, M.Z.; Zhang, M.Q.; Kong, F. Self-healing of polymer in acidic water toward strength restoration through the synergistic effect of hydrophilic and hydrophobic interactions. *ACS Appl. Mater. Interfaces.* 2017, 9, 37300–37309.

20. Yan, B.; Huang, J.; Han, L.; Gong, L.; Li, L.; Israelachvili, J.N.; Zeng, H. Duplicating dynamic strain-stiffening behavior and nanomechanics of biological tissues in a synthetic self-healing flexible network hydrogel. *ACS Nano* 2017, 11, 11074–11081.

21. Wei, Z.; Yang, J.H.; Liu, Z.Q.; Xu, F.; Zhou, J.X.; Zrinyi, M.; Osada, Y.; Chen, Y.M. Novel biocompatible polysaccharide-based self-healing hydrogel. *Adv. Funct. Mater.* 2015, 25, 1352–1359.

22. Li, X.; Cui, K.; Sun, T.L.; Meng, L.; Gong, J.P. Mesoscale bicontinuous networks in self-healing hydrogels delay fatigue fracture. *Proc. Natl. Acad. Sci. USA* 2020, 117, 7606–7612.
23. Shao, C.; Wang, M.; Chang, H.; Xu, F.; Yang, J. A Self-Healing cellulose nanocrystal-poly(ethylene glycol) nanocomposite hydrogel via Diels–Alder click reaction. *ACS Sustain. Chem. Eng.* 2017, 5, 6167–6174.
24. Wei, Z.; Yang, J.H.; Du, X.J.; Xu, F.; Zrinyi, M.; Osada, Y.; Li, F.; Chen, Y.M. Dextran-based self-healing hydrogels formed by reversible diels-alder reaction under physiological conditions. *Macromol. Rapid. Commun.* 2013, 34, 1464–1470.
25. Mosaddegh, B.; Takalloo, Z.; Sajedi, R.H.; Shirin Shahangian, S.; Hassani, L.; Rasti, B. An inter-subunit disulfide bond of artemin acts as a redox switch for its chaperone-like activity. *Cell Stress Chaperon.* 2018, 23, 685–693.
26. Li, T.; Hu, J.; Tian, R.; Wang, K.; Li, J.; Qayum, A.; Bilawal, A.; Gantumur, M.A.; Jiang, Z.; Hou, J. Citric acid promotes disulfide bond formation of whey protein isolate in non-acidic aqueous system. *Food Chem.* 2021, 338, 127819.
27. Black, S.P.; Sanders, J.K.; Stefankiewicz, A.R. Disulfide exchange: Exposing supramolecular reactivity through dynamic covalent chemistry. *Chem. Soc. Rev.* 2014, 43, 1861–1872.
28. Steinman, N.Y.; Domb, A.J. Instantaneous degelling thermoresponsive hydrogel. *Gels* 2021, 7, 169.
29. Xu, K.; Yao, H.; Fan, D.; Zhou, L.; Wei, S. Hyaluronic acid thiol modified injectable hydrogel: Synthesis, characterization, drug release, cellular drug uptake and anticancer activity. *Carbohydr. Polym.* 2021, 254, 117286.
30. Barcan, G.A.; Zhang, X.; Waymouth, R.M. Structurally dynamic hydrogels derived from 1,2-dithiolanes. *J. Am. Chem. Soc.* 2015, 137, 5650–5653.
31. Deng, G.; Li, F.; Yu, H.; Liu, F.; Liu, C.; Sun, W.; Jiang, H.; Chen, Y. Dynamic hydrogels with an environmental adaptive self-healing ability and dual responsive Sol-Gel transitions. *ACS Macro Lett.* 2012, 1, 275–279.
32. Wu, H.-D.; Yang, J.-C.; Tsai, T.; Ji, D.-Y.; Chang, W.-J.; Chen, C.-C.; Lee, S.-Y. Development of a chitosan–polyglutamate based injectable polyelectrolyte complex scaffold. *Carbohydr. Polym.* 2011, 85, 318–324.
33. Sun, T.L.; Kurokawa, T.; Kuroda, S.; Ihsan, A.B.; Akasaki, T.; Sato, K.; Haque, M.A.; Nakajima, T.; Gong, J.P. Physical hydrogels composed of polyampholytes demonstrate high toughness and viscoelasticity. *Nat. Mater.* 2013, 12, 932–937.
34. Lu, J.; Gu, J.; Hu, O.; Fu, Y.; Ye, D.; Zhang, X.; Zheng, Y.; Hou, L.; Liu, H.; Jiang, X. Highly tough, freezing-tolerant, healable and thermoplastic starch/poly(vinyl alcohol) organohydrogels for flexible electronic devices. *J. Mater. Chem. A* 2021, 9, 18406–18420.
35. Sijbesma, R.P. Reversible polymers formed from self-complementary monomers using quadruple hydrogen bonding. *Science* 1998, 29, 1601–1604.
36. Ma, C.; Pang, H.; Liu, H.; Yan, Q.; Zhang, S. A tough, adhesive, self-healable, and antibacterial plant-inspired hydrogel based on pyrogallol–borax dynamic cross-linking. *J. Mater. Chem. B* 2021, 9, 4230–4240.
37. Caprioli, M.; Roppolo, I.; Chiappone, A.; Larush, L.; Magdassi, S. 3D-printed self-healing hydrogels via Digital Light Processing. *Nat. Commun.* 2021, 12, 1234567890.

38. Wang, Z.; Zhang, Y.; Yin, Y.; Liu, J.; Li, P.; Zhao, Y.; Bai, D.; Zhao, H.; Han, X.; Chen, Q. High-strength and injectable supramolecular hydrogel self-assembled by monomeric nucleoside for tooth-extraction wound healing. *Adv. Mater.* 2022, 34, e2108300.

39. Appel, E.A.; Tibbitt, M.W.; Webber, M.J.; Mattix, B.A.; Veiseh, O.; Langer, R. Self-assembled hydrogels utilizing polymer-nanoparticle interactions. *Nat. Commun.* 2015, 6, 6295.

40. Tuncaboylu, D.C.; Sari, M.; Oppermann, W.; Okay, O. Tough and self-healing hydrogels formed via hydrophobic interactions. *Macromolecules* 2011, 44, 4997–5005.

41. Chang, X.; Geng, Y.; Cao, H.; Zhou, J.; Tian, Y.; Shan, G.; Bao, Y.; Wu, Z.L.; Pan, P. Dual-crosslink physical hydrogels with high toughness based on synergistic hydrogen bonding and hydrophobic interactions. *Macromol. Rapid Commun.* 2018, 39, e1700806.

42. Tuncaboylu, D.C.; Argun, A.; Sahin, M.; Sari, M.; Okay, O. Structure optimization of self-healing hydrogels formed via hydrophobic interactions. *Polymer* 2012, 53, 5513–5522.

43. Gulyuz, U.; Okay, O. Self-healing poly(acrylic acid) hydrogels: Effect of surfactant. *Macromol. Symp.* 2015, 358, 232–238.

44. Liu, L.; Xiang, Y.; Wang, Z.; Yang, X.; Yu, X.; Lu, Y.; Deng, L.; Cui, W. Adhesive liposomes loaded onto an injectable, self-healing and antibacterial hydrogel for promoting bone reconstruction. *NPG Asia Mater.* 2019, 11, 81.

45. Harrington, M.J.; Masic, A.; Holten-Andersen, N.; Waite, J.H.; Fratzl, P. Iron-clad fibers: A metal-based biological strategy for hard flexible coatings. *Science* 2010, 328, 216–220.

46. Shafiq, Z.; Cui, J.; Pastor-Pérez, L.; San Miguel, V.; Gropeanu, R.A.; Serrano, C.; del Campo, A. Bioinspired underwater bonding and debonding on demand. *Angew. Chem. Int. Ed.* 2012, 51, 4332–4335.

47. Liang, Y.; Li, Z.; Huang, Y.; Yu, R.; Guo, B. Dual-dynamic-bond cross-linked antibacterial adhesive hydrogel sealants with on-demand removability for post-wound-closure and infected wound healing. *ACS Nano* 2021, 15, 7078–7093.

48. Shi, Y.; Wang, M.; Ma, C.; Wang, Y.; Li, X.; Yu, G. A conductive self-healing hybrid gel enabled by metal-ligand supramolecule and nanostructured conductive polymer. *Nano Lett.* 2015, 15, 6276–6281.

49. Shi, L.; Zhao, Y.; Xie, Q.; Fan, C.; Hilborn, J.; Dai, J.; Ossipov, D.A. Moldable hyaluronan hydrogel enabled by dynamic metal–bisphosphonate coordination chemistry for wound healing. *Adv. Healthc. Mater.* 2018, 7, 1700973.

50. Zhang, K.; Yuan, W.; Wei, K.; Yang, B.; Chen, X.; Li, Z.; Zhang, Z.; Bian, L. Highly dynamic nanocomposite hydrogels self-assembled by metal ion-ligand coordination. *Small* 2019, 15, 1900242.

51. Kapoor, S.; Kundu, S.C. Silk protein-based hydrogels: Promising advanced materials for biomedical applications. *Acta Biomater.* 2016, 31, 17–32.

52. Roy, C.K.; Guo, H.L.; Sun, T.L.; Ihsan, A.B.; Kurokawa, T.; Takahata, M.; Nonoyama, T.; Nakajima, T.; Gong, J.P. Self-adjustable adhesion of polyampholyte hydrogels. *Adv. Mater.* 2015, 27, 7344–7348.

53. Sujan, M.I.; Sarkar, S.D.; Sultana, S.; Bushra, L.; Tareq, R.; Roy, C.K.; Azam, M.S. Bi-functional silica nanoparticles for simultaneous enhancement of mechanical strength and swelling capacity of hydrogels. *RSC Adv.* 2020, 10, 6213–6222.

54. Zhang, A.; Liu, Y.; Qin, D.; Sun, M.; Wang, T.; Chen, X. Research status of self-healing hydrogel for wound management: A review. *Int. J. Biol. Macromol.* 2020, 164, 2108–2123.

55. Fu, F.; Chen, Z.; Zhao, Z.; Wang, H.; Shang, L.; Gu, Z.; Zhao, Y. Bio-inspired self-healing structural color hydrogel. *Proc. Natl. Acad. Sci. USA* 2017, 114, 5900–5905.

56. Stammen, J.A.; Williams, S.; Ku, D.N.; Guldberg, R.E. Mechanical properties of a novel PVA hydrogel in shear and unconfined compression. *Biomaterials* 2001, 22, 799–806.

57. Zheng, H.; Zuo, B. Functional silk fibroin hydrogels: Preparation, properties and applications. *J. Mater. Chem. B* 2021, 9, 1238–1258.

58. Talebian, S.; Mehrali, M.; Taebnia, N.; Pennisi, C.P.; Kadumudi, F.B.; Foroughi, J.; Hasany, M.; Nikkhah, M.; Akbari, M.; Orive, G. Self-healing hydrogels: The next paradigm shift in tissue engineering? *Adv. Sci.* 2019, 6, 1801664.

59. Ou, Y.; Tian, M. Advances in multifunctional chitosan-based self-healing hydrogels for biomedical application. *J. Mater. Chem. B* 2021, 9, 7955–7971.

60. Agrawal, D.K.; Siddique, A. Rejuvenation of "broken heart" with bioengineered gel. *J. Thorac. Cardiovasc. Surg.* 2018, 157, 1491–1493.

61. Loebel, C.; Rodell, C.B.; Chen, M.H.; Burdick, J.A. Shear-thinning and self-healing hydrogels as injectable therapeutics and for 3D-printing. *Nat. Protoc.* 2017, 12, 1521–1541.

62. Loebel, C.; D'Este, M.; Alini, M.; Zenobi-Wong, M.; Eglin, D. Precise tailoring of tyramine-based hyaluronan hydrogel properties using DMTMM conjugation. *Carbohydr. Polym.* 2015, 115, 325–333.

63. Yang, B.; Wei, K.; Loebel, C.; Zhang, K.; Feng, Q.; Li, R.; Wong, S.H.D.; Xu, X.; Lau, C.; Chen, X. Enhanced mechanosensing of cells in synthetic 3D matrix with controlled biophysical dynamics. *Nat. Commun.* 2021, 12, 3514.

64. Dankers, P.Y.W.; Hermans, T.M.; Baughman, T.W.; Kamikawa, Y.; Kieltyka, R.E.; Bastings, M.M.C.; Janssen, H.M.; Sommerdijk, N.A.J.M.; Larsen, A.; Van Luyn, M.J.A. Hierarchical formation of supramolecular transient networks in water: A modular injectable delivery system. *Adv. Mater.* 2012, 24, 2703–2709.

65. Schotman, M.J.G.; Dankers, P.Y.W. Factors influencing retention of injected biomaterials to treat myocardial infarction. *Adv. Mater. Interfaces.* 2022, 9, 2100942.

66. Bastings, M.M.C.; Koudstaal, S.; Kieltyka, R.E.; Nakano, Y.; Pape, A.C.H.; Feyen, D.A.M.; Van Slochteren, F.J.; Doevendans, P.A.; Sluijter, J.P.G.; Meijer, E.W. A fast pH-switchable and self-healing supramolecular hydrogel carrier for guided, local catheter injection in the infarcted myocardium. *Adv. Healthc. Mater.* 2014, 3, 70–78.

67. Koudstaal, S.; Bastings, M.; Feyen, D.A.M.; Waring, C.D.; Van Slochteren, F.J.; Dankers, P.Y.W.; Torella, D.; Sluijter, J.P.G.; Nadal-Ginard, B.; Doevendans, P.A. Sustained delivery of insulin-like growth factor-1/hepatocyte growth factor stimulates endogenous cardiac repair in the chronic infarcted pig heart. *J. Cardiovasc. Transl. Res.* 2014, 7, 232–241.

68. Tseng, T.C.; Tao, L.; Hsieh, F.Y.; Wei, Y.; Chiu, I.M.; Hsu, S.h. An injectable, self-healing hydrogel to repair the central nervous system. *Adv. Mater.* 2015, 27, 3518–3524.

69. Liu, Y.; Hsu, S.-h. Synthesis and biomedical applications of self-healing hydrogels. *Front. Chem.* 2018, 6, 449.

70. Tottoli, E.M.; Dorati, R.; Genta, I.; Chiesa, E.; Pisani, S.; Conti, B. Skin wound healing process and new emerging technologies for skin wound care and regeneration. *Pharmaceutics* 2020, 12, 735.

71. Hasan, M.M.; Uddin, M.F.; Zabin, N.; Shakil, M.S.; Alam, M.; Achal, F.J.; Ara Begum, M.H.; Hossen, M.S.; Hasan, M.A.; Morshed, M.M. Fabrication and characterization of chitosan-polyethylene glycol (Ch-Peg) based hydrogels and evaluation of their potency in rat skin wound model. *Int. J. Biomater.* 2021, 2021, 4877344.

72. Tang, N.; Zheng, Y.; Cui, D.; Haick, H. Multifunctional dressing for wound diagnosis and rehabilitation. *Adv. Healthc. Mater.* 2021, 10, e2101292.

73. Shawan, M.; Islam, N.; Aziz, S.; Khatun, N.; Sarker, S.R.; Hossain, M.; Hossan, T.; Morshed, M.; Sarkar, M.; Shakil, M.S.J.M.A.S. Fabrication of xanthan gum: Gelatin (xnt: Gel) hybrid composite hydrogels for evaluating skin wound healing efficacy. *Mod. Appl. Sci.* 2019, 13, 101–111.

74. Guo, B.; Qu, J.; Zhao, X.; Zhang, M. Degradable conductive self-healing hydrogels based on dextran-graft-tetraaniline and N-carboxyethyl chitosan as injectable carriers for myoblast cell therapy and muscle regeneration. *Acta Biomater.* 2019, 84, 180–193.

75. Mao, X.; Cheng, R.; Zhang, H.; Bae, J.; Cheng, L.; Zhang, L.; Deng, L.; Cui, W.; Zhang, Y.; Santos, H.A.; et al. Self-healing and injectable hydrogel for matching skin flap regeneration. *Adv. Sci.* 2019, 6, 1801555.

76. Lin, C.; Gao, W.; Xu, H.; Lei, B.; Mao, C. Engineering bioactive self-healing antibacterial exosomes hydrogel for promoting chronic diabetic wound healing and complete skin regeneration. *Theranostics* 2019, 9, 65–76.

77. Chouhan, G.; Moakes, R.J.A.; Esmaeili, M.; Hill, L.J.; DeCogan, F.; Hardwicke, J.; Rauz, S.; Logan, A.; Grover, L.M. A self-healing hydrogel eye drop for the sustained delivery of decorin to prevent corneal scarring. *Biomaterials* 2019, 210, 41–50.

78. Shakil, M.S.; Mahmud, K.M.; Sayem, M.; Niloy, M.S.; Halder, S.K.; Hossen, M.S.; Uddin, M.F.; Hasan, M.A. Using chitosan or chitosan derivatives in cancer therapy. *Polysaccharides* 2021, 2, 795–816.

79. Wang, S.; Urban, M.W. Self-healing polymers. *Nat. Rev. Mater.* 2020, 5, 562–583.

80. Zhang, Z.; Zhang, R.; Chen, L.; Tong, Q.; McClements, D.J. Designing hydrogel particles for controlled or targeted release of lipophilic bioactive agents in the gastrointestinal tract. *Eur. Polym. J.* 2015, 72, 698–716.

81. Kajdič, S.; Planinšek, O.; Gašperlin, M.; Kocbek, P. Electrospun nanofibers for customized drug-delivery systems. *J. Drug Deliv. Sci. Technol.* 2019, 51, 672–681.

82. Singh, A.P.; Biswas, A.; Shukla, A.; Maiti, P. Targeted therapy in chronic diseases using nanomaterial-based drug delivery vehicles. *Signal Transduct. Target. Ther.* 2019, 4, 33.

83. Vaishya, R.; Khurana, V.; Patel, S.; Mitra, A.K. Long-term delivery of protein therapeutics. *Expert Opin. Drug Deliv.* 2015, 12, 415–440.

84. Tam, K. The roles of doxorubicin in hepatocellular carcinoma. *ADMET DMPK* 2013, 1, 29–44.

85. Qu, J.; Zhao, X.; Ma, P.X.; Guo, B. pH-responsive self-healing injectable hydrogel based on N-carboxyethyl chitosan for hepatocellular carcinoma therapy. *Acta Biomater.* 2017, 58, 168–180.

86. Jalalvandi, E.; Shavandi, A. In situ-forming and pH-responsive hydrogel based on chitosan for vaginal delivery of therapeutic agents. *J. Mater. Sci. Mater. Med.* 2018, 29, 158.

87. Malarvizhi, G.L.; Retnakumari, A.P.; Nair, S.; Koyakutty, M. Transferrin targeted core-shell nanomedicine for combinatorial delivery of doxorubicin and sorafenib against hepatocellular carcinoma. *Nanomed. Nanotechnol. Biol. Med.* 2014, 10, 1649–1659.

88. Qi, X.; Wei, W.; Li, J.; Liu, Y.; Hu, X.; Zhang, J.; Bi, L.; Dong, W. Fabrication and characterization of a novel anticancer drug delivery system: Salecan/poly (methacrylic acid) semi-interpenetrating polymer network hydrogel. *ACS Biomater. Sci. Eng.* 2015, 1, 1287–1299.

89. Gao, B.; Luo, J.; Liu, Y.; Su, S.; Fu, S.; Yang, X.; Li, B. Intratumoral administration of thermosensitive hydrogel co-loaded with norcantharidin nanoparticles and doxorubicin for the treatment of hepatocellular carcinoma. *Int. J. Nanomed.* 2021, 16, 4073.

90. Wang, S.; Zheng, H.; Zhou, L.; Cheng, F.; Liu, Z.; Zhang, H.; Zhang, Q. Injectable redox and light responsive MnO2 hybrid hydrogel for simultaneous melanoma therapy and multidrug-resistant bacteria-infected wound healing. *Biomaterials* 2020, 260, 120314.

91. Shakil, M.S.; Niloy, M.S.; Mahmud, K.M.; Kamal, M.A.; Islam, M.A. Theranostic potentials of gold nanomaterials in hematological malignancies. *Cancers* 2022, 14, 3047.

92. Woodward, W.A.; Strom, E.A.; Tucker, S.L.; Katz, A.; McNeese, M.D.; Perkins, G.H.; Buzdar, A.U.; Hortobagyi, G.N.; Hunt, K.K.; Sahin, A. Locoregional recurrence after doxorubicin-based chemotherapy and post-mastectomy: Implications for breast cancer patients with early-stage disease and predictors for recurrence after postmastectomy radiation. *Int. J. Radiat. Oncol. Biol. Phys.* 2003, 57, 336–344.

93. Morales-Vásquez, F.; Gonzalez-Angulo, A.M.; Broglio, K.; Lopez-Basave, H.N.; Gallardo, D.; Hortobagyi, G.N.; De La Garza, J.G. Adjuvant chemotherapy with doxorubicin and dacarbazine has no effect in recurrence-free survival of malignant phyllodes tumors of the breast. *Breast J.* 2007, 13, 551–556.

94. Li, Q.; Wen, J.; Liu, C.; Jia, Y.; Wu, Y.; Shan, Y.; Qian, Z.; Liao, J. Graphene-nanoparticle-based self-healing hydrogel in preventing postoperative recurrence of breast cancer. *ACS Biomater. Sci. Eng.* 2019, 5, 768–779.

95. An, H.; Yang, Y.; Zhou, Z.; Bo, Y.; Wang, Y.; He, Y.; Wang, D.; Qin, J. Pectin-based injectable and biodegradable self-healing hydrogels for enhanced synergistic anticancer therapy. *Acta Biomater.* 2021, 131, 149–161.

96. Qiao, Y.; Xu, S.; Zhu, T.; Tang, N.; Bai, X.; Zheng, C. Preparation of printable double-network hydrogels with rapid self-healing and high elasticity based on hyaluronic acid for controlled drug release. *Polymer* 2020, 186, 121994.

97. Pishavar, E.; Khosravi, F.; Naserifar, M.; Rezvani Ghomi, E.; Luo, H.; Zavan, B.; Seifalian, A.; Ramakrishna, S. Multifunctional and self-healable intelligent hydrogels for cancer drug delivery and promoting tissue regeneration in Vivo. *Polymers* 2021, 13, 2680.

98. Tian, R.; Qiu, X.; Yuan, P.; Lei, K.; Wang, L.; Bai, Y.; Liu, S.; Chen, X. Fabrication of self-healing hydrogels with on-demand antimicrobial activity and sustained biomolecule release for infected skin regeneration. *ACS Appl. Mater. Interfaces.* 2018, 10, 17018–17027.

99. Pandit, A.H.; Nisar, S.; Imtiyaz, K.; Nadeem, M.; Mazumdar, N.; Rizvi, M.M.A.; Ahmad, S. Injectable, Self-Healing, and biocompatible N,O-Carboxymethyl chitosan/multialdehyde guar gum hydrogels for sustained anticancer drug delivery. *Biomacromolecules* 2021, 22, 3731–3745.

100. Sarkar, S.D.; Uddin, M.M.; Roy, C.K.; Hossen, M.J.; Sujan, M.I.; Azam, M.S. Mechanically tough and highly stretchable poly (acrylic acid) hydrogel cross-linked by 2D graphene oxide. *RSC Adv.* 2020, 10, 10949–10958.

101. Rammal, H.; GhavamiNejad, A.; Erdem, A.; Mbeleck, R.; Nematollahi, M.; Diltemiz, S.E.; Alem, H.; Darabi, M.A.; Ertas, Y.N.; Caterson, E.J. Advances in biomedical applications of self-healing hydrogels. *Mater. Chem. Front.* 2021, 5, 4368–4400.

102. Hoare, T.R.; Kohane, D.S. Hydrogels in drug delivery: Progress and challenges. *Polymer* 2008, 49, 1993–2007.

103. Qiu, Y.; Park, K. Environment-sensitive hydrogels for drug delivery. *Adv. Drug Deliv. Rev.* 2001, 53, 321–339.

104. Madduma-Bandarage, U.S.K.; Madihally, S.V. Synthetic hydrogels: Synthesis, novel trends, and applications. *J. Appl. Polym. Sci.* 2021, 138, 50376.

105. Wang, Y.; Adokoh, C.K.; Narain, R. Recent development and biomedical applications of self-healing hydrogels. *Expert Opin. Drug Deliv.* 2018, 15, 77–91.

106. Gong, Z.; Zhang, G.; Zeng, X.; Li, J.; Li, G.; Huang, W.; Sun, R.; Wong, C. High-strength, tough, fatigue resistant, and self-healing hydrogel based on dual physically cross-linked network. *ACS Appl. Mater. Interfaces.* 2016, 8, 24030–24037.

107. Rumon, M.M.H.; Sarkar, S.D.; Uddin, M.M.; Alam, M.M.; Karobi, S.N.; Ayfar, A.; Azam, M.S.; Roy, C.K. Graphene oxide based crosslinker for simultaneous enhancement of mechanical toughness and self-healing capability of conventional hydrogels. *RSC Adv.* 2022, 12, 7453–7463.

108. Zhao, X.; Wu, H.; Guo, B.; Dong, R.; Qiu, Y.; Ma, P.X. Antibacterial antioxidant electroactive injectable hydrogel as self-healing wound dressing with hemostasis and adhesiveness for cutaneous wound healing. *Biomaterials* 2017, 122, 34–47.

109. Wang, S.; Liu, R.; Fu, Y.; Kao, W.J. Release mechanisms and applications of drug delivery systems for extended-release. *Expert Opin. Drug Deliv.* 2020, 17, 1289–1304.

110. Gil, E.S.; Hudson, S.M. Stimuli-reponsive polymers and their bioconjugates. *Prog. Polym. Sci.* 2004, 29, 1173–1222.

111. Blum, A.P.; Kammeyer, J.K.; Rush, A.M.; Callmann, C.E.; Hahn, M.E.; Gianneschi, N.C. Stimuli-responsive nanomaterials for biomedical applications. *J. Am. Chem. Soc.* 2015, 137, 2140–2154.

112. Han, Y.; Jiang, Y.; Hu, J. Collagen incorporation into waterborne polyurethane improves breathability, mechanical property, and self-healing ability. *Compos. Part A Appl. Sci. Manuf.* 2020, 133, 105854.

High-Energy Beam-Based Surface Texturing on Advanced Engineering Materials Used in Bioimplants

*D. Chinmoyee, T.N. Deepu Kumar,
R.R. Ravi, and D.S. Srinivasu*

8.1 INTRODUCTION

Surface modifications using top-down manufacturing approaches for securing specific functional properties in various industrial applications have been exploited abundantly since their inception. Among such modification techniques, a journey to improve patients' lives through surface texturing on bioimplants made of advanced engineering biocompatible materials (AEBMs) has become popular in the bioimplant field. Nowadays, genetic abnormalities, aging, or accidents have led to the impaired functionality of biological tissues in the human body. Towards this, biocompatible implant replacements have become a prevalent alternative to natural bone. Researchers estimated that over a quarter of all implants demonstrate that aseptic loosening is the primary cause of joint replacement failure, a critical issue in the bioimplant industry. Furthermore, loss of the bioimplants is associated with low osseointegration ability, i.e., the formation of bone at the implant surface affected by chemical and physical processes and mechanical aspects [1].

To overcome the challenges mentioned above, a proven surface texturing technology in other industrial applications, such as aerospace and automotive, has been considered a potential approach to improve the functional properties of AEBMs in the bioimplant field. Incorporating various micro-features (channels or porous structures) increases the contact area and mechanical interlocking, positively resulting in bone ingrowth [2]. On the other hand, the nanoscale texture features can further enhance these effects depending on specific turnover processes in bone biology [3]. Although surface texturing aids in enhancing the human life's quality by improving the functionality, biocompatibility, and longevity of tailor-made AEBMs, difficult-to-machine AEBMs (e.g., titanium alloys, 316LVM, Co-Cr-Mo, and cobalt-chromium alloys) is a challenging task with the existing conventional machining processes that demand advanced manufacturing technologies in bioimplant industry.

DOI: 10.1201/9781003470311-8

Towards this, unconventional technologies in bioimplant manufacturing are reported as an alternative. Among them, the electrochemical-, electric discharge-, and ultrasonic- machining process is suitable for fabricating various features simultaneously. However, they have limitations with target material properties. On the other hand, employing mechanical and thermal based high-energy beams (HEBs)- laser beam (LB), electron beam (EB), focused ion beam (FIB), abrasive air jet (AAJ), abrasive waterjet (AWJ), and abrasive suspension jet (ASJ) processes, enable multi-scaled texturing at high material removal rate (MRR) on AEBMs on a single manufacturing station with minimum adjustments by suitably manipulating the process conditions and systematically manoeuvring the HEBs on the target. Hence, this chapter reviews the potential of HEB-based surface texturing methods employed for AEBMs, their unique features, drawbacks, and future research trends to meet the industrial standards for various applications in bioimplant manufacturing. The commonly used AEBMs for manufacturing bioimplants having excellent biocompatibility and osseointegration with the human body are discussed in the following.

8.2 COMMONLY USED BIOCOMPATIBLE ADVANCED ENGINEERING MATERIALS

In recent decades, tailor-made bioimplants made of advanced engineered materials are increasing rapidly in the biomedical field. The increasing demand for human implants made of AEBMs has gained researchers' attention in materials and metallurgy. In the recent findings, researchers have identified several promising alternative advanced engineering materials for bone tissue that exhibit favorable biocompatibility. Acceptance of biomaterials for implant manufacturing must fulfill the following criteria: (i) biocompatibility, (ii) be non-toxic to the human body, preventing the occurrence of inflammatory or allergic reactions, and (iii) improved mechanical properties. The commonly employed metallic-based advanced engineering biomaterials used for various applications that meet the earlier-mentioned requirements are presented in Table 8.1.

Bioimplants made of AEBMs involve continuous mechanical motion during their functionality in the human body and generally have higher failure rates due to different wear mechanisms. Towards this, manufacturers in the biomedical field are putting constant effort into improving patient comfort and implant performance through various surface modification techniques. The basic texture shapes and patterns employed for enhancing the bioimplant performance are discussed in the following.

Table 8.1   Commonly employed biocompatible materials and their applications

AEBMs	Applications	Remarks
Stainless steel (316 series)	Total Hip Arthroplasty, screws, bone plates, pins, and steel threads in fixation of fractures	Low fabrication cost, low fracture strength, biocompatibility, high Young's modulus; however, low fatigue strength, low poor corrosion, and wear resistance
Cobalt alloys (Co-Cr-Mo, Co-Ni-Cr-Mo)	Prostheses for knee, shoulder, ankle, hip, in femoral stem	Favorable strength, corrosion, and wear characteristics, Young's modulus greater than titanium alloys, and high-stress shielding
Titanium alloys (Ti-6Al-4V, Ti–13Nb–13Zr, Ti-6Al-7Nb)	Stem and acetabular cement- less components of Total Hip Arthroplasty, total knee replacement, bone plates, screws	Highly biocompatible, excellent corrosion resistance, high strength-to-weight ratio, and high osseointegration; however, poor wear resistance, low Young's modulus, and expensive
Magnesium alloys (AZ91, ZE41)	Cardiovascular stents and bone repair, mesh cage for segmental defect in long bone	Enables optimal healing by gradually being absorbed into the human body as surrounding tissue replaces the implant, biodegradable, no-stress shielding

8.3 BASIC SHAPES OF TEXTURED FEATURES AND PATTERNS

Creating surfaces that lessen biofouling is highly desirable for biomedical applications since the term "biofouling" may threaten public health by resulting in medical device malfunctions, infections, and diseases. Towards this, creating various patterns or mimicking the characteristics of surfaces seen in nature may enable the creation of surfaces that improve the control over the adhesion of bacteria. According to the literature, orthopedic biomaterials with textured surfaces (Figure 8.1) provide better lubrication, which lowers wear and friction in prosthetic hip implants. To this end, Sawano *et al.* [4] examined the tribological performance of surface texture with circular patterns at a depth of 1 µm and discovered that the wear reduction of these patterns was 57.1% compared to polished samples. Studies are being conducted on different pattern shapes besides circular dimple patterns. Furthermore, a study on the tribological performance of the surface texture with micro-grooves with 40 µm width, 375 µm pitch, and various shapes is conducted, yielding a favorable result of 38% lower coefficient of friction [5]. Crosshatched texturing on a surface has been shown to enhance the tribological performance of metal-on-polymer bio-implants in another work [6]. Zhang *et al.* [7] examined a petaloid-like pattern's frictional performance and found it performed better during the

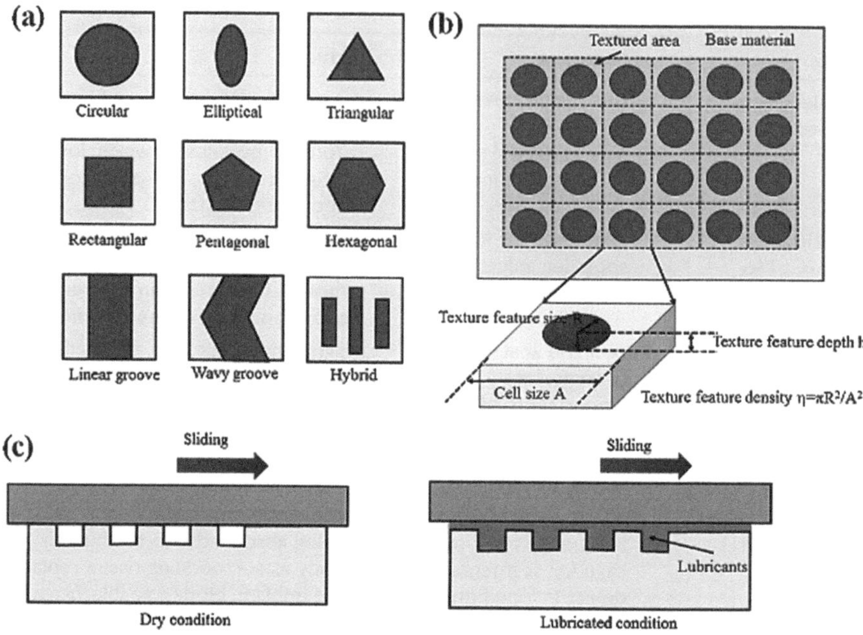

Figure 8.1 Schematic of (a) basic texture shapes, (b) texture features and their parameters, and (c) effect of textured design on tribological performance. (From Mao *et al.* [8], Copyright 2023 with permission from Elsevier.)

first running stage. Furthermore, the structures (pillars, ripples, spikes, and laser-induced periodic surface structures (LIPSS)) at various sizes, from macro- to nanoscale dimensions, are used to study and regulate the antibacterial behavior, cell adhesion, and implant proliferation.

For generating those textures on AEBMs, potential HEB-based methods with their unique features, drawbacks, and future research trends to meet the industrial standards for various applications in bioimplant manufacturing are discussed in detail in the following.

8.4 CLASSIFICATION OF HIGH-ENERGY BEAMS

In this section, high-energy beam processes are classified according to the energy type employed for machining (Figure 8.2) and their use in surface texturing on difficult-to-machine AEBMs in biomedical applications. Section 8.4.1 presents the thermal-based energy beam processes, pulsed LB, FIB, and EB. Following this, Section 8.4.2 discusses the mechanical-based energy beam processes, such as AAJs, AWJs, and ASJs, in detail.

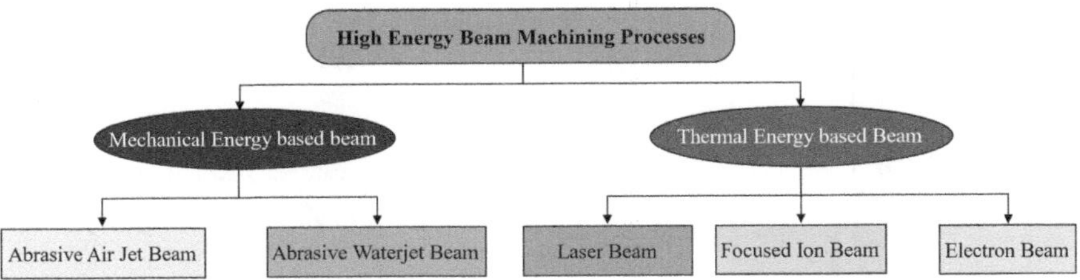

Figure 8.2 Classification of high-energy beam-based machining processes.

8.4.1 Thermal Energy-Based Beam

Thermal-based high-energy beam machining processes represent a cutting-edge realm of advanced manufacturing techniques, harnessing the power of intense thermal energy to shape and manipulate materials at the micro and nanoscale levels. The thermal machining processes of material removal employ a heat source to remove material from the workpiece surface. The different thermal processes use a wide range of heat sources. The heat sources can be categorized into four basic types: thermal sources, radiation, and electric arcs. The heat source used for surface texturing determines how the energy is transferred between the workpiece and the source. Sections 8.4.1.1 to 8.4.1.3 discuss the different thermal processes: laser beam machining, focussed ion beam machining, and electron beam machining for surface texturing applications.

8.4.1.1 Laser Surface Texturing

Employing laser surface texturing (LST) has proven to be a prominent and widespread strategy for surface modification aimed at enhancing the lubrication, controlling friction, and wear resistance of engineered materials. In 1967, the first operational laser treatments were documented in the literature for dental components and teeth structure in vitro and in vivo to stop the gradual rise in temperature in other areas. The LST process involves creating micro or nano-features, such as tiny dimples or constructed geometry, that are exclusively applied to a portion of the material's surface and are often distributed in a specific pattern. Laser ablation, or LST, removes material by heating and melting the target material with an irradiation laser pulse, which produces nanoparticles. LST has drawn much interest because of its unique advantages over other texturing techniques, such as being more rapid, efficient, ecologically friendly, and controllable. The three mechanical LST taxonomies that are most frequently employed are nanosecond (ns), picosecond (ps), and femtosecond (fs) (Figure 8.3). These taxonomies provide improved reliability, precision, and intricacy over texturing patterns. Recent advancements in LST have led to the classification of surface texturing procedures

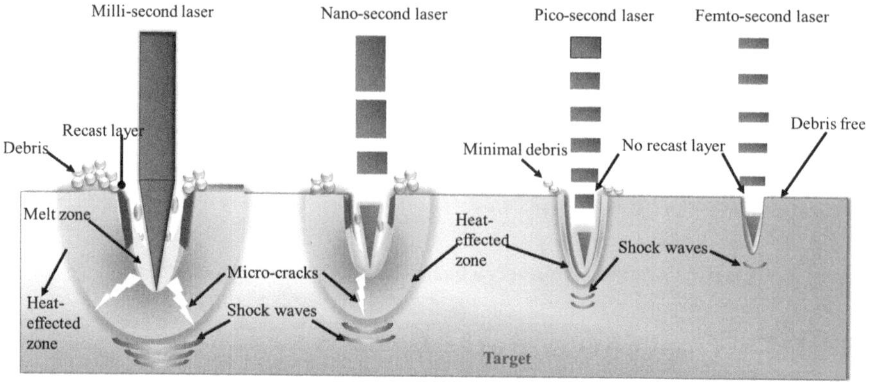

Figure 8.3 Material removal with different laser beam-based ablation.

can be classified into three categories depending on the pulse duration. First, ns laser texturing produces longer-lasting pulses than any other method, interacting with the substrate's lattice, heating the target material, melting the intended surface, and finally evaporating. Secondly, producing accurate micro-texturing and micromachining is well suited to picosecond lasers of short pulse duration. Thirdly, the ultra-short pulses emitted by the fs laser are ideal for creating high-precision texturing with almost minimal burr formation. With significantly better-defined features, the femtosecond laser source has nearly no topside burr. It may also generate picosecond laser beams with appropriate parameter selection, such as laser power, beam intensity, and frequency. Selecting a laser type requires careful consideration of the surface morphological behavior, pattern size, textural depth modification, precision level, pulse repetition rate, and laser fluence during the LST process to achieve the desired tribological performance of the processed material.

Furthermore, a proper selection of appropriate parametric levels and the best possible design of the LST pattern depend on a knowledge of the impact of the parameters as mentioned above. Among the various uses for laser surface texturing, the biomedical industry is seeing a rise in its application as micromanipulation of materials aids in bone replacement, the repair of synovial joints such as the hip, knee, and shoulder, and dental implants. The research began in the late 1990s, and since 2011, significant advancements have been made. To address this, the sections from 8.4.1.1.1 to 8.4.1.1.4 summarise the most current developments in the various laser texturing techniques used in bioimplant applications.

8.4.1.1.1 Millisecond Surface Texturing

The conceptualization of lasers initially emerged in the 1950s, and Theodore Maiman showed the ruby laser, the world's first operational laser, in 1960.

These early lasers' pulses usually lasted a thousandth of a second and were measured in milliseconds. These lasers are appropriate for macroscopic applications requiring controlled exposure periods [9]. The ms laser's energy cumulative impact is apparent, and this causes the material's surface to take on novel morphologies [10]. The pulse duration of a millisecond laser is approximately 10^{-3} seconds (1 millisecond). As a result, the millisecond laser pulses have enough time to re-deposit the molten material rim around the textured features with a lot of spatter, melting a sizable portion of the surface material [11]. According to the research findings, titanium samples can acquire a texture similar to shark skin if pulses overlap during the laser processing. This is because distinct textures are produced with varied laser processing parameters [12]. A review of the tribological properties of the textures that emerged from the literature revealed that the average value associated with the friction coefficient decreased dramatically during the millisecond laser processing [13]. Nevertheless, adding millisecond laser processing results in a significant amount of heat input on the workpiece, eventually creating many cracks in the target areas.

Moreover, its primary disadvantage is that the highest thermal stresses must be appropriately cleaned afterward. Spranger *et al.* have demonstrated that hardness of less than 900 HV of bioimplants can be obtained at the focal spot since a pulsed millisecond laser can cause dispersal and partial dissolution of the initial particles that happens depending on the laser's intensity. Particle impact on melt dispersion results in significantly different weld pool profiles in the implanted regions compared to the laser-remelted areas. As a result, the implant's morphology changes from dome-shaped to ring-shaped [14].

8.4.1.1.2 Nanosecond Surface Texturing

A low-intensity, prolonged pulse from a ns laser source comes into contact with the target's material structure when it is subjected to radiation. When exposed to nanosecond laser pulses, the thermal wave has adequate time to penetrate the metallic substrate and create a comparatively larger molten layer. Due to vaporization, a rebound pressure is created in this case, which ejects the substrate material as liquid and vapours. Creating superhydrophobic surfaces with nanosecond lasers has drawn attention as a new study area for functional surface analysis. On an aluminium substrate, Jagdheesh et al. [15] created micro- and nano features to produce superhydrophobic surfaces that were modelled after natural surfaces (Figure 8.4). In contrast to traditional chemical procedures, the creation of micro-holes and walls using ns laser processing is found to be a significant factor in the fabrication of superhydrophobic surfaces throughout his research. Nanostructuring is developed on metal alloys utilizing a two-stage process that includes chemical immersion treatment and nanosecond laser texturing. As a result, observed an exceptional wettability. An investigation

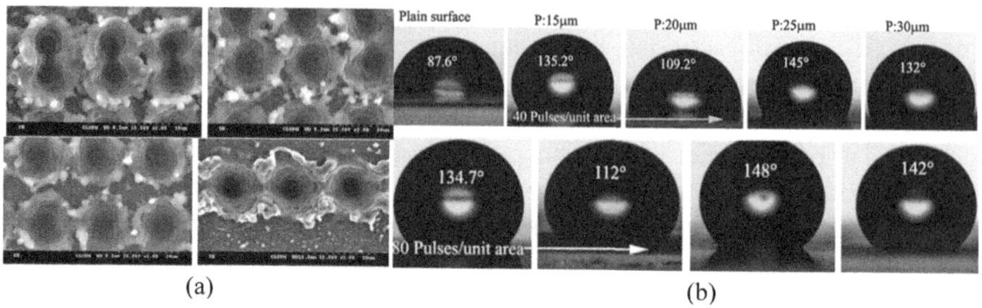

Figure 8.4 Surface texturing by nanosecond laser processing: (a) microholes fabricated at different pitches, and (b) Contact angle measured and compared with the plain surface. (From Jagdheesh *et al.* [15], Copyright 2023 with permission from Elsevier.)

by Zhao *et al.* [16] examines two distinct designs to create a non-wetting surface: a single horizontal pattern measuring 20 μm in width and 20 μm grid size on the target material. The specimens were found to be hydrophilic at the time of texturing; nevertheless, it is interesting to observe that the textured pattern became hydrophobic following a 20-day exposure to the surrounding environment.

Furthermore, developing a stochastic pattern by nanosecond laser treatment is a more effective way to improve the adhesive resiliency and coated layer than the conventional sandblasting approach to surface roughening. Moreover, a surface wettability transition from hydrophilic to superhydrophobic is achieved in a nanosecond pulsed laser on the Ti-6Al-4V surface. Several bacterial cells are dispersed across the superhydrophobic surface [17]. Conversely, a nanosecond pulsed laser is focused through a cylindrical lens onto type 316 L SS, commonly used as a biomaterial, to create micro-groove patterns through broad-area surface texturing. This texturing resulted in a considerable improvement in the sample's anti-corrosion performance and a noticeable decrease in pitting corrosion. Although surface modification with ns lasers has been the subject of numerous articles, one of the most prevalent challenges with this technique is that, in the case of square textural modification, the texture pattern becomes an oval shape, and in other textured patterns, it is barely destroyed when a material melts or evaporates from the targeted surface. Furthermore, the surface ablation caused by the ns laser treatment causes the material's top layer to grow large holes and cracks. Nevertheless, limited processing efficiency and expensive equipment maintenance costs are drawbacks of using a nanosecond laser [18].

8.4.1.1.3 Picosecond Surface Texturing

An optical pulse with a duration of around 10 ps, or slightly more than one trillionth (10-12) of a second, is emitted by a picosecond laser. During laser surface texturing, the free electrons interact with the laser pulses before they are irradiated on the substrate surface. Following electron excitation, heat energy is transferred to the lattice of the intended substrate through heat conduction, causing the material to melt and be removed when the matrix temperature reaches the critical temperature of the target surface. The ps laser has a high peak power of 1-100 kW and an incredibly short pulse duration of 10-12s. Its advantages include great precision, no chemical contamination of the surface, practically negligible heat-affected zone, and lack of cracks. LIPSS is consistently highlighted during ablation, and the structures generated on various materials by laser irradiation can typically be either nanoscale or microscale in size.

Furthermore, samples are exposed to a picosecond laser to determine the optimum process conditions for controlled grooves, structured textures, and enhanced osteoblast adhesion and proliferation (Figure 8.5). According to the study, the surfaces of the chromium-Ti nitride (CrTiN) thin films developed periodic corrugated nanopod shapes as a result of ultrafast laser processing with a picosecond pulsed laser. This finding suggests that cells can quickly increase on these kinds of surfaces. This technique can improve cell activation and proliferation by inducing the creation of periodic corrugated nanopod structures on the surfaces of these films [19]. Analysis of surface characteristics revealed that, as opposed to composition, LST altered the material's morphology. In addition, the material's hydrophobicity is enhanced by the laser-textured groove array, and the wetting behavior showed a notable directivity since the groove

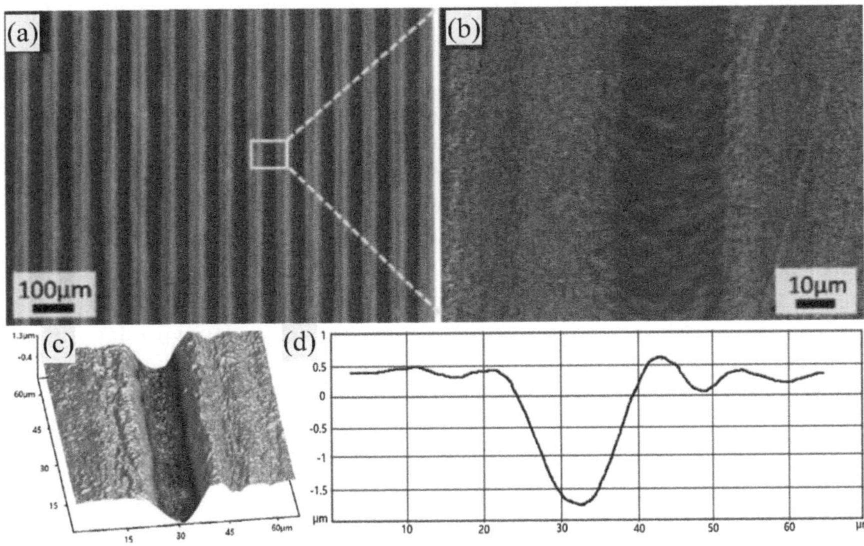

Figure 8.5 Surface texturing by picosecond laser processing on titanium alloy: (a) grooved pattern, (b) enlarged view, (c) 3D surface topography, and (d) 2D profile of groove. (From Yu *et al.* [21], Copyright 2023 with permission from Elsevier.)

array is anisotropic. Furthermore, Schultz et al. [20] evaluated the texturing taxonomy of ps and ns pulses according to three criteria: (1) suitable processing windows, (2) pulses for total material removal, and (3) associated ablation treatments. Debris generated during the picosecond laser treatment process is significantly smaller.

8.4.1.1.4 Femtosecond Surface Texturing

Femtosecond laser ablates materials using high-intensity ultrashort pulses lasting less than one picosecond, which allows for the machining of high-precision features at the micro and nanoscales in a highly controlled and localized way. Similar to other laser texturing technologies, femtosecond laser technology has certain advantages. These include the ability to texturize non-planar surfaces, texture nearly any material, and texturize materials quickly in one step while maintaining normal ambient conditions- all without the need for masks. Ultra-short pulse durations are produced by fs laser texturing, which is most suitable for high-precision texturing and machining with nearly no burr development. This method can improve tissue contact, cellular adherence, and biocompatibility with medical implants and equipment. Femtosecond laser surface texturing can significantly enhance the surface properties of biomaterials by forming complex micro and nanostructures, which can improve wear resistance, decrease bacterial adherence, and boost biological responses. According to the study, the incorporation of fs laser micromachining improved the quality of the soft-tissue integration around implants by creating micropores on the surfaces of Ti alloy (Ti6Al4V, Ti64) that are vertically aligned. This investigation has used optimized settings of 2×104 pulses per spot, 100 kHz, and 220 fs laser pulse duration to create highly accurate micropore texturing on Ti64 substrates. The research findings showed that on the Ti64 surfaces, the fs micromachining approach yields unique topological features of highly systematic vertically aligned micropores (7 and 15 µm) [22].

Moreover, using a femtosecond laser, Lutey *et al.* [23] have created laser-textured antibacterial surfaces on 316L stainless steel (Figure 8.6). On the surface of the stainless steel, many surface structures, such as spikes, nano-pillars, and LIPSS, are generated with a wavelength of 1030 nm lasting 250 fs, and with varying laser energies of 1.01 µJ, 19.1 µJ, and 1.46 µJ, respectively. After 30 days in the atmosphere, the artificially created hydrophilic spike formations turned superhydrophobic (CA = 160°), which may have resulted from airborne organic contamination. Additionally, Sarbada and Shin [24] used a high-speed femtosecond laser to create superhydrophobic contoured surfaces on metal to decrease the roll-off angle and improve the water contact angle. The surface nanostructures have significantly influenced the contact angle of laser-textured surfaces; periodic nano-ripples are shown to be less effective than nano-bumps for identical surface microstructures. It has been demonstrated that the fs laser is a potential tool in precise micro and nano machining for various biomaterials.

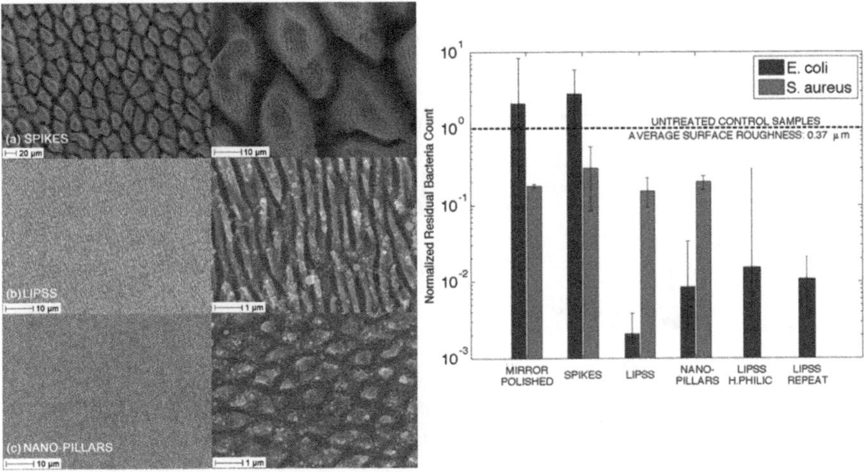

Figure 8.6 Surface texturing by femtosecond laser processing of different patterns: (a) spikes, (b) LIPSS, and (c) nano-pillars. (From Lutey *et al.* [22], an open-access article.)

8.4.1.2 *Focused-Ion Beam Texturing*

The focused ion beam uses focused charged particles to remove, add, or modify the target surface [25], and at first, Kubena et al. [26] reported that FIB can be used for micromachining. The FIB is well-established process in semiconductor industries for polishing and texturing. Figure 8.7 shows the working principle of the focused ion beam machining [27]. The FIB system has three main components: ion source, ion column, and beam writing mechanism. Gallium ions are primarily used in FIB machining and are commonly extracted from liquid metal. Furthermore, the extracted Gallium ions are accelerated with a vacuum chamber's accelerated voltage in the 5-30 keV range [25]. Figure 8.7a presents a focused ion beam column schematic, where the aperture removes multiple charged ions and clusters that originate from the point. Mainly focused ion beam used for the following process: milling, deposition, implantation, and imaging. In the "milling" process, the irradiation of an ion beam onto a solid surface result in the imparting of energy to all surface atoms. The surface atoms become sputtered if this energy surpasses the surface binding energy, and this is the primary material removal mechanism (Figure 8.7b). On the other hand, for material addition, as seen in the "deposition" process, when an ion beam bombards the target, surface atoms receiving energy lower than the surface binding energy do not undergo sputtering. Instead, they remain excited at the surface and can subsequently release their energy to interact with adsorbed gas molecules and form thin solid films on the substrate (Figure 8.7c) [28].

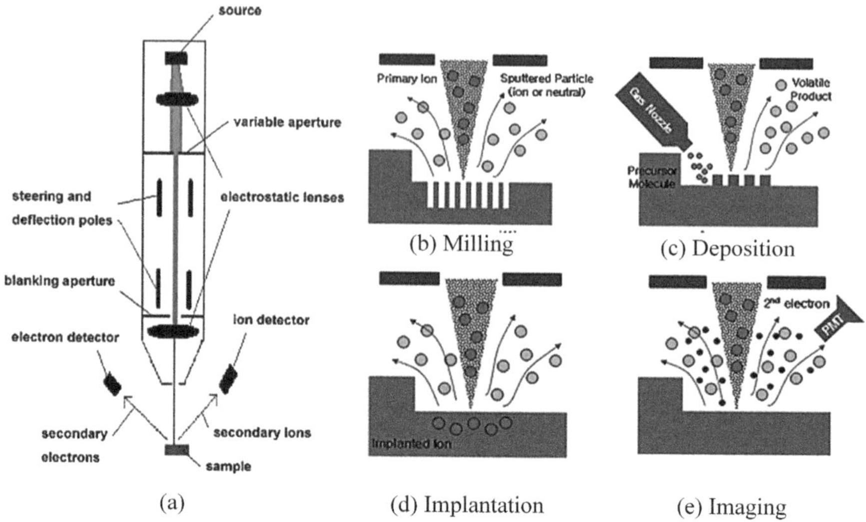

Figure 8.7 Schematic diagram of (a) FIB column, (b) FIB milling principle, (c) FIB deposition, (d) FIB implantation, and (e) FIB imaging. (From Refs. [27, 28], Copyright 2023 with permission from Elsevier.)

In the case of implantation, the accelerated ions are directed to bombard the substrate target with significant kinetic energy, leading to implantation (Figure 8.7d) [28]. The secondary electrons are collected through a photomultiplier tube while the ion beams are scanned over the substrate target surface for imaging. This approach enables the characterization of micro/nanoscale materials and is valuable for tissue engineering failure analysis (Figure 8.7e) [28]. The ease of manipulating the ion beam also enables polishing in various directions [29], which can be very resourceful in modifying medical materials. In 1990, ion implantation was used to coat the biomedical implants to improve biocompatibility [30]. The detailed schematic of the ion beam-assisted deposition process is stated in Figure 8.8 [31]. In a conventional ion implantation process, ions are subjected to acceleration via a significant potential difference and precisely directed toward a substrate material. As these accelerated ions dissipate energy, they integrate into the substrate due to interactions with the solid material [30]. Ion-beam therapy has demonstrated the potential to improve the surface properties of titanium bioimplants coated with hydroxyapatite (HA), leading to increased wear resistance [30]. The ion-beam deposition is explored to form a TiP phase on the titanium surface to enhance the corrosion resistance of the biomaterials made from titanium. In this direction, Krupa *et al.* [32] show the titanium implanted biocompatibility with phosphorus ions.

Additionally, ion-beam implantation influences the biocompatibility by increasing crystallinity and reducing the dissolution rate of apatite [33]. Chen *et al.* [34] investigated Ca ion deposition's effects on porous titanium's

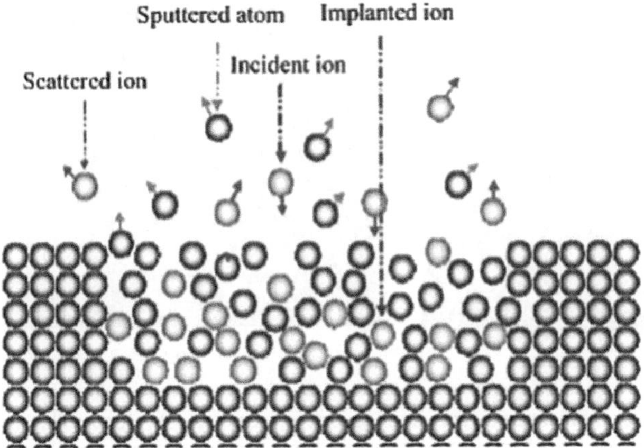

Figure 8.8 Schematic of the ion-beam-assisted deposition process. (From Ref. [42], an open-access article.)

capacity to induce apatite formation. The results support that pretreatment of porous titanium with calcium ions can enhance its bioactivity, making it suitable for bone tissue engineering. Furthermore, research indicates that ion implantation of ions such as calcium (Ca), nitrogen (N), and fluorine (F) can enhance the antibacterial properties of specific titanium surfaces [35]. Ion implantation represents a precise and tunable method for improving biomaterials' mechanical, chemical, and biological characteristics. Currently, ion-beam-based treatments are primarily employed in high-value-added applications rather than ordinary manufacturing processes, and they are less suitable for components with complex geometries [36]. Shape memory alloys have various applications in microelectronics and biomedical. Focused ion beams can produce nanostructures desirable for biomedical implants. In this context, polycrystalline NiTi pillars are fabricated using the FIB method, analyzed its influence on the material properties, and found that increasing the size of the pillars enhances the transformation stress and strain (Figure 8.9a) [37]. A focused ion beam, in combination with the chemical vapor deposition method, is employed to fabricate the cell wall-cutting tool, which can cut the cell wall without injuring the subcellular organelles (Figure 8.9b) [38]. In addition, FIB chemical vapor deposition is utilized to fabricate the nonchemical devices (Figure 8.9c) [39].

Furthermore, the ion implantation method is used for the surface enhancement of the bioimplants with desirable properties to improve the wear resistance of the artificial joints [40]. The corrosion resistance of the shape memory alloy (NiTi) improves with the help of ion implantation [41]. The mechanical, chemical, and biological properties of Titanium alloys are enhanced by ion implantation, and results show that its wear resistance and antibacterial properties are improved [42]. Figure 8.10 shows the surface

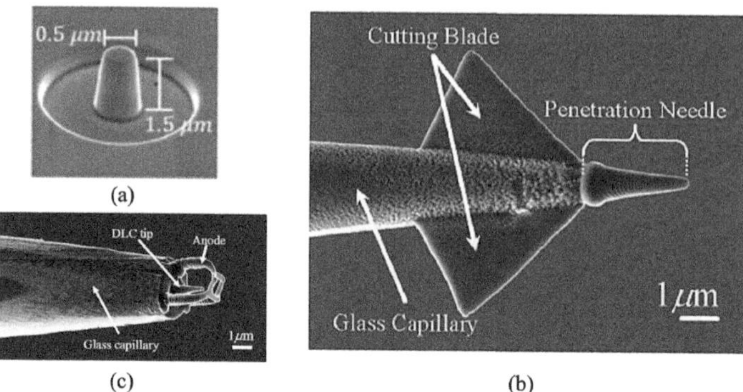

Figure 8.9 Parts fabricated by focused ion beam method: (a) micro-pillar, (b) cell wall cutting tool, and (c) glass capillary-based local field emitter. (From Ref. [36–37], Copyright 2023 with permission from Elsevier, [38] an open-access article.)

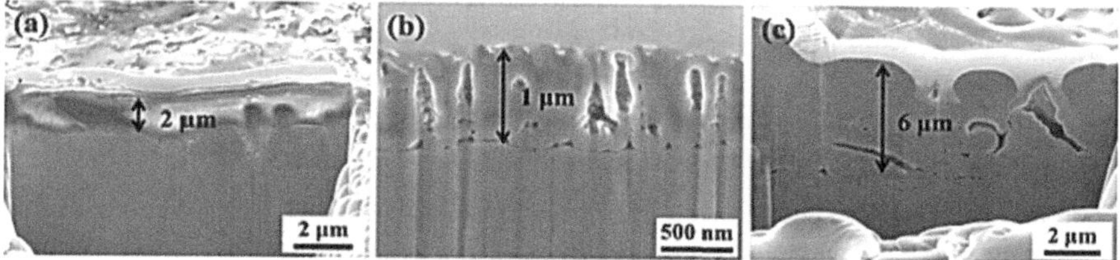

Figure 8.10 Focused ion beam images of surface-modified Ti: (a) HA, (b) SLA/AO, and (c) SLA/MAO. (From Ref. [43], an open-access article.)

modification to enhance the osseointegration of titanium and its alloy for orthopedic application by various coating processes. The FIB imaging process is used to analyze the effectiveness of the coating layers on Ti surfaces treated with HA, sandblasting, acid etching/anodic oxidation (SLA/AO), and SLA/MAO (micro-arc oxidation) [43].

The ion beam-assisted deposition (IBAD) process is a more practical approach for generating a gradual transition layer that blends the substrate material with the deposited material at the interface between them. In the case of IBAD, the coating forms with a relatively higher adhesive strength to the substrate [44]. In a similar line, Chen *et al.* [45] conducted a study in which they prepared calcium phosphate thin film coatings on pure titanium using IBAD; this process was employed to control the precipitation processes and improve the biocompatibility of the coating. Furthermore, FIB etching fabricates the nanoneedles for drug delivery (Figure 12.11). In this process, FIB mills physically individual microneedles to increase their aspect ratio [46].

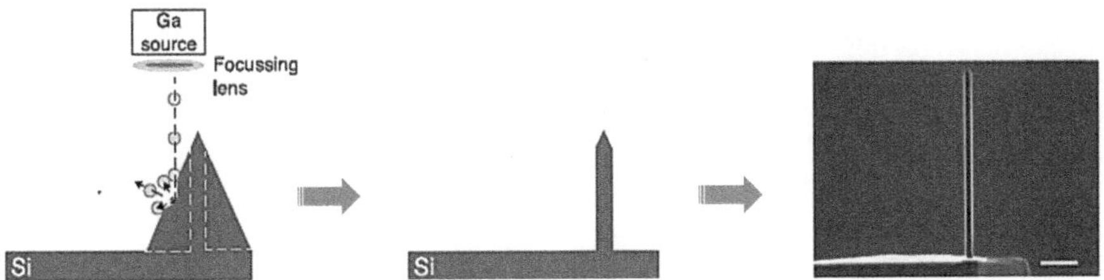

Figure 8.11 Fabrication of the nanoneedles by FIB milling. (From Ref. [46], Copyright 2023 with permission from Elsevier.)

- Y. Fu and L. Wang [47] show that ripples can be spontaneously generated at the nanoscale during ion bombardment, which can be used as nanowires for biomedical sensing. These ripples can be converted into different structures by controlling the ion beam's overlap percentage. Nano dots can be generated with the FIB bombardment, and the high-intensity FIB can produce nanofibers on the material surface.

8.4.1.3 Electron Beam Texturing

Electron beam machining falls in the thermal process category, which removes the material through melting and vaporization. The basic principle of EBM is an electron gun, mainly a cathode made of tungsten filament shown in Figure 8.12 heated between 2500 to 3000°C in a vacuum chamber to emit the electron. The cathode cartridge is maintained at a notably strong negative bias, effectively repelling thermo-ionic electrons away from the cathode. Just following the cathode, an annular bias grid is situated. An elevated negative bias is applied to this grid to prevent the divergence of the electrons generated by the cathode and direct them toward the subsequent element, the annular anode, forming a concentrated electron beam. The annular anode serves to attract and gradually accelerate the electron beam. Subsequent to the anode, the electron beam proceeds through a sequence of magnetic lenses and apertures. The magnetic lenses serve the dual purpose of shaping the beam and reducing its divergence. Following this, the electron beam focused on the desired target spot progresses through the final segment of deflection coils [48].

Electron beam machining is used to texture medical materials due to its capability to machine a wide range of materials, smaller sport size, and highly localized heat, making it more suitable for fine texturing required for various applications in medical implants. In this direction, the electron beam is used to create the cones on the Ti-6Al-4V by the surf-sculpt process [49]. Furthermore, an electron beam was used to texture the acetabular cup used in uncemented total hip replacements and found that it is faster, and costs less than hydroxyapatite coating commonly used for orthopedic

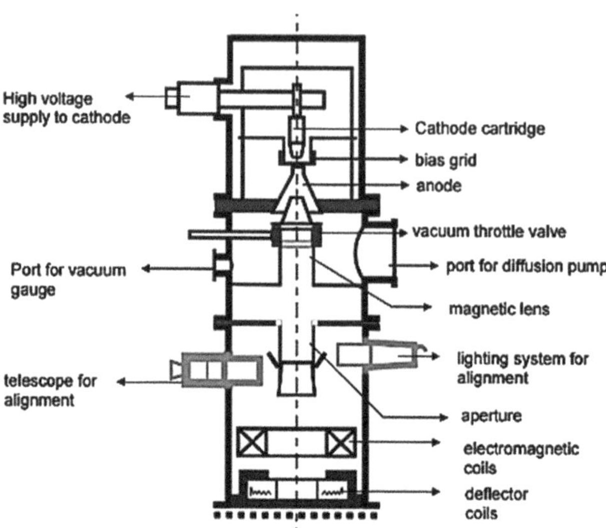

Figure 8.12 Schematic of the electron beam gun. (From Ref. [48], an open-access article.)

implants [50]. Furthermore, implants fabricated of dense metals such as titanium tend to be considerably heavier than natural bone. The implant is made of titanium twice as heavy as the natural bone it replaces. In a healthy individual, bone can remodel itself in response to the mechanical stress it encounters. However, when the high modulus of titanium leads to a reduction in the stresses transmitted to the adjacent bone, it can trigger a phenomenon known as "stress shielding". In turn, it can result in bone resorption and aseptic loosening of the implant, impacting its long-term performance.

Moreover, implants often necessitate complex geometries with variable mechanical properties in diverse areas of a single implant. Different mechanical requirements are needed for load-bearing implants like hip and mandible implants to effectively reduce weight without compromising functionality. The introduction of voids into the inner architectural design mainly reduces the part's mass, albeit with a trade-off in strength [51]. Towards this, Figure 8.13 shows the custom Ti-6Al-4V parts to meet the bioimplant requirement with controlled porosity fabricated by layer-by-layer pattern deposition using a rapid EBM manufacturing process [51].

Figure 8.14 shows custom bioimplant parts fabricated using EBM melting in a similar line. The weight and density of the custom parts are distributed according to their load-bearing requirements and capacity. This process improves the stress shielding and influences the plants' longevity.

Different scaffold structures (Figure 8.15) made from Ti-6Al-4V for the orthopedic application by EBM melting process. The designs are tested in different conditions, and results show that the cubic scaffold structure and

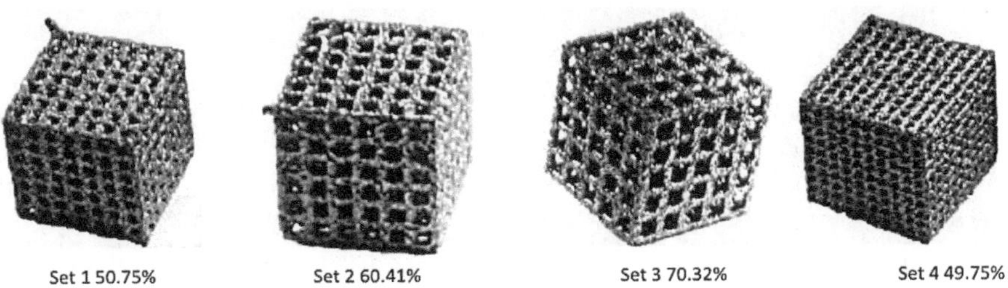

Figure 8.13 Ti-6Al-4V parts fabricated by EBM. (From Ref. [51], Copyright 2023 with permission from Elsevier.)

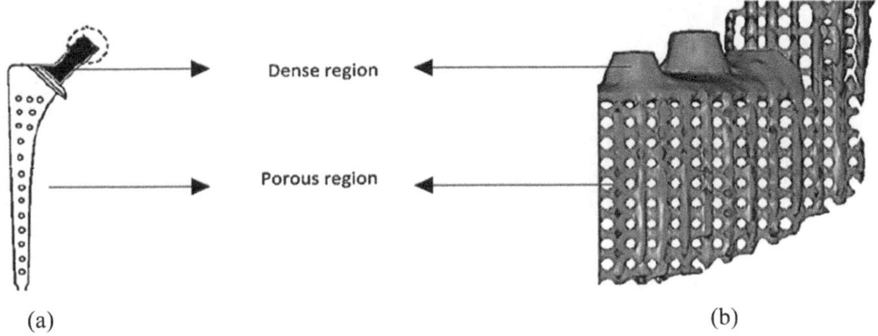

Figure 8.14 Bioimplants fabricated by EBM: (a) pours stem and dense head region of the hip implant, and (b) part of a mandible with dense dental abutments structure and porous body. (From Ref. [52], Copyright 2023 with permission from Elsevier.)

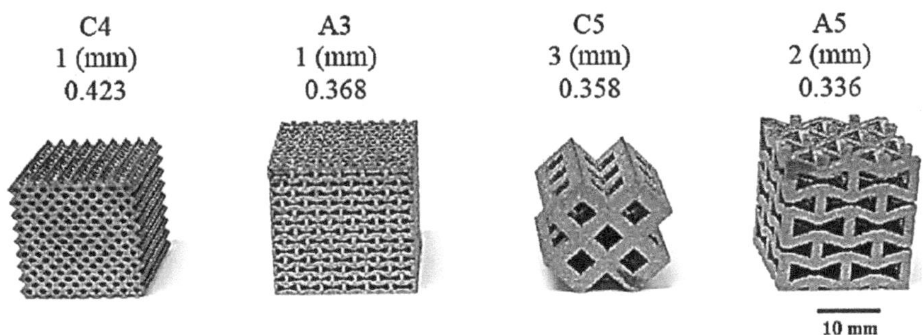

Figure 8.15 Electron beam machined Ti-6Al-4V lattice structures. (From Ref. [53], Copyright 2023 with permission from Elsevier.)

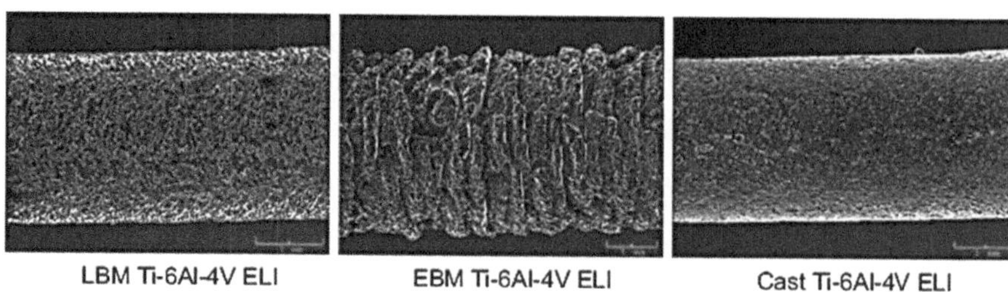

Figure 8.16 Comparison of the cylinder made from the different methods. (From Ref. [54], Copyright 2023 with permission from Elsevier.)

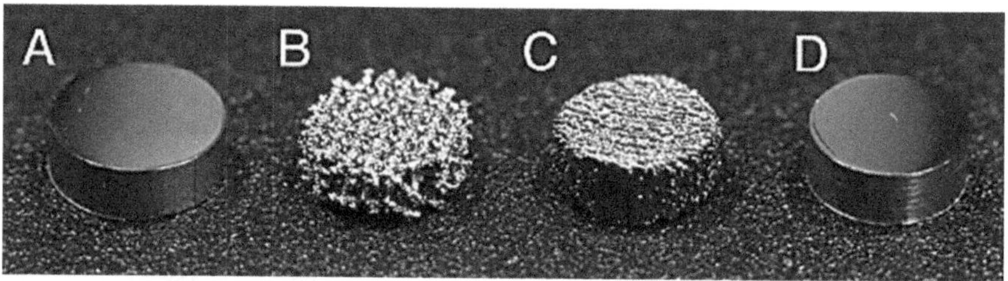

Figure 8.17 Photographs of the EBM machine Ti-6Al-4V discs: (a) solid polished discs, commercially available, (b) porous unpolished EBM discs, (c) solid unpolished EBM discs, and (d) solid polished EBM discs made using EBM melting additive manufacturing. (From Ref. [55], Copyright 2023 with permission from Elsevier.)

structure with a strut thickness of more than 0.5 demonstrate higher stiffness and compression load [53].

The parts made of Ti-6Al-4V for biomedical implant applications (Figure 8.16) from different methods, such as LBM, casting, and electron beam machining, are analyzed [54]. The findings from this study revealed that the parts manufactured by the EBM process have higher surface roughness compared to the LBM and casting processes.

Transdermal osseointegrated prostheses have emerged as a compelling alternative to traditional socket prostheses, and titanium alloy Ti-6Al-4V is widely recognized as a biocompatible material for biomedical implants. Research conducted by Jessica Collins Springer *et al.* [55] focused on the in vitro evaluation of transdermal osseointegrated prostheses (Figure 8.17). Their findings revealed that the survival and proliferation of dermal and epidermal cells on smooth Ti-6Al-4V surfaces, processed using EBM, with a surface roughness of less than 0.5 μm, met acceptable standards. Additionally, their study indicated that the survival and proliferation of dermal and epidermal cells were enhanced on electron-beam-processed Ti-6Al-4V surfaces compared to solid or porous Ti-6Al-4V surfaces.

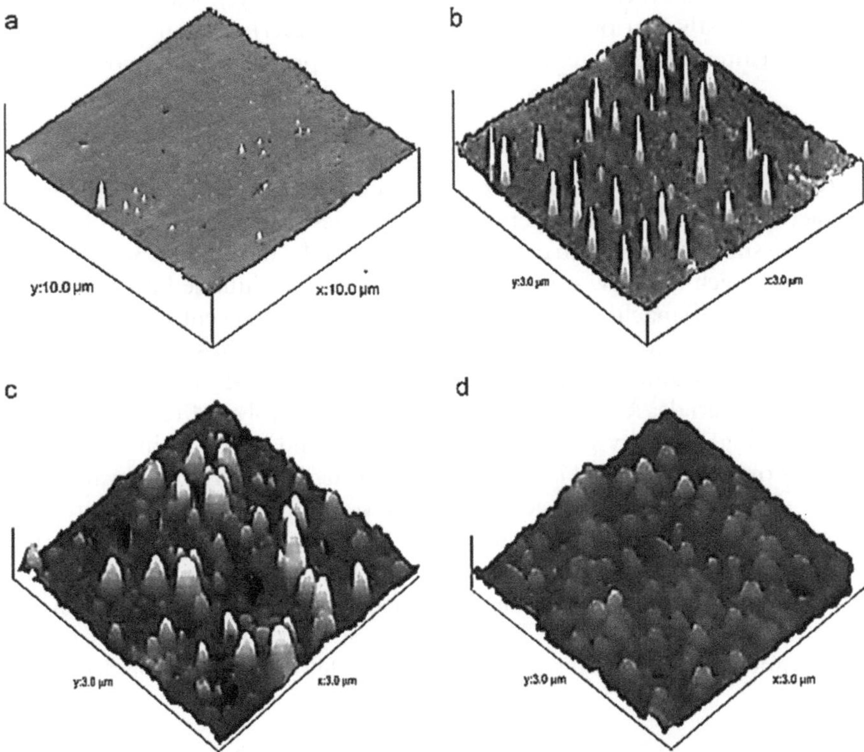

Figure 8.18 AFM images for electron beam treated PET film with different electron fluences: (a) pristine, (b) ϕ = 1.3 × 10^{19} e/cm2, (c) ϕ = 4 10^{19} e/cm2 and (d) ϕ = 6.6 10^{19} e/cm². (From Ref. [56], Copyright 2023 with permission from Elsevier.)

The PET (polyethylene terephthalate) polymer surface is treated with low-energy electrons with varying fluences (Figure 8.17) to improve biocompatibility, wettability, and adhesion, and the results show that the process improves the wettability and adhesion properties [56].

However, the advancements in difficult-to-machine biocompatible materials demand alternative machining technologies to overcome such challenges. Towards this, detailed literature on mechanical-based HEBs (AAJ, AWJ, and ASJ) employed for surface texturing on any softer-to-harder AEBMs, irrespective of their properties from the macro-to-micro scale, is discussed in the following.

8.4.2 Mechanical-Based Beams

This section presents the utilization and capabilities of mechanical-based beam energy for surface texturing applications on biomaterials. Section

8.4.2.1. focuses on the abrasive air jet beams employed for texturing bio-implants. Lastly, various formats of abrasive waterjet beams utilized as a potential alternative for texturing purposes are presented in section 8.4.2.2.

8.4.2.1 Abrasive Air Jet for Surface Texturing

In the late 20th century, research on erosion was driven by the "solid particle impact" issue in the oil and aerospace industries. The historical evolution of freeform surface generation can be attributed to the influence of solid particle impacts, which has now evolved into the modern technique known as abrasive air jet (AAJ) machining. At the beginning of the 21st century, micro-manufacturing technology using AAJ beams received significant attention from various sectors and demonstrated the generation of 3D micro-features on different materials. AAJ machining (Figure 8.19) involves directing a nozzle-propelled high-velocity stream of solid particles and gas or air in a controlled manner over the targets (Figure 8.19b), resulting in material removal (Figure 8.19c) through an erosion mechanism (micro-cutting or brittle fracture). The pressurized gas or air in AAJ is used as a carrier medium, and converting that to kinetic energy results in a high-velocity abrasives beam. The erosion by the AAJ beam on the target is controlled by adjusting the process parameters (Figure 8.19c) suitably for a fixed type of abrasive particles (Figure 8.19d) and nozzle diameter to achieve desirable three-dimensional features.

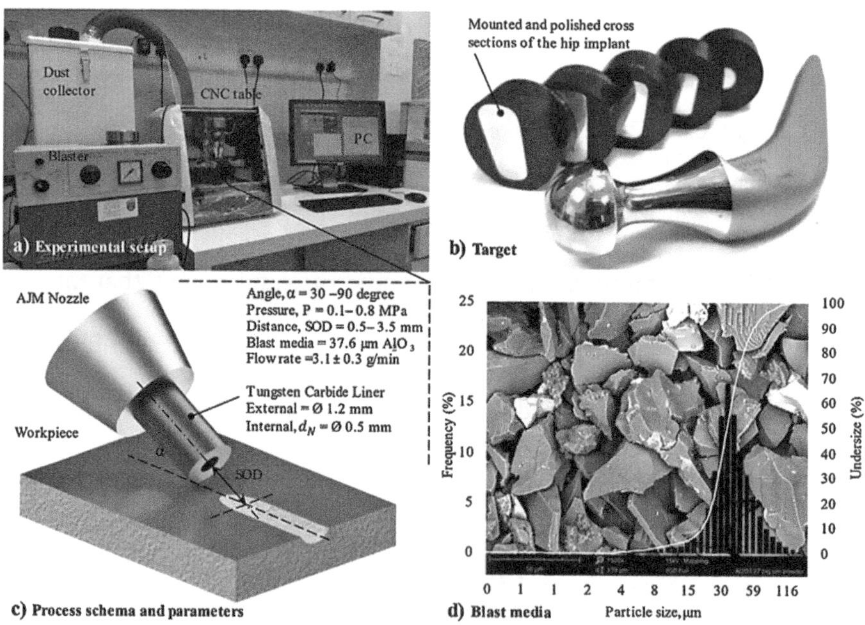

Figure 8.19 Experimental details. (From Melentiev and Fang [64], an open-access article.)

In this regard, pioneered researchers' work [57–63] played an essential role in developing the Dutch microelectronics industry, where the texture resolution ranges from 50 to 500 µm was achieved using a circular nozzle of diameter 1.5 mm by directing the high-velocity abrasive particles through patterned erosion-resistant masks docked over the target. Masking aids in protecting the remaining surface of the target from the erosion of stray particles in the divergent AAJ beam. Metal masks are widely regarded as the most appropriate choice among various masks due to their highest erosion resistance capability. However, masking the target for surface texturing applications is a highly complex and involved process for generating controlled features, resulting in increased manufacturing steps and production costs. In addition, the pattern transfer accuracy issue contributes to dimensional errors of up to 20% [64], which is also a concern in generating micro-features by AAJs using masks.

An alternative solution to address the challenges mentioned above was found in the form of maskless machining using AAJ beam methodologies. Among such, Nouhi *et al.* [65] attempted to attach the mask to the nozzle instead of the target to gain control over the shape/size of the AAJ beam. On the other hand, Sookhak *et al.* [66] developed a rotational disk mask with specific pattern holes separating the target and nozzle in which the AAJ beam passes through to impinge on the target at a given location and time. On the other hand, maskless milling strategies with micro-AAJ beams gained the attention of various industries due to the commercially available small-diameter nozzles of 125 µm [67, 68]. Machining using micro-scale beams is called micromachining; in the present context, it is called micro-AAJ (µ-AAJ) milling. Notably, there is an essential distinction between AAJ and µ-AAJ processes, where the former process uses masks with micro-opening, while the latter employs micro-beams to generate micro-scale features.

Regarding µ-AAJ milling of biomedical alloy, Ally et al. [69] studied the evolution of microchannels on biomaterials (SS 316 L and Ti-6Al-4V alloy) up to an aspect ratio (depth/width) of 1.25 under without and with masking (hardened steel sheets) conditions. The rate of volumetric erosion in these alloys is ten times lower than that observed in glass and polymers and suggests that this approach is suitable for machining shallow features or controlled etching operations. These are prominent characteristics of surface textures, where shallow features and reproducibility are essential. Furthermore, observed an embedment of particles in the target that is significant in the SS 316 L biomaterial.

On the other hand, by exploiting the potential benefits of the µ-AAJ milling, Melentieve et al. [64] are the first to investigate the possibility of generating tribological shallow microchannels in maskless milling conditions or the µ-AAJ direct writing approach. This study attempted to solve a production case through experimental work on the influence of operating parameters, such as air pressure (0.1–0.8 MPa), jet impingement angle (90°–30°), standoff distance (0.5–3.5 mm), on the microchannels characteristics

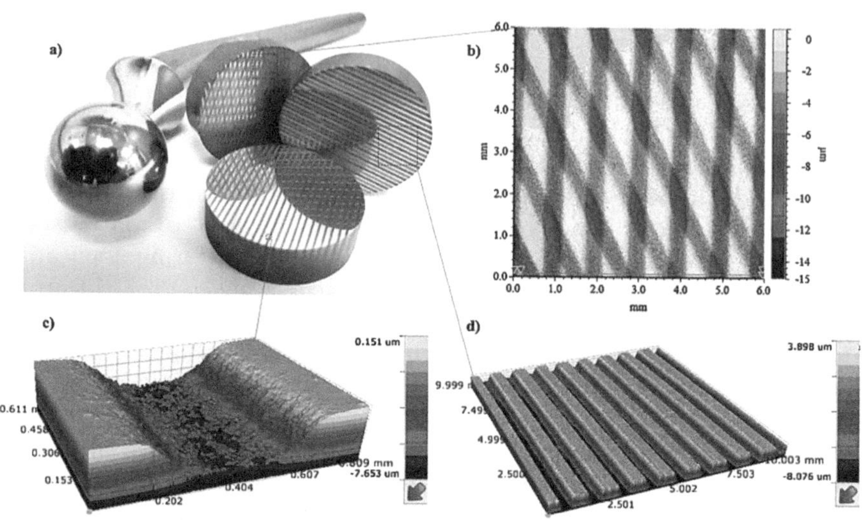

Figure 8.20 Surface texturing on 30 mm diameter of Co-Cr-Mo disks: (a) crosshatched 550 μm × 5 μm pattern, (b) straight 550 μm × 10 μm channels, (c) exaggerated view of straight channels in (a), and (d) depicts the (c) after polishing. (From Melentiev and Fang [64], an open-access article.)

(depth, width, and profile) fabricated in Co-Cr-Mo alloy (vitallium) based bioimplant (Figure 8.20). The results show that a wide variety of bottom surface-shaped U, V, and W microchannels milled on the hip joint's femoral head within a few minutes using a circular shape nozzle and one gram of abrasive particles.

On the other hand, Shen *et al.* [54] studied the tribological performance of CoCrMo-on-ultra-high molecular-weight-polyethylene with three distributions modes of micro-dimple-textured patterns of aspect ratio (depth/diameter) 0.01 using μ-AAJs (Figure 8.21). The study demonstrated that surface texturing enhanced the tribological performance and concluded that an evenly distributed array of micro-dimples is ideal for the CoCrMo-UHMWPE bioimplant.

In recent decades, bioimplant manufacturers have shifted their attention from metal alloys to bioceramics to mimic the structures they intend to replace due to their excellent durability and superior strength. Towards this, Kang *et al.* [71] generated various shapes (flat, arched, conical, and W) micro-dimples with different aspect ratios on alumina-based ceramics (pure alumina and zirconia-toughened alumina) using μ-AAJs under varying process conditions (Figure 8.22). The pin-on-disk experiment verified that μ-AAJs is a practical approach to enhancing the wear resistance in lubricating systems. To achieve sub-micro or nanoscale textures, more sophisticated nozzles must be developed and require finer abrasive particles.

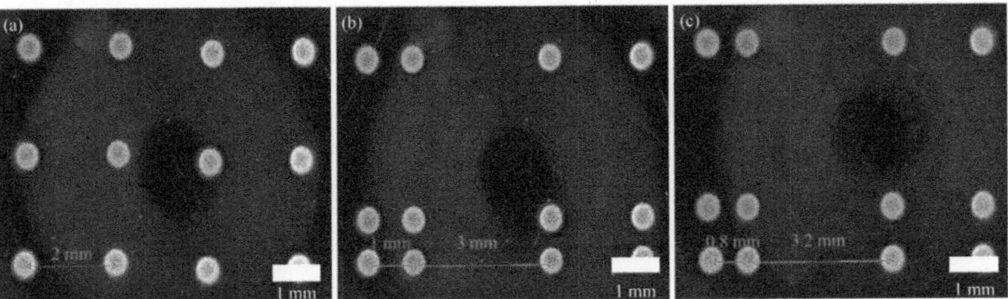

Figure 8.21 Photographs of three modes of micro-dimple distributions: (a) even distribution with a pitch length of 2 mm, (b) uneven distribution with a pitch length of 1 and 3 mm, and (c) uneven distribution with a pitch length of 0.8 and 3.2 mm. (From Shen *et al.* [70], an open-access article.)

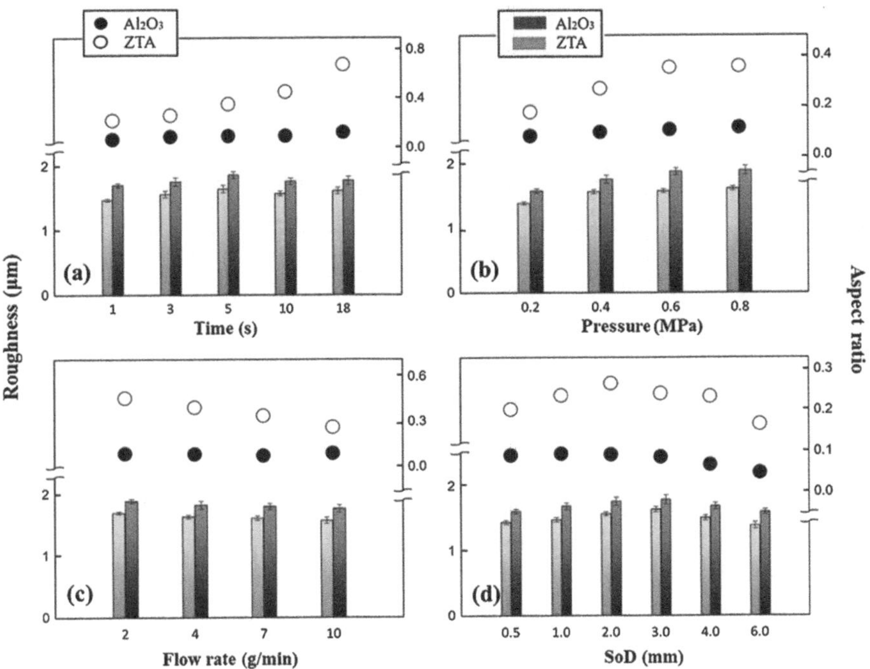

Figure 8.22 Correlation between aspect ratio/added bottom surface roughness and micro-abrasive air jet process parameters. (From Kang *et al.* [71], Copyright 2023 with permission from Elsevier.)

8.4.2.2 *Waterjet-Based Surface Texturing*

Ultra-high-pressure waterjet (UHPW) beams with or without abrasive particles are considered *universal flexible tools* that preserve structural integrity and are preferred as an alternative potential machining process for producing macro-to-micro features on various AEBMs. In recent

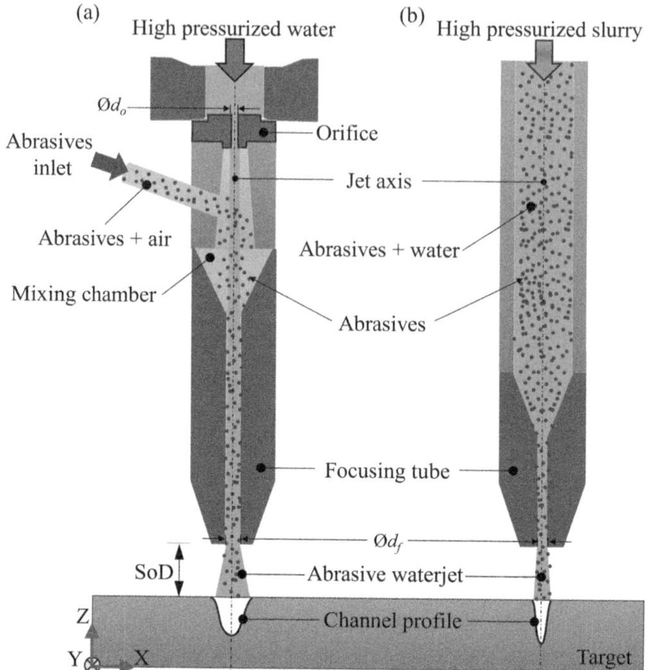

Figure 8.23 Schematic of (a) injection jets, and (b) suspension jets.

decades, the pressurized waterjet beams technology has been competing equally with other slow, expensive, and material constraints processes, such as conventional CNCs, lasers, and wire-EDM. This is possible due to the inherent unique capabilities of the UHPW beams, such as eco-friendly, no heat-affected zone, minimum force exertion on parts needs simple fixtures, no tooling, machining of high-aspect-ratio features (blind/through), and capability for micromachining. Nevertheless, with these unique capabilities, this technology has gained the attention of various industries, such as aerospace, automotive, and biomedical for machining freeform surfaces on AEMs. Figure 8.23 presents the schematic of UHPW beams operating in three different configurations: (1) *plain waterjets* (PWJs) without abrasive particles, (2) *abrasive injection waterjets* – abrasive particles injected into a high-velocity waterjet, and (3) *abrasive suspension jets* – premixed slurry made of abrasives, water, and some additives pumped through the nozzle.

The UHPW beams, *i.e.*, AWJs and ASJs, behave similarly after leaving the focusing tube. However, the significant difference between the two beam types is that the ASJs expand slower than AWJs/PWJs due to the lack of air in the jet. The UHPW beams can operate beyond 600 MPa in the case of the PWJs/AWJs, while the ASJs are limited to only 70 to 140 MPa to minimize the components' wear along the high abrasive slurry flow [72].

The MRR with ASJs is higher than the PWJs/AWJs generated at the same pressure [73]. In preventing undesired erosion using the UHPW beams, it is necessary to understand their penetration behavior into the target. Studies on the material removal mechanism (MRM) in various AEBMs were reported for all the beams mentioned above [73, 74]. In the case of PWJs impingement on general materials such as rigid, ductile, brittle, and composite, Adler [77] introduced the four modes of MRM to explain damaging effects: (i) stress wave propagation, (ii) direct deformation, (iii) lateral out-flow jetting, and (iv) hydraulic penetration. Whereas, the MRM in the case of AWJs/ASJs impingements in machining (i) ductile materials is mainly by ploughing and micro-cutting at low impact angles and plastic failure material at high impact angles, and (ii) brittle materials is due to crack initiation and propagation. The capability of AWJ cutting in the biomedical field has been demonstrated against laser cutting techniques in generating structures like stents in thin NiTi shape memory alloy sheets [75]. However, the real challenging task of getting control over the jet penetration is of paramount importance in achieving the desired freeform surface texturing on AEBMs for specific biomedical applications. A vast published literature shows studies on milling low-to-high aspect ratio (*i.e.*, depth/width) channels on bio-materials (*e.g.*, Ti-6Al-4V, NiTi alloy) using conventional UHPW beams (over Ø1 mm jet diameter) [76–85]. The source of concern in biomedical applications is the residual abrasives embedded in the machined zone when AWJs/ASJs are used. For this purpose, Kong *et al.* [76] suggested that AWJ milling is utilized first, followed by PWJ milling is an effective way to remove the embedded particles. However, in the biomedical field, the noncontaminating soluble abrasives in UHPW beams generated by injection/suspension systems for processing the AEBMs are yet to be explored.

Fabrication of damage-free micro features or textures on difficult-to-machine AEBMs is a pressing need of the biomedical industry, which demands a reduction in the scale of the macro-UHPW beam technology. A scaled-down of this technology according to beam diameter has been classified into two types: (i) fine abrasive jets (Ø100-Ø300 μm), and (ii) microfabrication abrasive jets (under Ø100 μm). The working principles of these technologies remain the same for injection and suspension jet systems. Moreover, these technologies can even be employed with/without masking the target or machining the target by submerging beams to gain control over the jet divergence as it emerges from the focusing tube enable to achieve the precision for micromachining. Towards this, Miller [86] explored waterjet technology's potential and future possibilities for micromachining applications using various waterjet beams and compared the multiple configurations of UHPW beams with lasers. As depicted in Figure 8.24, it is evident that PWJs can achieve beam diameters similar to laser beams; however, they are limited to machine-soft and thin materials. On the contrary, AWJs result in larger beam diameters, and ASJs are smaller-diameter beams. With the advent of miniaturized micro-tubes of diameter Ø254 μm, Haghbin

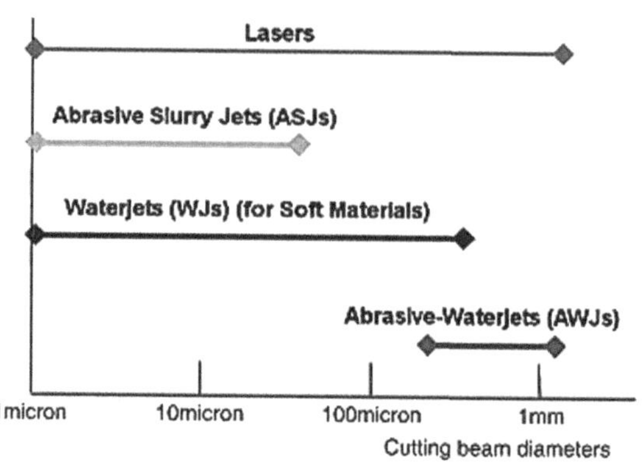

Figure 8.24 Comparison of ultra-high pressure waterjet beams with a laser beam. (From H.-T. Liu [89], Copyright 2023 with permission from Elsevier.)

et al. [87] demonstrated micro-milling of channels of aspect ratio 3 in SS 316 L and Al 60601-T6 alloys under in-air and submerged conditions. The results show that machining with submerged AWJs yields narrower features than machining in-air without reducing the centerline erosion rate. In line with this, Haghbin *et al.* [88] demonstrated the feasibility of using metal masks to generate micromachining channels as narrow as ~150 μm wide in glass and Al6061-T6 by utilizing micro-AWJs. This demonstration opened opportunities to utilize UHPW beams in micromachining applications for fabricating microchannels of width 600 μm and microholes of 660 μm diameter. Nevertheless, micromachining necessitates beam diameters less than 100 μm, so the current generation of injection-type AWJ systems cannot be used for micromachining applications.

Downsizing the currently available micro-sized injection jets presents challenges [89, 90]: (i) insufficient waterjet pressure in a microjet system to generate the required vacuum to entrain for entraining the particles in a high-velocity jet, (ii) it demands precision alignment between the orifice and focusing tube, particles-agglomeration effect, (iii) blockage of flow in focusing tube, and (iv) inconsistent in abrasive feed rate. For this purpose, Miller [91] developed a micro-ASJs system (Figure 8.25a), which operates at a pressure under 70 MPa with a 58 μm diameter nozzle for micro-milling applications for ductile to brittle materials. Further, demonstrated the drilling of a square array pattern of a 33 × 33 array of holes in 50 μm thick stainless steel (Figure 8.25b). This technology captivated the attention of various researchers for generating various micro-features for various industrial applications [92–96].

In the technology mentioned above, sufficient pressure is maintained to overcome the erosion of focusing tubes having a diameter of about a

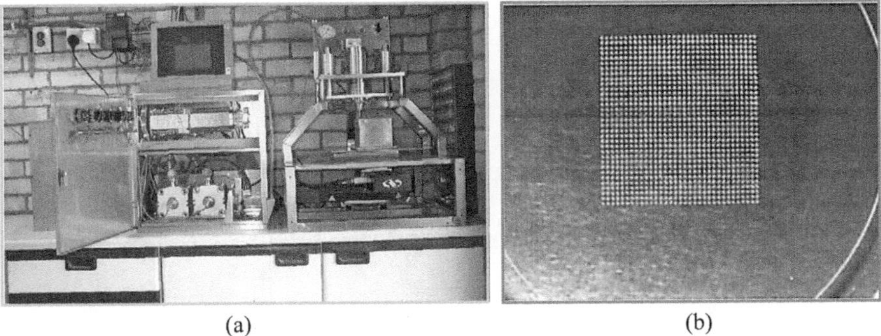

(a)   (b)

Figure 8.25 Photographs of (a) micro-abrasive suspension jet system, and (b) fabrication of micro-holes of diameter 85 µm with a 250 µm pitch. (From D. S. Miller [91], Copyright 2023 with permission from Elsevier.)

hundred micrometers while the slurry flows through them, which also possesses enough energy to initiate the erosion by multiple particle impact on the target. Nevertheless, the micro-ASJ systems mentioned above involve the high-pressure slurry being forced through crucial components, leading to premature damage to the slurry valve and significant wear in nozzles and valves [97, 98]. Hence, demands a new technology to overcome such challenges.

By considering the challenges in exiting micro-ASJs, Haghbin *et al.* [99, 100] developed a high-pressure (up to 250 MPa) abrasive slurry micromachining (HASJM) system in which the slurry is entrained after the high-pressure waterjet passes through an orifice into the mixing chamber (Figure 8.26). By employing a single pass at a jet traverse rate of 40 mm/min, the HASJM system can produce symmetric micro-channels of aspect ratios > 0.9 with a centerline waviness below 6.9 µm and a centerline roughness below 1.1 µm. On the other hand, using a multipass at a jet traverse rate of 1000 mm/min in the HASJM system, asymmetric microchannels of aspect ratios < 0.9 could be generated. Overall, using HASJM technology with micro-tubes of diameter Ø254 µm, roughness and waviness of 19% and 44 % smaller than those machined with conventional AWJ micromachining can be achieved. This enhancement was observed due to the improved consistency in the abrasive mass flow rate and the elimination of air bubbles in the generated high-pressure abrasive slurry beams.

The high-energy beam-based processes employed for surface texturing discussed in section 8.4 yield various surface structures. The characteristics of the textured features corresponding to the specific machining processes are tabulated (Table 8.2), allowing the surface structures to be optimized for the intended use.

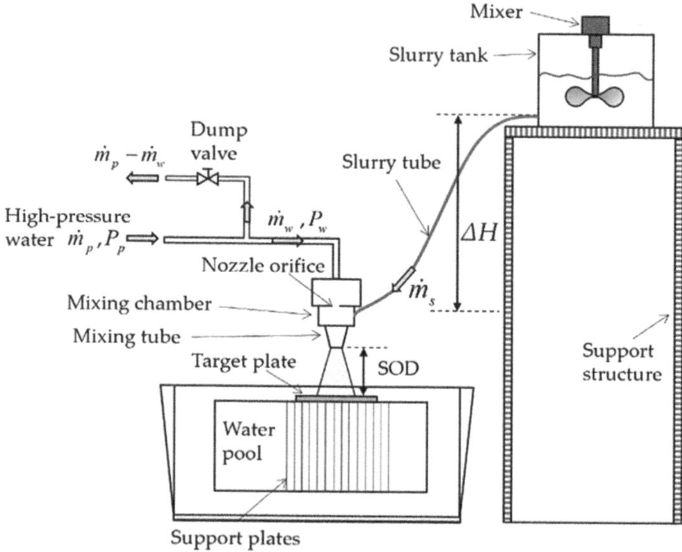

Figure 8.26 Schematic of abrasive suspension jet system. (From Moghaddam *et al.* [101], Copyright 2023 with permission from Elsevier.)

Table 8.2 Surface texture features, scale of respective structures, and corresponding machining processes

Process	Sub-processes	Geometrical patterns	Scales
LST	Milliseconds Nanoseconds Picoseconds Femtoseconds	Grooves, dimples, pillars (circular, squared, hexagonal, pyramid), channels, crosshatched patterns, LIPSS, moats, hybrid patterns, and bio-inspired pattern	Features of width can be achieved between less than 5 μm to 50 μm and beyond
FIB	Chemical vapor deposition	Pillars (conical, hexagonal etc.,), grooves, dimples, ripples	Features achieved of width less than 1 μm
AAJ	Macro-AAJ, and Micro-AAJ with/ without masking the target	Dimples, pillars, and channels of different geometrical patterns	Features width/diameter can be achieved between 50 μm to 1000 μm and beyond.
WJ	PWJ, AWJ, and ASJ with/without masking the target	Dimples, Pillars, hexagonal patterns, channels, crosshatched patterns of different shapes	Features width/diameter can be achieved between 1 μm to 1000 μm and beyond.

8.5 CONCLUSION

This chapter presents an overview of surface texturing of advanced engineering biocompatible materials (AEBMs) using high-energy beam-based (LB, FIB, EB, AAJ, AWJ, and ASJ) machining processes employed for generating multiscale (macro-to-micro) features of texture. The discussed high-energy beams (HEBs) hold significant promise in enhancing the performance and longevity of bioimplants. Furthermore, to advance the field of bioimplant manufacturing, the HEB-based machining processes offer a pathway to address critical issues, such as aseptic loosening due to different wear mechanisms and poor osseointegration, paving the way for improved patient outcomes (best lives with better quality and increased life expectancy) by enhancing the bioimplants' functionality, biocompatibility, and longevity through surface texturing. The literature survey on thermal-based HEBs (LB, FIB, and EB) for surface texturing shows that, at present, they have become potential methods for surface modification of biomaterial in implant applications. Through their utilization, different scales (macro-to-nano) of surface texture patterns using dimples, pillars, grooves, moats, and hybrid textures can be created on the target implant surface. These patterns have been shown to enhance the micro-hardness, texture feature, and oxidization of the implant material, resulting in improved wettability and wear properties to the implant material compared to the plain target surface. Hence, finding more suitable options for bioimplant applications currently. In the category of thermal-based HEBs, new processes, such as waterjet-guided lasers and gas-assisted waterjet-guided lasers, have recently been reported in the literature, which is not mature enough and is yet to be explored critically in biomedical applications.

On the other hand, the advancements in biocompatible materials, which are difficult to machine, demand alternative technologies. Towards this, detailed literature on mechanical-based HEBs (AAJ, AWJ, and ASJ) employed for surface texturing on AEBMs reveals that these processes show promising results in generating suitable surface textures on any softer-to-harder materials irrespective of their properties from macro- to micro- meter scale. However, in these waterjet-based HEBs, the embedment of harder particles in the textured surface is a critical issue yet to be addressed to meet the standards of bioimplant manufacturing for acceptance. Some possible ways to avoid particle embedment are (i) developing/employing other novel processing techniques for removing embedded particles, (ii) traversing a plain waterjet over the textured surface in a controlled way to remove only the embedded particles instead of target material, and (iii) selecting suitable biocompatible abrasive particles for eroding the target that does not affect the performance of the textured implant during its functionality in the human body. Furthermore, to achieve textures at a sub-micrometer or nanometre scale, more sophisticated nozzles must be developed with finer abrasive particles, which demands further technological advancement in the existing cutting heads for generating HEBs at that scale.

ABBREVIATIONS

AAJ:	Abrasive air jet
AEBMs:	Advanced engineering biocompatible materials
ASJ:	Abrasive suspension jets
AWJ:	Abrasive waterjet
EB:	Electron beam
fs:	Femtoseconds
FIB:	Focused-Ion beam
HEBs:	High energy beams
HPASMM:	High pressure abrasive slurry micromachining
LB:	Laser beam
LIPSS:	Laser-induced periodic surface structures
LST:	Laser surface texturing
ms:	Milliseconds
MRM:	Material removal model
ns:	Nanoseconds
ps:	Picoseconds
PWJ:	Pure waterjet
THA:	Total hip arthroplasty
UHMWP:	Ultra-high-molecular-weight-polyethylene
UHPW:	Ultra high-pressure waterjet
μ-AAJ:	Micro abrasive waterjet

REFERENCES

1. A.F. Mavrogenis, R. Dimitriou, J. Parvizi, and G.C. Babis, Biology of implant osseointegration, *J. Musculoskelet. Neuron. Interact.*, vol. 9, pp. 61–71, 2009. https://doi.org/10.1016/j.joms.2007.05.013

2. B. Jetté, V. Brailovski, C. Simoneau, M. Dumas, P. Terriault, Development and invitro validation of a simplified numerical model for the design of a biomimetic femoral stem, *J. Mech. Behav. Biomed. Mater.*, vol. 77, pp. 539–550, 2018. https://doi.org/10.1016/j.jmbbm.2017.10.019

3. D.M.D. Ehrenfest, P.G. Coelho, B.S. Kang, Y.T. Sul, T. Albrektsson, Classification of osseointegrated implant surfaces: Materials, chemistry and topography, *Trends Biotechnol.*, vol. 28, pp. 198–206, 2010. https://doi.org /10.1016/j.tibtech.2009.12.003

4. H. Sawano, S. Warisawa, and S. Ishihara, Study on long life of artificial joints by investigating optimal sliding surface geometry for improvement in wear resistance, *Precis. Eng.*, vol. 33, pp. 492–498, 2009. https://doi.org/10.1016/j .precisioneng.2009.01.005

5. D. Choudhury, R. Walker, T. Roy, S. Paul, and R. Mootanah, Performance of honed surface profiles to artificial hip joints: An experimental investigation, *Int. J. Precis. Eng. Manuf.*, vol. 14, pp. 1847–1853, 2013. https://doi.org/10 .1007/s12541-013-0247-z

6. V. Kashyap and P. Ramkumar, Comprehensive analysis of geometrical parameters of crosshatched texture for enhanced tribological performance under biological environment, *Proc. Inst. Mech. Eng. Part J J. Eng. Tribol.*, vol. 235, pp. 434–452, 2021. https://doi.org/10.1177/1350650120915136

7. H. Zhang, L. G. Qin, M. Hua, G. N. Dong, and K. S. Chin, A tribological study of the petaloid surface texturing for Co-Cr-Mo alloy artificial joints, *Appl. Surf. Sci.*, vol. 332, 557–564, 2015. https://doi.org/10.1016/j.apsusc.2015.01.215

8. B. Mao, A. Siddaiah, Y. Liao, and P. L. Menezes, Laser surface texturing and related techniques for enhancing tribological performance of engineering materials: A review, *J. Manuf. Process.*, vol. 53, pp. 153–173, 2020. https://doi.org/10.1016/j.jmapro.2020.02.009

9. Sixty years of lasers, *Nat. Rev. Phys.*, vol. 2, pp. 221, 2020. https://doi.org/10.1038/s42254-020-0181-9

10. C. Y. Cui, X. G. Cui, Q. Zhao, J. D. Hu, Y. H. Liu, and Y. M. Wang, Investigation of different surface morphologies formed on AISI 304 stainless steel via millisecond Nd: YAG pulsed laser oxidation, *Opt. Laser Technol.*, vol. 44, pp. 815–820, 2012. https://doi.org/10.1016/j.optlastec.2011.11.025

11. R. Bathe, V. Sai Krishna, S. K. Nikumb, and G. Padmanabham, Laser surface texturing of Gray cast iron for improving tribological behavior, *Appl. Phys. A Mater. Sci. Process.*, vol. 117, pp. 117–123, 2014. https://doi.org/10.1007/s00339-014-8281-y

12. P. Pou, *et al.*, Laser surface texturing of Titanium for bioengineering applications, *Procedia Manuf.*, vol. 13, pp. 694–701, 2017. https://doi.org/10.1016/j.promfg.2017.09.102

13. S.P. Murzin, V.B. Balyakin, A.A. Melnikov, N.N. Vasiliev, and P.I. Lichtner, Determining ways of improving the tribological properties of the silicon carbide ceramic using a pulse-periodic laser treatment, *Comput. Opt.*, vol. 39, pp. 64–69, 2015. https://doi.org/10.18287/0134-2452-2015-39-1-64-69

14. F. Spranger, S. Schirdewahn, M.D.O Lopes, M. Merklein, and K. Hilgenberg, Investigations on TaC localized dispersed X38CrMoV5-3 surfaces with regard to the manufacturing of wear resistant protruded surface textures, *Lasers Manuf. Mater. Process.*, vol. 7, pp. 38–58, 2020. https://doi.org/10.1007/s40516-019-00106-x

15. R. Jagdheesh, J.J. García-Ballesteros, and J.L. Ocaña, One-step fabrication of near superhydrophobic aluminum surface by nanosecond laser ablation, *Appl. Surf. Sci.*, vol. 374, pp. 2–11, 2016. https://doi.org/10.1016/j.apsusc.2015.06.104

16. J. Zhao, J. Guo, P. Shrotriya, Y. Wang, Y. Han, Y. Dong, and S. Yang, A rapid one-step nanosecond laser process for fabrication of super-hydrophilic aluminum surface, *Opt. Laser Technol.*, vol. 117, pp. 134–141, 2019. https://doi.org/10.1016/j.optlastec.2019.04.015

17. Y. Wang, X. Zhao, C. Ke, J. Yu, and R. Wang, Nanosecond laser fabrication of superhydrophobic Ti-6Al-4V surfaces assisted with different liquids, *Colloids Interface Sci. Commun.*, vol. 35, p. 100256, 2019. https://doi.org/10.1016/j.colcom.2020.100256

18. S. Böhm, A. Ahsan, J. Kröger, and J. Witte, Additive surface texturing of cutting tools using pulsed laser implantation with hard ceramic particles, *Prod. Eng.*, vol. 14, pp. 733–742, 2020. https://doi.org/10.1007/s11740-020-00984-7

19. Z. Chen, T. Chang, Q. Wu, C. Liu, H. Chen, and C. Huang, Surface modification of bio-orderly CrTiN thin films with periodic corrugated nanopod structures by picosecond laser ablation, *J. Alloys Compd.*, vol. 938, pp. 168–193, 2023. https://doi.org/10.1016/j.jallcom.2022.168193

20. C. Schultz, M. Fenske, J. Dagar, A. Zeisera, A. Bartelta, R. Schlatmanna, E. Unger, and B. Stegemann, Ablation mechanisms of nanosecond and picosecond laser scribing for metal halide perovskite module interconnection – An experimental and numerical analysis, *Sol. Energy*, vol. 198, pp. 410–418, 2019. https://doi.org/10.1016/j.solener.2020.01.074

21. Z. Yu, G. Yang, W. Zhang, and J. Hu, Investigating the effect of picosecond laser texturing on microstructure and biofunctionalization of titanium alloy, *J. Mater. Process. Technol.*, vol. 255, pp. 129–136, 2018. https://doi.org/10.1016/j.jmatprotec.2017.12.009

22. A. Abdal-hay, R. Staples, A.Alhazaa, B. Fournier, M. Al-Gawati, R.S.B. Lee, and S. Ivanovsk, Fabrication of micropores on titanium implants using femtosecond laser technology: Perpendicular attachment of connective tissues as a pilot study, *Opt. Laser Technol.*, vol. 148, p. 107624, 2021. https://doi.org/10.1016/j.optlastec.2021.107624

23. A.H.A. Lutey, L. Gemini, L. Romoli, G. Lazzini, F. Fuso, M. Faucon, and R. Kling, Towards laser-textured antibacterial surfaces, *Sci. Rep.*, vol. 8, pp. 1–10, 2018. https://doi.org/10.1038/s41598-018-28454-2

24. S. Sarbada and Y.C. Shin, Superhydrophobic contoured surfaces created on metal and polymer using a femtosecond laser, *Appl. Surf. Sci.*, vol. 405, pp. 465–475, 2017. https://doi.org/10.1016/j.apsusc.2017.02.019

25. S. Reyntjens and R. Puers, A review of focused ion beam applications in microsystem technology, *J. Micromech. Microeng.*, vol. 11, pp. 287–300, 2001. https://doi.org/10.1088/0960-1317/11/4/301

26. R.L. Kubena, R.L. Seliger, and E.H. Stevens, High resolution sputtering using a focused ion beam, *Thin Solid Films*, vol. 92, pp. 165–169, 1981. https://doi.org/10.1016/0040-6090

27. D.M. Allen, P. Shore, R.W. Evans, C. Fanara, W. O'Brien, S. Marson, W. O'Neill, Ion beam, focused ion beam, and plasma discharge machining, *CIRP Annals*, vol. 58, pp. 647–662, 2009. https://doi.org/10.1016/j.cirp.2009.09.007

28. C.-S. Kim, S.-H. Ahn, D.-Y. Jang, Review: Developments in micro/nanoscale fabrication by focused ion beams, *Vacuum*, vol. 86, pp. 1014–1035, 2012. https://doi.org/10.1016/j.vacuum.2011.11.004

29. K. Watanabe, J. Schrauwen, A. Leinse, D. V. Thourhout, R. Heideman, and R. Baets, Total reflection mirrors fabricated on silica waveguides with focused ion beam, *Electron. Lett.*, vol. 45, p. 883, 2009. https://doi.org/10.1049/el.2009.0473

30. T.R. Rautray, R. Narayanan, K.-H. Kim, Ion implantation of titanium based biomaterials, *Prog. Mater. Sci.*, vol. 56, pp. 1137–1177, 2011. https://doi.org/10.1016/j.pmatsci.2011.03.002

31. C.W. Kang, F.Z. Fang, State of the art of bioimplants manufacturing: Part II, *Adv. Manuf.*, Vol. 6, pp. 137–154, 2018. https://doi.org/10.1007/s40436-018-0218-9

32. D. Krupa, J. Baszkiewicz, J.A. Kozubowski, A. Barcz, J.W. Sobczak, A. Biliński, M. Lewandowska-Szumieł, B. Rajchel, Effect of phosphorus-ion implantation on the corrosion resistance and biocompatibility of titanium, *Biomaterials*, vol. 23, pp. 3329–3340, 2002. https://doi.org/10.1016/S0142-9612(02)00020-0

33. J.-M. Choi, H.-E. Kim, I.-S. Lee, Ion-beam-assisted deposition (IBAD) of hydroxyapatite coating layer on Ti-based metal substrate, *Biomaterials*, vol. 21, pp. 469–473, 2000. https://doi.org/10.1016/S0142-9612(99)00186-6

34. X.-B. Chen, Y.-C. Li, J.D. Plessis, P.D. Hodgson, Cui'e Wen, Influence of calcium ion deposition on apatite-inducing ability of porous titanium for biomedical applications, *Acta Biomaterialia*, vol. 5, pp. 1808–1820, 2009. https://doi.org/10.1016/j.actbio.2009.01.015

35. M. Yoshinari, Y. Oda, T. Kato, K. Okuda, Influence of surface modifications to titanium on antibacterial activity in vitro, *Biomaterials*, vol. 22, pp. 2043–2048, 2001. https://doi.org/10.1016/S0142-9612(00)00392-6

36. H. Hornberger, S. Virtanen, A.R. Boccaccini, Biomedical coatings on magnesium alloys – A review, *Acta Biomaterialia*, vol. 8, pp. 2442–2455, 2012. https://doi.org/10.1016/j.actbio.2012.04.012

37. P. Kabirifar, K. Chu, F. Ren, and Q. Sun, Effects of grain size on compressive behavior of NiTi polycrystalline superelastic macro- and micropillars, Mater. Lett., vol. 214, pp. 53–55, 2018. https://doi.org/10.1016/j.matlet.2017.11.069

38. R. Kometani, R. Funabiki, T. Hoshino, K. Kanda, Y. Haruyama, T. Kaito, J. Fujita, Y. Ochiai, S. Matsui, Cell wall cutting tool and nano-net fabrication by FIB-CVD for subcellular operations and analysis, *Microelectron. Eng.*, vol. 83, pp. 1642–1645, 2006. https://doi.org/10.1016/j.mee.2006.01.217

39. R. Kometani and S. Ishihara, Nanoelectromechanical device fabrications by 3-D nanotechnology using focused-ion beams, *Sci. Technol. Adv. Mater.*, vol. 10, p. 034501, 2009. https://doi.org/10.1088/1468-6996/10/3/034501

40. F.Z. Cui and Z.S. Luo, Biomaterials modification by ion-beam processing, *Surf. Coat. Technol.*, vol. 112, pp. 278–285, 1999. https://doi.org/10.1016/S0257-8972(98)00763-4

41. L. Tana, R.A. Dodd, and W.C. Cronec, Corrosion and wear-corrosion behavior of NiTi modified by plasma source ion implantation, *Biomaterials*, vol. 24, pp. 3931–3939, 2003. https://doi.org/10.1016/S0142-9612(03)00271-0

42. T.R. Rautray, R. Narayanan, and K. Kim, Ion implantation of titanium based biomaterials, *Prog. Mater. Sci.*, vol. 56, pp. 1137–1177, 2011. https://doi.org/10.1016/J.PMATSCI.2011.03.002

43. J. Kim, H. Lee, T.-S. Jang, D. Kim, C.-B. Yoon, G. Han, H.-E. Kim, H.-D. Jung, Characterization of titanium surface modification strategies for osseointegration enhancement, *Metals*, vol. 11, p. 618, 2021. https://doi.org/10.3390/met11040618

44. Z.Y. Qiu, C. Chen, X.M. Wang, I.S. Lee, Advances in the surface modification techniques of bone-related implants for last 10 years. Regen. *Biomater.*, vol. 1, pp. 67–79, 2014. https://doi.org 10.1093/rb/rbu007

45. C. Chen, I.S. Lee, S. M. Zhang, I.S. Lee, Biomimetic fibronectin/ mineral and osteogenic growth peptide/mineral composites synthesized on calcium phosphate thin films, *Chem. Commun.*, vol. 47, pp. 11056–11058, 2011. https://doi.org/10.1039/C1CC13480A

46. C. Chiappini, C. Almeida, Silicon nanoneedles for drug delivery, In: J.L. Coffer (ed), *Semiconducting Silicon Nanowires for Biomedical Applications*, Woodhead Publishing, pp. 144–167, 2014. ISBN 9780857097668. https://doi.org/10.1533/9780857097712.2.144

47. Y. Fu, L. Wang, Focused ion beam machining and deposition. In: R. Hellborg, H. Whitlow, Y. Zhang, (eds) *Ion Beams in Nanoscience and Technology, Particle Acceleration and Detection*, Springer, Berlin, Heidelberg, 2009. https://doi.org/10.1007/978-3-642-00623-4_20

48. A. Moarrefzadeh, Finite-element simulation of electron beam machining (EBM) process, *Int. J. Multidiscip. Sci. Eng.*, vol. 2, pp. 51–56, 2011.

49. T. Pinto, A. Buxton, K. Neailey, S. Barnes, Surface engineering improvements and opportunities with electron beams. *J. Electrotech. Electron. (E+E)*, vol. 49, pp. 221–225, 2014. ISSN: 0861-4717 (Print), 2603-5421

50. T.M. Pinto, *Development of Novel Applications for the Electron Beam Texturing and Surfi-Sculpt® Processes*, Ph.D. Thesis, University of Warwick, October 2020, http://webcat.warwick.ac.uk/record=b3679348

51. J. Parthasarathy, B. Starly, S. Raman, and A. Christensen, Mechanical evaluation of porous titanium (Ti6Al4 V) structures with electron beam melting (EBM). *J. Mech. Behav. Biomed. Mater.*, vol. 3, pp. 249–259, 2010. https://doi.org/10.1016/j.jmbbm.2009.10.006

52. J. Parthasarathy, B. Starly, S. Raman, A design for the additive manufacture of functionally graded porous structures with tailored mechanical properties for biomedical applications, *J. Manuf. Proc.*, vol. 13, pp. 60–170, 2011. https://doi.org/10.1016/j.jmapro.2011.01.004

53. I. Eldesouky, O. Harrysson, H. West, H. Elhofy, Electron beam melted scaffolds for orthopedic applications, *Addit. Manuf.*, vol. 17, pp. 169–175, 2017. https://doi.org/10.1016/j.addma.2017.08.005

54. A. Ataee, Y. Li, G. Song, C. Wen, 3 - Metal scaffolds processed by electron beam melting for biomedical applications, *Metallic Foam Bone*, pp. 83–110, 2017. https://doi.org/10.1016/B978-0-08-101289-5.00003-2

55. J. Collins Springer, O.L.A. Harrysson, D.J. Marcellin-Little, S.H. Bernacki, In-vitro dermal and epidermal cellular response to titanium alloy implants fabricated with electron beam melting, *Med. Eng. Phys.*, vol. 36, pp. 1367–1372, 2014. https://doi.org/10.1016/j.medengphy.2014.07.004

56. A.A. El-Saftawy, A. Elfalaky, M.S. Ragheb, S.G. Zakhary, Electron beam induced surface modifications of PET film, *Radiat. Phys. Chem.*, vol. 102, pp. 96–102, 2014. https://doi.org/10.1016/j.radphyschem.2014.04.025

57. P.J. Slikkerveer, P.C.P. Bouten, and F.C.M.D. Haas, High quality mechanical etching of brittle materials by powder blasting. *Sensors Actuators, A. Phys.*, vol. 85, pp. 296–303, 2000. https://doi.org/10.1016/S0924-4247(00)00343-5

58. H. Wensink and M.C. Elwenspoek, A closer look at the ductile-brittle transition in solid particle erosion, *Wear*, vol. 253, pp. 1035–43, 2002. https://doi.org/10.1016/S0043-1648(02)00223-5

59. M. Achtsnick, J. Drabbe, A.M. Hoogstrate, and B. Karpuschewski, Erosion behaviour and pattern transfer accuracy of protecting masks for micro-abrasive blasting, *J. Mater. Process. Technol.*, vol. 149, pp. 43–9, 2004. https://doi.org/10.1016/j.jmatprotec.2003.10.037

60. M. Achtsnick, A.M. Hoogstrate, and B. Karpuschewski, Advances in high performance micro abrasive blasting, *CIRP Ann. - Manuf. Technol.*, vol. 54, pp. 281–4, 2005. https://doi.org/10.1016/S0007-8506(07)60103-6

61. E. Belloy, A.G. Pawlowski, A. Sayah, and MAM Gijs, Microfabrication of high-aspect ratio and complex monolithic structures in glass, *J. Microelectromechanical Syst.*, vol. 11, pp. 521–7, 2002. https://doi.org/10.1109/JMEMS.2002.803418

62. E. Belloy, A. Sayah, and M.A.M. Gijs, Powder blasting for three-dimensional microstructuring of glass, *Sensors Actuators, A. Phys.*, vol. 86, pp. 231–237, 2000. https://doi.org/10.1016/S0924-4247(00)00447-7

63. F. Ahmadzadeh, S.S.H. Tsai, M. Papini, Effect of curing parameters and configuration on the efficacy of ultraviolet light curing self-adhesive masks used for abrasive jet micromachining, *Precis. Eng.*, vol. 49, pp. 354–64, 2017. https://doi.org/10.1016/j.precisioneng.2017.03.005

64. R. Melentiev and F. Fang, Fabrication of micro-channels on Co–Cr–Mo joints by micro-abrasive jet direct writing, *J. Manuf. Process.*, vol. 56, pp. 667–677, 2020. https://doi.org/10.1016/j.jmapro.2020.05.022

65. A. Nouhi, M.R. Sookhak Lari, J.K. Spelt, and M. Papini, Implementation of a shadow mask for direct writing in abrasive jet micromachining, *J. Mater. Process. Technol.*, vol. 223, pp. 232–9, 2015. https://doi.org/10.1016/j.jmatprotec.2015.04.007

66. M.R. Sookhak Lari, A. Ghazavi, and M. Papini, A rotating mask system for sculpting of three-dimensional features using abrasive jet micromachining, *J. Mater. Process. Technol.*, vol. 243, pp. 62–74, 2017. https://doi.org/10.1016/j.jmatprotec.2016.12.006

67. R. Melentiev, and F.Z. Fang, Recent advances and challenges of abrasive jet machining, *CIRP J. Manuf. Sci. Technol.*, vol. 22, pp. 1–20, 2018. https://doi.org/10.1016/j.cirpj.2018. 06.001

68. K. Abhishek, S.S. Hiremath, and S. Karunanidhi, A novel approach to produce holes with high degree of cylindricity through Micro-Abrasive Jet Machining (μ-AJM), *CIRP J. Manuf. Sci. Technol.*, vol. 21, pp. 110–119, 2018. https://doi.org/10.1016/J.CIRPJ.2018.02.002

69. S. Ally, J.K. Spelt, and M. Papini, Prediction of machined surface evolution in the abrasive jet micromachining of metals, *Wear*, vol. 292–293, pp. 89–99, 2012. https://doi.org/10.1016/j.wear.2012.05.029

70. G. Shen, J. Zhang, D. Culliton, R. Melentiev, and F. Fang, Tribological study on the surface modification of metal-on-polymer bioimplants, *Front. Mech. Eng.*, vol. 17, pp. 1–13, 2022. https://doi.org/10.1007/s11465-022-0682-6

71. C. Kang, F. Liang, G. Shen, D. Wu, and F. Fang, Study of micro-dimples fabricated on alumina-based ceramics using micro-abrasive jet machining, *J. Mater. Process Technol.*, vol. 297, p. 117181, 2021. https://doi.org/10.1016/j.jmatprotec.2021.117181

72. A.M. Hoogstrate, T. Susuzlu, and B. Karpuschewski, High performance cutting with abrasive waterjets beyond 400 MPa, *Ann. CIRP*, vol. 55, pp. 339–342, 2006. https://doi.org/10.1016/S0007-8506(07)60430-2

73. R. Kovacevic, M. Hashish, R. Mohan, M. Ramulu, T. J. Kim, and E. S. Geskin, State of the art research and development in abrasive waterjet machining, *J. Manuf. Sci. Eng. Trans.*, vol. 119, pp. 776–785, 1997. https://doi.org/10.1115/1.2836824

74. M.C. Kong, D. Axinte, and W. Voice, Aspects of material removal mechanism in plain waterjet milling on gamma titanium aluminide, *J. Mater. Process Technol.*, vol. 210, pp. 573–584, 2010. https://doi.org/10.1016/j.jmatprotec.2009.11.009

75. M. Frotscher, F. Kahleyss, T. Simon, D. Biermann, and G. Eggeler, Achieving small structures in thin NiTi sheets for medical applications with water jet and micro machining: A comparison, *J. Materi. Eng. Perform.*, vol. 20, pp. 776–782, 2011. https://doi.org/10.1007/s11665-010-9789-8

76. M.C. Kong, D. Axinte, and W. Voice, Challenges in using waterjet machining of NiTi shape memory alloys: An analysis of controlled-depth milling, *J. Mater. Process Technol.*, vol. 211, pp. 959–971, 2011. https://doi.org/10.1016/j.jmatprotec.2010.12.015

77. W.F. Adler, The mechanics of liquid impact, In: C. M. Preece (ed), *Treatise on Materials Science and Technology*, Academic Press Inc., London, UK, pp. 132–140, 1979.

78. P.H. Shipway, G. Fowler, and I.R. Pashby, Characteristics of the surface of a titanium alloy following milling with abrasive waterjets, *Wear*, vol. 258, pp. 23–13, 2005. https://doi.org/10.1016/j.wear.2004.04.005

79. G. Fowler, P.H. Shipway, and I.R.Pashby, Abrasive waterjet controlled depth milling of Ti-6Al-4V alloy-an investigation of the role of jet-workpiece traverse speed and abrasive grit size on the characteristics of the milled material, *J. Mater. Process Technol.*, vol. 161, 407–414, 2005. https://doi.org/10.1016/j.jmatprotec.2004.07.069

80. M.C. Kong, S. Anwar, J. Billingham, and D. Axinte, Mathematical modelling of abrasive waterjet footprints for arbitrarily moving jets: Part I - Single straight paths, Int. J. Mach. Tools Manuf., vol. 53, pp. 58–68, 2012. https://doi.org/10.1016/j.ijmachtools.2011.09.010

81. J. Billingham, C.B. Miron, D. Axinte, and M.C. Kong, Mathematical modelling of abrasive waterjet footprints for arbitrarily moving jets: Part II - Overlapped single and multiple straight paths, *Int. J. Mach. Tools Manuf.*, vol. 68, pp. 30–39, 2013. https://doi.org/10.1016/j.ijmachtools.2013.01.003

82. Y.W. Seo, M. Ramulu, and D. Kim, Machinability of titanium alloy (Ti-6Al-4V) by abrasive waterjets, *Proc. Inst. Mech. Eng. Pt B J. Eng. Manuf.*, vol. 217, pp. 1709–1721, 2003. https://doi.org/10.1243/095440503772680631

83. T.N. Deepu Kumar, and D.S. Srinivasu, A generic model for prediction of kerf cross-sectional profile in multipass abrasive waterjet milling at macroscopic scale by considering the jet flow dynamics, *Int. J. Adv. Manuf. Technol.*, vol. 127, pp. 2815–2841, 2023. https://doi.org/https://doi.org/10.1007/s00170-023-11683-9

84. T.N. Deepu Kumar and D.S. Srinivasu, Integration of CFD simulated abrasive waterjet flow dynamics with the material removal model for kerf geometry prediction in overlapped erosion on Ti-6Al-4V alloy, *Simul. Model. Pract. Theory*, vol. 127, p. 102788, 2023. https://doi.org/10.1016/j.simpat.2023.102788

85. Y. Yuan, J. Chen, and H. Gao, Surface profile evolution model for titanium alloy machined using abrasive waterjet, *Int. J. Mech. Sci.*, vol. 240, p. 107911, 2023. https://doi.org/10.1016/j.ijmecsci.2022.107911

86. D.S. Miller, Developments in abrasive waterjets for micromachining, In: *Proceedings of the 2003 WJTA American Waterjet Conference*, Houston. https://doi.org/10.1016/j.jmatprotec.2004.02.041

87. N. Haghbin, J. K. Spelt, and M. Papini, Abrasive waterjet micromachining of channels in metals: Comparison between machining in air and submerged in water, *Int. J. of Mac. Tools and Manuf.*, vol. 88, pp. 108–117, 2015. http://dx.doi.org/10.1016/j.ijmachtools.2014.09.012

88. N. Haghbina, F. Ahmadzadeha, and M. Papini, Masked micro-channel machining in aluminum alloy and borosilicate glass using abrasive water jet micromachining, *J. Manuf. Processes*, vol. 35, pp. 307–316, 2018. https://doi.org/10.1016/j.jmapro.2018.08.017

89. H.-T. Liu, Waterjet technology for machining fine features pertaining to micromachining, *J. Manuf. Processes.*, vol. 12, pp. 8–18, 2010. https://doi.org/10.1016/j.jmapro.2010.01.002

90. H.-T. Liu and E. Schubert, Micro abrasive-waterjet technology, In: M. Kahrizi (ed), *Micromachining Techniques for Fabrication of Micro-and Nanostructures*, Manhattan, New York, USA: InTech; pp. 206–34, 2012. https://doi.org/10.5772/30409

91. D.S. Miller, Micromachining with abrasive waterjets, *J. Mater. Process. Technol.*, vol. 149, pp. 37–42, 2004. https://doi.org/10.1016/j.jmatprotec.2004.02.041

92. T. Nguyen, K. Pang, J. Wang, A preliminary study of the erosion process in micromachining of glasses with a low pressure slurry jet. *Key Eng. Mater.*, vol. 389, pp. 375–380, 2009. https://doi.org/10.4028/www.scientific.net/KEM.389-390.375

93. T. Nguyen and J. Wang, A review on the erosion mechanisms in abrasive waterjet micromachining of brittle materials, *Int. J. Extrem. Manuf.*, vol. 1, p. 012006, 2019. https://doi.org/10.1088/2631-7990/ab1028

94. J. Wang, T. Nguyan, and K.L. Pang, Mechanism of microhole formation on glasses by an abrasive slurry jet, *J. Appl. Sci.*, vol. 105, p. 044906, 2009. https://doi.org/10.1063/1.3079802

95. K.L. Pang, T. Nguyen, J.M. Fan, and J. Wang, Machining of micro-channels on brittle glass using an abrasive slurry jet, *Key Eng. Mater.*, vol. 443, pp. 639–644, 2010. https://doi.org/10.4028/www.scientific.net/KEM.443.639

96. H. Nouraei, A. Wodoslawsky, M. Papini, and J.K. Spelt, Characteristics of abrasive slurry jet micromachining: A comparison with abrasive air jet micromachining, *J. Mater. Process. Technol.*, vol. 213, pp. 1711–1724, 2013. https://doi.org/10.1016/j.jmatprotec.2013.03.024

97. M. Hashish, Performance of high-pressure abrasive suspension jet system, *Am. Soc. Mech. Eng. Prod. Eng. Div. Pub.*, vol. 67, pp. 199–207, 1993. https://doi.org/10.1007/s00170-015-7769-8

98. H.-T. Liu, Near-net shaping of optical surfaces with abrasive suspension jets, *14th Int. Conference on Jetting Technology, Brugge*, pp. 285–294, 1998. https://doi.org/10.1016/j.procir.2019.03.228

99. N. Haghbin, F. Ahmadzadeh, J.K. Spelt, and M. Papini, Micromachining of channels using a high pressure abrasive slurry jet machine (HASJM), *The 4M/ICOMM2015 Conference on Micro Manufacturing, Milan*, pp. 459–462, 2015. https://doi.org/10.3850/978-981-09-4609-8_110

100. N. Haghbin, F. Ahmadzadeh, J. K. Spelt, and M. Papini, High pressure abrasive slurry jet micromachining using slurry entrainment, *Int. J. Adv. Manuf. Technol.*, vol. 84, pp. 1031–1043, 2016. https://doi.org/10.1007/s00170-015-7769-8

101. M. Moghaddam, I. Hajiyev, and M. Papin, Prediction and mechanism of surface evolution in high-pressure slurry jet micromachining of channels, *Precis. Eng.*, vol. 82, pp. 251–269, 2023. https://doi.org/10.1016/j.precisioneng.2023.04.003

Chapter 9

Nanocomposites in Cytotoxicity and Targeted Drug Delivery Applications

Jitender Kumar, Hemant Kumar, Rajesh Kumar, and Pramod Kumar

9.1 INTRODUCTION

Nanocomposites represent a class of materials composed of more than two different components at the nanometer scale, where at least one component is a nanoparticle. These nanomaterials have garnered significant attention because of their exceptional thermal, electrical, mechanical and optical properties, which often surpass those of conventional materials. They can be either organic or inorganic and their physicochemical features, which include shape, dimension, chemical composition, and functionality, can be easily modified. When nanoparticles are incorporated into a matrix material such as carbon-based materials, polymers, or ceramics, nanocomposites are created that have better or more synergistic qualities than the sum of their separate parts (Omanović-Mikličanin et al. 2020).

The fact that nanocomposites can potentially be customized to fulfil certain performance standards by altering the type, size, and concentration of the nanofillers is one of its main advantages. Nanoparticles that are frequently employed as reinforcements in nanocomposites include metal oxides, carbon nanotubes, graphene, nanoclays, and quantum dots (QDs). The homogeneous dispersion of these nanoparticles inside the matrix creates a three-dimensional network that strengthens the material at the nanoscale. The unique features and a wide range of uses of nanocomposites, which are made up of nanoparticles scattered throughout a matrix material, have attracted a lot of interest in a number of sectors, including biomedicine (J. Kumar and Roy 2024; Hassan et al. 2021; Mohan, Kumar, and Roy 2023). In particular, their use in cytotoxicity assessment and targeted drug delivery has shown promising results, offering potential solutions to challenges faced in conventional therapeutic approaches.

Sol-gel processing, chemical vapour deposition, electrospinning, and in situ polymerization are some of the processes often used to precisely regulate the size, shape, content, and dispersion of nanoparticles inside the matrix material during the production of nanocomposites. By incorporating nanoparticles into the matrix, nanocomposites exhibit synergistic properties that surpass those of the individual components. Reducing material

DOI: 10.1201/9781003470311-9

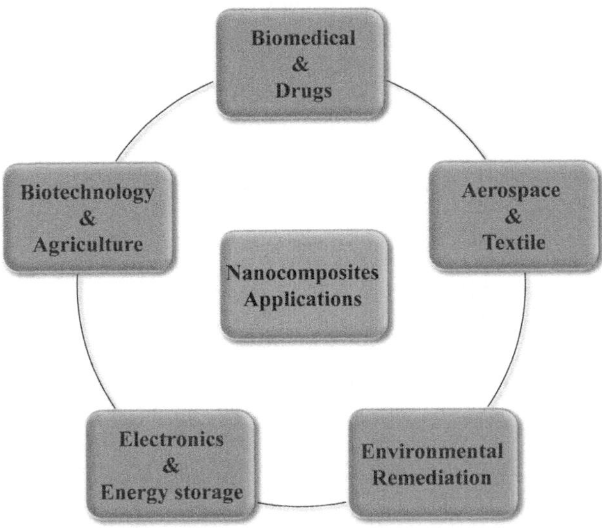

Figure 9.1 Various applications of nanocomposites.

dimensions to the nanometer scale generates phase interfaces crucial for enhancing material properties (Ravichandran et al. 2018). The relationship between the surface area-to-volume ratio of the reinforced material utilized in nanocomposite preparation directly contributes to comprehending the structure–property relationship. This ratio is essential to understanding how the material's nanoscale structure affects its qualities. Therefore, understanding and controlling this relationship is fundamental for optimizing the performance of nanocomposite materials.

Nanocomposites present novel opportunities across diverse sectors, including medical, pharmaceuticals, food packaging, electronics, and energy, as shown in Figure 9.1. They offer innovative solutions to various challenges by leveraging unique properties at the nanoscale. As an example, they have the potential to significantly impact a number of medical applications, including delivery of drugs, implanted devices, photothermal treatment, imaging for diagnosis, and nucleic acid delivery. Targeted and controlled release of therapeutic agents is made possible by nanocomposite-based drug delivery systems, which increase treatment effectiveness while reducing systemic toxicity and adverse effects (Hassan et al. 2021). Additionally, nanocomposites can serve as scaffolds for tissue regeneration, providing mechanical support and biochemical cues for cell growth and differentiation.

This book chapter aims to explore various aspects of nanocomposites; also it provides an overview of the potential cytotoxic effects associated with different nanocomposites used in biomedical applications. Furthermore, it discusses their potential applications in drug delivery systems, highlighting their significance in the field of medicine. Lastly, the chapter delves into future prospects and emerging trends in nanocomposite research, emphasizing the importance of understanding their properties and potential impact on human health for advancing biomedical technologies.

9.2 TYPES OF NANOCOMPOSITES

The presence or absence of a polymeric component divides nanocomposites into two categories. Those containing polymers are termed polymer-based nanocomposites, while those lacking polymeric material are referred to as non-polymer-based or inorganic nanocomposites. The latter is further subdivided into three classes, as illustrated in Figure 9.2.

9.2.1 Polymer Nanocomposites (PNCs)

These nanocomposites have become an intriguing category of materials, characterized by a distinct blend of properties resulting from the integration of nanoscale fillers into a polymer matrix. This integration provides superior mechanical, thermal, and barrier properties compared to pure polymers. The particular type of polymer matrix and nanoparticles included determines their classification. There are two primary categories of polymers: natural and synthetic (Feldman 2016; Fu et al. 2019). Natural polymers are sourced from natural materials and can be extracted for various applications. Examples of these polymers include silk, wool, cellulose, proteins, and DNA many of which are dependent on water. On the other hand, synthetic polymers are created artificially using chemical methods. Synthetic polymers encompass a variety of materials, such as nylon, polyester, Teflon, and epoxy. PNCs can be prepared by integrating several kinds of inorganic nanofillers into a polymer matrix, including metal nanoclays,

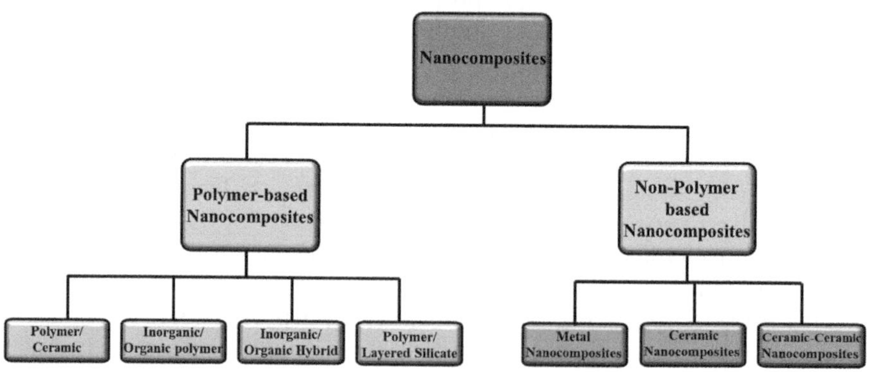

Figure 9.2 Schematic representation of classification of nanocomposites.

carbon nanomaterials and metal-oxide nanoparticles. The qualities of the composite material are improved by the addition of nanofillers, which customizes them to fit the demands of a certain application.

9.2.1.1 Clay–Polymer Nanocomposites (CPNs)

A family of cutting-edge materials known as CPNs is made up of clay nanoparticles scattered throughout a polymer matrix. In comparison to traditional polymers, these nanocomposites provide a special blend of mechanical, thermal, barrier, and flame-retardant qualities that come from both the clay nanoparticles and the polymer matrix. Typically, layered silicates such montmorillonite, kaolinite, and halloysite are utilized as clay nanoparticles in CPNs. Owing to their huge surface area and high aspect ratio, these nanoparticles can participate in extensive interactions with the polymer matrix. Improved mechanical qualities, such as greater stiffness, strength, and toughness, may result from the interaction between the clay nanoparticles and the polymer chains. This reinforcing effect results from the clay nanoparticles and polymer matrix forming a strong interface that limits the mobility of the polymer chains and stops fracture progression. CPNs are appropriate for applications needing gas and moisture barrier qualities because of their outstanding barrier qualities. Reduced permeability through the nanocomposite is caused by the high aspect ratio and layered structure of the clay nanoparticles, which meander gas molecules along convoluted diffusion paths (Kotal and Bhowmick 2015).

9.2.1.2 Carbon Nanotube (CNT) Polymer Nanocomposites

A family of cutting-edge materials known as CNT polymer nanocomposites combines the adaptability of polymers with the special qualities of carbon nanotubes. All CNTs are cylinder-shaped nanostructures with remarkable mechanical, thermal, and electrical characteristics. The process of integrating carbon nanotubes (CNTs) into polymer matrices can provide nanocomposites that possess improved mechanical strength, electrical conductivity, thermal stability, and other favourable attributes. Typically, solution mixing, melt blending, or in situ polymerization are used to disperse CNTs inside a polymer matrix in order to fabricate CNT polymer nanocomposites (Chen et al. 2018). For the final nanocomposite material to function at its best, the CNTs must be properly dispersed and aligned inside the polymer matrix. The tuneable features of CNT polymer nanocomposites are one of its main advantages. These qualities may be adjusted by varying the polymer matrix composition, dispersion technique, and CNT concentration. These nanocomposites have demonstrated potential in a variety of applications, including energy storage, automotive, electronics, and biomedicine, in addition to their mechanical and electrical qualities

The synthesis of bromine-terminated poly(styrene) and its grafting onto multi-walled carbon nanotubes (MWCNTs) were achieved by Chen et al. by the use of the atom transfer radical polymerization (ATRP) technology (Liu and Chen 2007). In the process of grafting, the bromine atoms from poly(styrene) were affixed to the carbon nanotube surface, acting as catalysts for further polymerization. The carbon nanotube–poly(styrene) surfaces were then used to commence a surface-initiated ATRP of poly(N-isopropylacrylamide).

9.2.1.3 Graphene–Polymer Nanocomposites

A hexagonally lattice of carbon atoms organized in two dimensions is scattered inside a polymer matrix to form graphene–polymer nanocomposites. With the processability and adaptability of polymers combined with the remarkable qualities of graphene – such as its vast surface area, great mechanical strength, and outstanding electrical conductivity – this combination is possible. Three common polymer matrices are polyvinyl alcohol (PVA), polycarbonate, and poly(methyl methacrylate) (PMMA). Mechanical strength, electrical conductivity, thermal conductivity, and barrier qualities are just a few of the features that may significantly improve the polymer's ability to incorporate graphene. Biomedical devices, electronics, energy storage, and coatings are just a few of the domains in which these nanocomposites have found use (K. Hu et al. 2014; Sun et al. 2021). In electronics, they are used for flexible and conductive substrates, electromagnetic interference shielding, and sensors. Thanks to their excellent electrical conductivity and huge surface area, graphene–polymer composites are used in energy storage devices such as batteries, fuel cells, and supercapacitors. They are being investigated for biosensors, scaffolds for tissue engineering, and drug delivery devices in the biomedical industry.

9.2.2 Ceramic Nanocomposites

Ceramic nanocomposites combine ceramic matrices with nanoscale reinforcing agents, offering a range of enhanced properties compared to traditional ceramics. Due to meticulous atomic and molecular engineering aimed at achieving specific capabilities, nanocomposites exhibit remarkable adaptability and find extensive applications across various sectors. These nanocomposites are created by incorporating nanoscale reinforcements, such as carbon nanotubes, graphene, or ceramic nanoparticles, into the ceramic matrix. This integration enhances the properties of the resulting composite material, allowing it to fulfill a wide array of applications. The presence of nanoscale reinforcements inhibits crack propagation and improves the overall fracture resistance of the composite, making it highly durable and damage-tolerant (Mera et al. 2015).

The composite's thermal conductivity can be greatly increased by adding high-thermal conductivity nanoscale fillers, such as boron nitride or alumina nanoparticles. This makes the composite appropriate for uses requiring effective heat dissipation, such as thermal management in electronics or aerospace components. Similarly, the incorporation of conductive nanomaterials like carbon nanotubes or graphene can impart electrical conductivity to the ceramic matrix, enabling applications in electronic devices, sensors, and electromagnetic shielding.

Advanced processing methods like sol-gel, chemical vapour deposition, or mechanical alloying are frequently used in the production of ceramic nanocomposites. These methods allow for exact control over the distribution, content, and structure of nanoparticles inside the ceramic matrix.

9.2.2.1 Ceramic-Matrix Nanocomposites (CMNCs)

Here ceramic matrices are reinforced with nanoscale fillers to enhance their mechanical, thermal, and functional properties such as alumina (Al_2O_3), zirconia (ZrO_2), or silicon carbide (SiC), within a ceramic matrix. Because of the special qualities that these nanocomposites provide, which come from both the ceramic matrix and the nanoscale reinforcements, they are very appealing for a variety of applications (Omanović-Mikličanin et al. 2020). They have improved mechanical qualities in addition to excellent thermal characteristics. Better heat transfer properties are produced by the high aspect ratio and dispersion of nanoscale fillers in combination with the high thermal conductivity of ceramic matrices. This makes CMNCs ideal for applications requiring thermal management, such as heat sinks in electronic devices, thermal barrier coatings, and high-temperature structural components.

9.2.3 Metal-Matrix Nanocomposites (MMNCs)

MMNCs combine the properties of metals with the unique characteristics of nanoscale reinforcements. To improve mechanical, thermal, electrical, and other functional qualities, these reinforcements, typically in the form of nanoparticles or nanofibers – are inserted into a metallic matrix. One common approach for fabricating MMNCs involves techniques such as powder metallurgy, mechanical alloying, and electrodeposition. During fabrication, the nanoscale reinforcements are uniformly dispersed within the metal matrix, ensuring intimate contact and strong bonding between the two phases. This dispersion is crucial for optimizing the properties of the resulting composite material. MMNCs exhibit several advantageous properties compared to conventional metal alloys or monolithic metals. To further increase the mechanical strength and stiffness of the composite, for example, nanoscale reinforcements with high strength-to-weight ratios, such graphene or carbon nanotubes, can be added. Additionally, the large surface area of nanoparticles can enhance thermal conductivity and electrical conductivity, making MMNCs suitable for applications requiring efficient heat dissipation or electrical conduction (Yoo et al. 2023; Z. Hu et al. 2016).

9.2.4 Hybrid Nanocomposites

The goal of hybrid nanocomposites is to spread metal, ceramic, polymer, carbon nanotube, and graphene nanoparticles as well as other nanoparticle kinds inside a single matrix material to produce synergistic characteristics and functions. Hybrid nanocomposites are made by layer-by-layer construction, chemical vapour deposition, electrospinning, in-situ polymerization, and solution mixing, among other techniques. Compared to typical composites or their separate components, they have improved mechanical, electrical, thermal, and optical characteristics. The synergistic interactions between different types of nanoparticles lead to unique functionalities, such as improved conductivity, thermal stability, and light absorption. By carefully selecting and controlling the composition, morphology, and dispersion of nanofillers, researchers can fine-tune the performance of hybrid nanocomposites for targeted applications (Sanchez et al. 2003). By incorporating bioactive nanoparticles or functionalized nanomaterials into biocompatible matrices, hybrid nanocomposites enable controlled drug release, enhanced cellular interactions, and improved imaging contrast for diagnostic purposes.

Li et al. used hematite as precursors and templates for magnetic iron oxide to create the hybrid nanocomposites (iron oxide@SiO_2-Au@C) in a variety of forms, such as peanut, ellipsoid, and pseudocube (Figure 9.3) (Li et al. 2015). The silica and carbon layers were equally distributed with small AuNPs, around 6 nm in size. Effective aggregation prevention and reduced metal nanocrystal loss during recycling procedures were achieved by the deliberate embedding of the nanoparticles into the two separate layers.

9.2.5 Bio-Nanocomposites

Bio-nanocomposites incorporate biodegradable nanoparticles, such as cellulose nanocrystals or chitosan nanoparticles, within a biopolymer matrix derived from natural sources. These nanocomposites are ideal for biomedical and ecological purposes because of their controlled release characteristics, long-term viability and biological compatibility. In tissue engineering and regenerative medicine, bio-nanocomposites are essential components in biomedical applications. These materials provide an environment that is perfect for cell adhesion, proliferation, and differentiation by imitating the extracellular matrix. Biopolymer matrices, such collagen

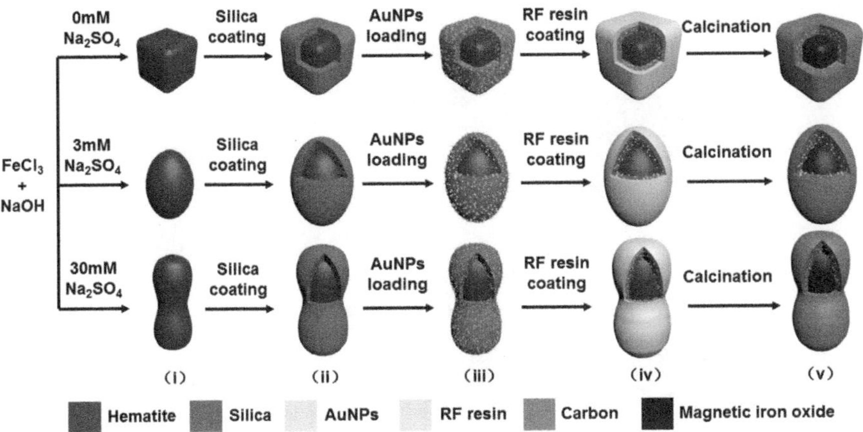

Figure 9.3 Diagrammatic representation of the synthesis of iron oxide@SiO$_2$–Au@C nanocomposites (reported with permission (Li et al. 2015), ©American Chemical Society).

and chitosan, which are reinforced with nanoparticles like graphene or hydroxyapatite, provide better mechanical strength and bioactivity, which makes them appropriate for use as scaffolds in the regeneration of bone and cartilage. Moreover, bio-nanocomposites serve as drug delivery systems, enabling controlled release of therapeutics to targeted sites (Kulkarni 2021). Nanoparticle-loaded biopolymers provide sustained release profiles, improving drug efficacy and reducing side effects in treatments for cancer, infections, and chronic diseases.

9.3 CYTOTOXICITY OF NANOCOMPOSITES

There are numerous applications of nanocomposites in different fields including biomedical and drug delivery as shown in Figure 9.4. Thus, the evaluation of cytotoxicity, or the toxic effects on cells or tissues, is crucial for assessing the biocompatibility and safety of nanocomposites intended for biomedical and other applications. Exposure to nanomaterials has been associated with various health issues including allergies, neurotoxicity, pulmonary toxicity, fibrosis, and haematological toxicity. These issues highlight how crucial it is to fully comprehend the potential hazards connected to exposure to nanomaterials. Many physicochemical properties of nanocomposites, such as shape, dimension, area of surface, chemical makeup, and stability, are hypothesized to affect their hazardous effects (Zhao et al. 2011; Lewinski, Colvin, and Drezek 2008). These characteristics have the potential to greatly affect how biological systems and nanomaterials interact, which in turn can affect the toxicity profiles of the latter. However,

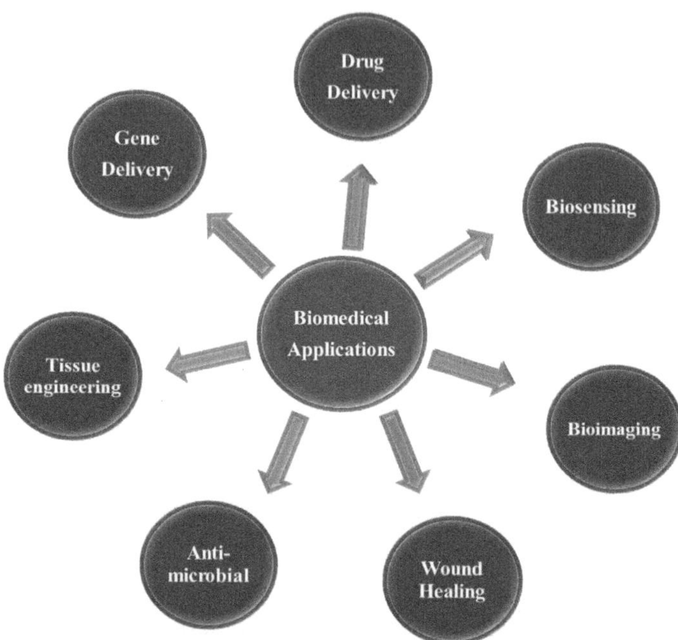

Figure 9.4 Various applications of nanocomposites in biomedicine.

determining a nanocomposite's toxicity in vitro (in a lab environment) and in vivo (in a living creature) can be difficult, costly, and time-consuming because of their complex and diverse nature. In vitro studies involve exposing cell cultures to nanomaterials and evaluating their effects on cellular viability, morphology, and function. In vivo studies, on the other hand, involve administering nanomaterials to living organisms and monitoring their physiological responses, organ function, and overall health.

Traditional cytotoxicity assays, such as the MTT assay and live/dead cell staining, have been adapted for use with nanocomposites to assess their impact on cell viability, proliferation, and morphology. Nanocomposites designed for biomedical applications must demonstrate minimal cytotoxicity to ensure their suitability for in vitro and in vivo use. Furthermore, the cytotoxicity profile and cellular interactions of nanocomposites can be influenced by their physicochemical features, such as dimensions, charge on the surface, and functionalization of the surface. There are various methods for determining the potential cytotoxicity of nanocomposites.

9.3.1 Cell Viability Assays

Cell viability assays measure the metabolic activity or membrane integrity of cells. It can be determined using a variety of techniques, each with unique

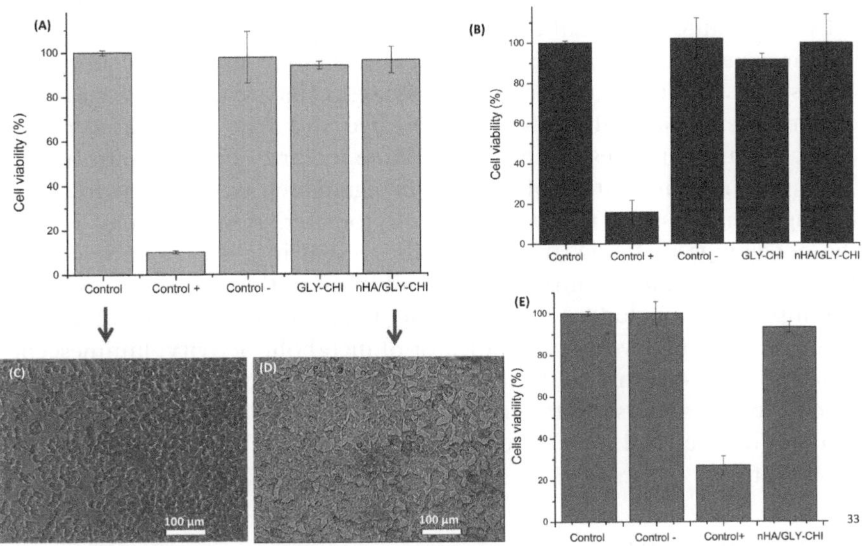

Figure 9.5 (A) SAOS (B) HEK293T cells' viability response as measured by the MTT test during a 24-hour incubation period in contact with the GLY-CHI extracts (C) nHA/GLY-CHI. nHA/GLY-CHI (200×) and (E) HBMS cells survival response by MTT test following 48 hours of incubation in close contact with the nHA/GLY-CHI (reported with permission (Dumont et al. 2016), ©Elsevier).

benefits, restrictions, and uses. The MTT (3-(4,5-dimethylthiazol-2-yl)-2,5-diphenyltetrazolium bromide) assay or the MTS (3-(4,5-dimethylthiazol-2-yl)-5-(3-carboxymethoxyphenyl)-2-(4-sulfophenyl)-2H-tetrazolium) assay are two of the most widely used assays for determining cell viability. The tetrazolium salt is transformed by living cells in these assays into a colored formazan product that can be measured by spectrophotometry. There exists a clear correlation between the quantity of viable cells in the culture and the intensity of color generated. Dumont et al. synthesized biocomposites using nano-hydroxyapatite (nHA) particles integrated into glycol chitosan (GLY-CHI) matrices (Dumont et al. 2016). Figure 9.5 illustrates the MTT test they used to examine cytotoxicity and cell viability evaluations on three different cell lines. The research results demonstrated the critical function of the GLY-CHI ligand in promoting the formation, expansion, and colloidal stability of calcium phosphate particles at nanoscale sizes, leading to a restricted size distribution with an average diameter of 74 ± 15 nm.

An additional often employed technique to evaluate cell viability is the trypan blue exclusion experiment. Trypan blue, a dye that only stains non-viable cells with damaged cell membranes, is used to stain the cells in this experiment. Under a microscope, live cells have unstained membranes that reject the dye, making them seem unstained, whereas non-viable cells look blue. One can then manually count the number of viable and non-viable cells or use automated cell counts.

Flow cytometry is another powerful technique used for cell viability assessment. In flow cytometry-based assays, cells are labeled with fluorescent markers that distinguish between live and dead cells based on specific cellular properties, such as membrane integrity or enzymatic activity. Through the examination of fluorescent signals released by individual cells during their passage through a flow cytometer, scientists may measure the percentage of living and dead cells present in a specimen (Goudarzi, Salavati-Niasari, and Amiri 2019). In addition to these methods, other cell viability assays include ATP (adenosine triphosphate) assays, which measure cellular ATP levels as an indicator of metabolic activity; luminescence-based assays, such as the CellTiter-Glo assay, which quantify ATP levels using a luminescent substrate; and impedance-based assays, which measure changes in electrical impedance caused by cell attachment, spreading, and proliferation.

9.3.2 Cell Proliferation Assays

The capacity of cells to divide and multiply in the presence of nanocomposites is evaluated using tests for cell proliferation. One common approach to cell proliferation assays is based on detecting cellular metabolic activity, which is often indicative of cell viability and proliferation. These assays typically utilize colorimetric, luminescent readouts to measure cellular metabolic activity indirectly, often through the conversion of a substrate into a detectable signal by viable cells (Koyanagi, Kawakabe, and Arimura 2016). For instance, resazurin-based assays (e.g., alamarBlue) and the MTT test, as well as the XTT (2,3-bis-(2-methoxy-4-nitro-5-sulfophenyl)-2H-tetr azolium-5-carboxanilide) assay, are frequently used to evaluate cell viability and proliferation based on metabolic activity.

Another approach to cell proliferation assays involves directly quantifying DNA synthesis, a key indicator of cell proliferation. It is possible to specifically identify proliferating cells by incorporating nucleotide analogs, such as 5-ethynyl-2′-deoxyuridine (EdU) or bromodeoxyuridine (BrdU), into freshly generated DNA. Subsequent detection of these labeled cells using immunocytochemistry or click chemistry-based assays enables researchers to assess cell proliferation and DNA synthesis with high specificity and sensitivity (Buck et al. 2008). In these assay, the amount of metabolically active cells is correlated with the intensity of the colored or fluorescent product that is produced when viable cells break down the colorless or faintly fluorescent substrate. By measuring the absorbance, fluorescence, or luminescence of the reaction product, researchers can quantify cell proliferation and viability in response to different experimental conditions, such as drug treatments, growth factors, or environmental stressors.

9.3.3 Morphological Analysis

One of the primary objectives of morphological analysis in nanocomposites cytotoxicity assessment is to examine the structural changes induced in cells upon exposure to nanocomposites. Techniques such as optical microscopy, fluorescence microscopy, and electron microscopy enable researchers to visualize and analyse alterations in cellular morphology, including changes in cell shape, size, organelle structure, and membrane integrity. For example, optical microscopy can provide insights into gross morphological changes such as cell rounding, shrinkage, or membrane blebbing, which are indicative of cytotoxic effects. Additionally, fluorescence microscopy coupled with fluorescent dyes or markers allows for the visualization of specific cellular structures or processes, such as cytoskeletal organization, nuclear morphology, or intracellular organelles. By labeling cells with fluorescent probes targeting specific cellular components, researchers can assess nanocomposite-induced changes at the subcellular level, providing detailed information on cellular responses and potential cytotoxic mechanisms. Hemant et al. prepared folic acid-conjugated mesoporous silica nanocomposites (FA/DOX@Silica) for targeted delivery of DOX, which is a fluorescent anticancer drug. They used fluorescent microscopy to determine the cell morphology and cellular uptake of the drug (H. Kumar, Kumar, et al. 2022). Strong morphological analysis methods are used to look at ultrastructural alterations in cells exposed to nanocomposites using transmission electron microscopy (TEM) and scanning electron microscopy (SEM). These techniques offer high-resolution imaging capabilities, allowing researchers to examine nanoscale alterations such as mitochondrial damage, endoplasmic reticulum stress, or nanoparticle internalization within cells.

9.3.4 Apoptosis and Necrosis Assays

Assays for necrosis and apoptosis evaluate the processes of cell death after exposure to nanocomposites. Programmed cell death, or apoptosis, is a highly controlled mechanism that keeps tissues in a homeostasis. Several assays are commonly employed to detect and quantify apoptosis in cells exposed to nanocomposites. TUNEL assay (terminal deoxynucleotidyl transferase dUTP nick end labeling) is the most widely used technique in apoptosis research. It is able to identify DNA fragmentation, which is a characteristic of apoptotic cell death. TUNEL tests mark the free 3′-OH ends of DNA strand breaks produced during apoptosis using fluorescently tagged nucleotides. Flow cytometry or fluorescence microscopy is then employed to measure the degree of DNA fragmentation in treated cells (Hasanzadeh, Shadjou, and de la Guardia 2017).

A different technique is called annexin V labeling, which uses a protein to attach to phosphatidylserine that is externalized on the outer membrane of dying cells. Annexin V staining assays utilize fluorescently labeled annexin V to detect apoptotic cells (Kuku et al. 2016). By combining annexin V staining with a viability dye such as propidium iodide (PI), different stages of apoptosis can be distinguished (early apoptosis vs. late apoptosis/necrosis) using flow cytometry. Caspase activity assays, here fluorogenic substrates specific for caspases, such as caspase-3, -8, and -9, can be used to measure caspase activity in treated cells. Upon cleavage by active caspases, these substrates release fluorescent signals that can be quantified using fluorescence microscopy or plate readers.

Next, the death of cells that exhibits enlargement of the cell, rupture of the plasma membrane, and discharge of the contents of the cell is called necrosis. Here, propidium iodide (PI) staining is commonly is used where PI is a membrane impermeable dye that binds to nucleic acids of dead or permeabilized cells. PI staining assays are commonly used to assess necrotic cell death. To determine the proportion of PI-positive cells after being exposed to nanocomposites, cells are labeled with PI and examined using fluorescence microscopy or flow cytometry (Wiemann et al. 2016).

An additional test is the release of the cytoplasmic enzyme lactate dehydrogenase (LDH), which is a characteristic of necrotic cell death and is released into the extracellular media when the plasma membrane is damaged (Oh et al. 2014). LDH release assays measure the activity of LDH in cell culture supernatants using colorimetric or fluorometric assays. Increased LDH activity indicates cellular necrosis.

9.3.5 Inflammatory Response Assays

Assays measuring inflammatory response are essential for assessing the possible cytotoxic effects of nanocomposites and providing insight into their immunomodulatory characteristics. These assays are indispensable tools for assessing the inflammatory response induced by nanocomposite exposure, as inflammation is a fundamental aspect of the body's defense mechanism against foreign substances.

One of the key assays used to assess the inflammatory response to nanocomposites is the measurement of cytokine release. Cytokines are signaling molecules secreted by immune cells in response to stimuli, including exposure to nanomaterials. The method known as enzyme-linked immunosorbent assay (ELISA) is frequently used to measure the production of pro-inflammatory cytokines from immune cells that have been exposed to nanocomposites, including interleukin (IL-1β), IL-6, and tumor necrosis factor-alpha (TNF-α) (Afsharnezhad et al. 2014). By quantifying cytokine levels in cell culture supernatants, researchers can discern the extent of the inflammatory response triggered by nanocomposite exposure. Moreover, multiplex cytokine assays enable the simultaneous quantification of multiple cytokines in a single sample, providing a comprehensive assessment of the inflammatory milieu. These assays offer insights into the intricate network of inflammatory mediators involved in the response to nanocomposites, allowing researchers to identify potential patterns or synergistic effects among different cytokines.

Apart from cytokine analysis, gene expression analysis offers significant insights about the transcriptional reaction of immune cells upon exposure to nanoparticles. To measure alterations in the expression levels of genes responsible for producing pro-inflammatory cytokines, chemokines, and other inflammatory mediators, researchers employ a technique known as quantitative real-time polymerase chain reaction, abbreviated as qRT-PCR. This method allows for precise quantification of gene expression levels in response to various stimuli or treatments. By examining the transcriptional profile of immune cells treated with nanocomposites, researchers can elucidate the underlying molecular mechanisms driving the inflammatory response.

Flow cytometry is another indispensable tool for evaluating the inflammatory response to nanocomposites. This technique allows for the quantitative analysis of immune cell populations and the expression of cell surface markers associated with inflammation. Major histocompatibility complex (MHC) class II, CD80, CD86, and other surface markers that are increased during activation and influence the inflammatory response may be identified on immune cells by staining them with fluorescently labeled antibodies (Maisanaba et al. 2015). Flow cytometry provides valuable insights into changes in immune cell phenotype and activation status following exposure to nanocomposites.

Furthermore, the measurement of nitric oxide (NO) production serves as a marker of inflammation and immune activation. NO is a key signaling molecule involved in various physiological processes, including inflammation. The Griess test is a colorimetric method that measures the amount of NO produced by immune cells when they come into contact with nanocomposites. By measuring NO levels in cell culture supernatants, researchers can assess the degree of immune cell activation and the intensity of the inflammatory response induced by nanocomposite exposure.

9.4 NANOCOMPOSITES IN DRUG DELIVERY

Ensuring that the drugs reaches to its target location within the body while limiting the possibility of harmful effects on healthy organs is one of the main challenges in drug delivery. This challenge becomes particularly daunting in cancer therapy, where tumors can manifest as discrete metastases in different organs. As systemic toxicity and off-target effects are reduced, drug delivery methods are being developed to maximize the effectiveness and selectivity of medicinal medicines. Given their capacity to encapsulate, shield, and administer medications to certain cellular or tissue targets, nano-composites have special benefits for targeted drug administration. In order to efficiently transport medications to specific tumor areas, the majority of them have the capacity to circulate in the circulation for lengthy periods of time without being eliminated.

A careful balance must be achieved by nanocomposites used in drug delivery systems: they must be sufficiently big to stop fast leaking into blood capillaries but tiny enough to avoid being picked up by stationary macro-phages in the reticuloendothelial system. In the vasculature of tumors with increased permeability, the size range of gap junctions between endothelial cells typically falls between 100 and 600 nm. In comparison, the sinusoids found in the spleen and fenestrae of Kupffer cells in the liver typically have a size range of around 150 nm. These variations in size play a crucial role in regulating the passage of molecules and cells across these endothelial barriers, influencing physiological processes such as immune surveillance and tumor progression. Hence, nanoparticles ideally should be sized up to 100 nm to effectively traverse these specific vascular structures and reach tumor tissues.

For nanocomposites to avoid being engulfed by macrophages, their sur-face should ideally be hydrophilic. Two approaches can be used to do this: either cover the surface of the nanocomposites with a hydrophilic poly-mer (PEG, PAA, etc.) that repels plasma proteins and protects them from opsonization, or build nanoparticles from block copolymers that have both hydrophilic and hydrophobic domains. Surface functionalization of nano-composites with targeting ligands, such as antibodies, peptides, or aptam-ers, enables selective recognition and binding to cell surface receptors, facilitating targeted drug delivery (Sofi et al. 2019; Cui, Li, and Decher 2016). Stimulus-responsive nanocomposites also have the ability to release medications in response to particular environmental signals, such pH, tem-perature, or enzymatic activity, which improves both their biocompatibility and therapeutic effectiveness.

9.4.1 Non-Covalent and Covalent Drug Delivery

The reversible connection between drug molecules and carrier materials by non-covalent forces such hydrogen bonding, electrostatic contacts, hydro-phobic interactions, and van der Waals forces is known as non-covalent drug delivery. In practical terms, non-covalent drug delivery utilizing nanocomposites typically involves either encapsulating the drug within the nanostructure or creating a stabilizing pocket for the drug (encapsulation refers to the process of entrapping the drug molecules within the interior space or matrix of the nanoparticle). This can be accomplished in a number of ways, including solvent evaporation, emulsion-based approaches, and self-assembly procedures, in which the drug molecules are encircled and shielded by the nanoparticle material. On the other hand, a stabilizing pocket involves embedding the drug molecules onto the surface or within the structure of the nanoparticle, creating a protective environment that stabilizes the drug and prevents degradation or premature release (Doane and Burda 2013). This approach ensures that the drug remains intact and effectively delivered to the target site when administered to the patient.

This method has a number of advantages, such as ease of preparation, flexibility in selecting carrier materials, and the capacity to administer a broad variety of medications with different physicochemical characteristics. Among the non-covalent drug delivery methods are cyclodextrin-based carriers, liposomes, micelles, and nanoparticles. These systems can encapsulate drugs within their structures or adsorb drugs onto their surfaces, providing protection from degradation, improved solubility, and controlled release kinetics. The therapeutic efficacy of drugs can be maintained by creating non-covalent drug delivery methods without actually changing the drug molecule. This approach ensures that the drug retains its inherent properties and pharmacological activity, which is crucial for achieving desired therapeutic outcomes. Lastly, drugs attached to nanoparticles without covalent bonds can be released from the nano-platform without the need for outside stimulation. Rather, shifts in the physiological milieu nearby, including fluctuations in pH, temperature, or enzyme concentration, are what cause them to release. This inherent responsiveness to environmental cues enables precise control over drug release kinetics and ensures targeted delivery to specific tissues or cells, enhancing the therapeutic efficacy and minimizing off-target effects.

On the other hand, covalent drug delivery involves the formation of chemical bonds (such as ester bonds, amide bonds, or disulfide bonds) between the drug molecules and nanocomposites. For covalent drug delivery to occur, the chemical bond securing the drug molecule to the nanocomposites must be directly broken. While covalent bonding offers the advantage of enhanced stability and decreased risk of premature drug release, it requires external stimuli to break the covalent linkages and release the drug payload. Despite the need for external triggers, such as changes in pH or temperature, covalent binding can reduce non-specific drug release, thereby improving the precision and efficiency of drug delivery. Moreover, covalent drug conjugation allows for precise control over drug loading and release kinetics, enabling tailored therapeutic interventions with minimal off-target effects.

9.4.2 Hydrophobicity-Induced Drug Delivery

Hydrophobicity-induced drug release using nanocomposites is a sophisticated approach in drug delivery that capitalizes on the properties of hydrophobic materials to control the release of therapeutic agents. Hydrophobic and hydrophilic forces are predominantly relevant in the context of drugs that are primarily bound non-covalently. This means that hydrophobic drug molecules are encapsulated or loaded into the hydrophobic regions of the nanocomposite matrix. The drug cargo is stabilized by these hydrophobic contacts between the drug molecules and the nanocomposite, which prevents premature release and improves drug loading efficiency. Common hydrophobic materials used in nanocomposites include lipids, polymers, and hydrophobic nanoparticles (Ianchis et al. 2017). Drug release from hydrophobic nanocomposites can be initiated by local environmental changes, including pH, temperature, and the presence of certain biomolecules. There are several benefits to delivering drugs by hydrophobicity-induced drug release utilizing nanocomposites. Drugs can be released at the target location under regulated and triggered conditions, reducing systemic adverse effects and enhancing therapeutic efficacy. Moreover, precise spatiotemporal control over drug release is made possible by the stimulus-responsive nature of hydrophobic nanocomposites, which supports customized medicine techniques.

9.4.3 pH-Induced Drug Delivery

In this strategy, the release of therapeutic agents is caused by variations in the pH of the surrounding environment in drug delivery system. Polymers which are pH-responsive play a crucial for nanocomposites-based drug delivery carriers reliant on encapsulation. The mechanism behind controlled and triggered release relies on the contrast between the physiological pH level (around pH 7.4) and the acidic environment found in endosomes and lysosomes (with a pH range of 5 to 6).

The mechanism of behind this in respect of nanocomposites relies on the pH-dependent swelling or degradation. At specific pH levels, the nanocomposite undergoes structural changes, leading to the release of encapsulated drugs. This pH responsiveness can be attributed to the presence of pH-sensitive moieties, such as acidic or basic functional groups, within the nanocomposite structure. Additionally, tumor tissues exhibit a lower pH compared to healthy tissues, a characteristic that proves advantageous for drug delivery specific to cancer treatment. As cancer cells rapidly metabolize glucose to sustain their growth and proliferation, they produce significant amounts of lactic acid, leading to a decrease in pH levels within the tumor tissue (Zhu and Chen 2015). This discrepancy in pH levels enables nanocomposites to release drugs selectively in acidic environments, such as those found in tumor tissues, thereby enhancing the efficacy of cancer therapy while minimizing adverse effects on healthy cells. One of the key advantages of pH-induced drug release systems is their ability to target specific physiological environments within the body.

To minimize side effects and maximize treatment efficiency, anticancer medicines can be selectively released from pH-responsive nanocomposites into tumor cells by taking advantage of the acidic pH environment present in these tissues.

Acidic pH-responsive drug-eluting nanocomposite (pH-DEN) was created by Park et al. specifically for MRI-guided transcatheter administration of sorafenib (Park et al. 2016). The magnetic iron oxide nanocubes and pH-sensitive synthetic peptides coupled with lipid tails (octadecylamine–p(API-l-Asp)10) compose up the pH-DEN. In addition to their exceptional sensitivity to MR contrast effects, the produced sorafenib-loaded pH-DENs exhibit unique pH-dependent drug release features, which are especially noticeable in acidic environments (Figure 9.6A). At pH 6.5, the pH-DENs demonstrated a notably accelerated drug release rate, with approximately 80% cumulative drug release observed within 96 hours. On the other hand, as Figure 9.6B and C illustrates, the release of sorafenib from the pH-DENs at pH 7.4 was significantly reduced. Also the percentage cell viability reduced significantly in the acidic environment.

Similarly, Hemant et al. prepared silica encapsulated iron oxide nanocomposites (DOX/IO@Silica) for the pH-responsive release of drug. They investigated release of DOX with respect to pH dependence, revealing notable release particularly at lower pH levels (H. Kumar, Pani, et al. 2022).

9.4.4 Temperature-Induced Drug Delivery

A potential method that takes use of temperature variations to cause the release of therapeutic drugs at certain locations inside the body is temperature-induced drug delivery using nanocomposites. This strategy relies on the design and engineering of nanomaterials with temperature-responsive properties, allowing for precise control over drug release kinetics (Ding et al. 2017). Three distinct categories of thermoresponsive drug delivery strategies have been documented, each offering unique mechanisms for controlled drug release: (1) diffusion from temperature-sensitive hydrogels and polymers, (2) triggered rupture of encapsulated drugs, and (3) thermally induced release from nanocomposites. In these schemes, inorganic nanoparticles, particularly metal and magnetic nanoparticles, play dual roles by serving as a source of thermal stimulation via external stimuli and providing a scaffold for drug delivery system. Nanocomposites typically consist of a thermoresponsive polymer matrix combined with drug molecules tailored for temperature-induced drug delivery has gained significant attention. The lower critical solution temperature (LCST) or upper critical solution temperature (UCST), depending on the specific polymer, refers to the transition of these polymers between hydrophilic and hydrophobic states in response to changes in temperature. This phenomenon involves

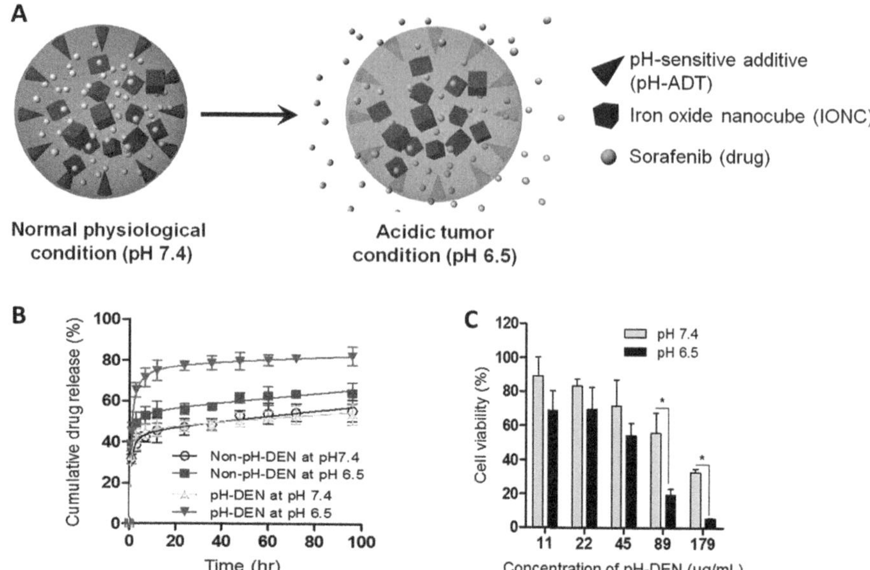

Figure 9.6 (A) Diagrammatic representation of pH-responsive drug-eluting nanocomposites (pH-DENs), showcasing their structure and mechanism of action in releasing therapeutic agents in response to changes in pH levels within the surrounding environment. (B) pH-dependent sorafenib release characteristics in both pH-DEN and non-pH-DEN samples and (C) percentage viability of McA-RH7777 hepatoma cells to survive treatment with different pH-DEN concentrations at pH 7.4 or 6.5 (reported with permission (Park et al. 2016), ©American Chemical Society).

a shift in the polymer's solubility behavior, typically triggered by alterations in temperature. At temperatures below the LCST or above the UCST, the polymer chains are either predominantly hydrophilic or hydrophobic, respectively. However, when the temperature crosses the LCST or UCST threshold, the polymer undergoes a phase transition, leading to a change in its solubility properties. The encapsulated medication can get liberated from the nanocomposite matrix as a result of this transition causing structural variations in the structure of the polymer.

Thermoresponsive hydrogel nanocomposite with drug-loaded micelles and water-dispersible ferrimagnetic iron oxide nanocubes (wFIONs) was described by Kang et al. and is injected into the surgically removed tumor location after surgery (Kang et al. 2023). Upon exposure to body temperature, the hydrogel nanocomposite rapidly undergoes gelation, forming a soft, deeply penetrating intracortical drug reservoir (Figure 9.7). To minimize premature drug release, the drug-loaded micelles are designed to preferentially target remaining glioblastoma multiforme (GBM) cells.

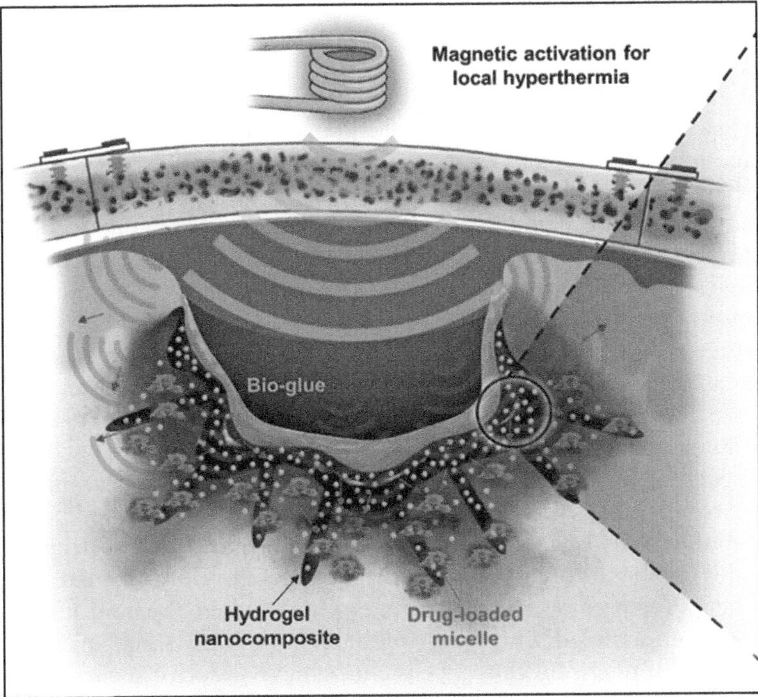

Figure 9.7 An illustration showing how moderate heat may be used to promote penetrative and sustained medication delivery to deep brain tumors through the use of an intracortical hydrogel nanocomposite (reported with permission (Kang et al. 2023), ©American Chemical Society).

9.4.5 Biomolecular-Assisted Drug Delivery

Targeted controlled release of drugs can be achieved via biomolecular-assisted drug delivery with nanocomposites, which take advantage of the complex interactions between biomolecules and nanoparticles. This method directs the delivery of medicinal drugs to certain cells, tissues, or organs by taking use of the selectivity and affinity of biomolecules, such as peptides, proteins, antibodies, and nucleic acids.

This method may be roughly divided into three basic mechanisms: chemical reduction-based release, enzymatic release, and ligand exchange-mediated release. In these mechanisms, nanocomposites primarily serve as carriers and are not directly involved in drug release. Still, altering their structure is essential to the effectiveness of biomolecular-assisted drug administration because it affects how the biomolecules and nanocomposites interact. One of the key strategies in biomolecular-induced drug delivery involves the functionalization or conjugation of biomolecules onto the surface of nanoparticles. This can be achieved through various techniques, including covalent binding, electrostatic interactions, and affinity-based conjugation. By attaching biomolecules to the nanoparticle surface, researchers can enhance the targeting capability of the nanocomposite and promote selective uptake by target cells or tissues. In addition to surface functionalization, biomolecular-induced drug delivery can also leverage biomolecular recognition and signaling pathways to trigger drug release in response to specific biological cues. For instance, the design of the nanocomposite can integrate stimulus-responsive biomolecules, such as aptamers, pH-sensitive peptides, and enzymes, to allow for on-demand drug release in response to certain molecular triggers or modifications in the physiological environment.

Furthermore, biomolecular-induced drug delivery systems can exploit biological processes, such as receptor-mediated endocytosis and intracellular trafficking, to facilitate the internalization and intracellular delivery of therapeutic agents. When biomolecular targeting ligands, such antibodies or receptor ligands, are built into nanocomposites, they can bind to cell surface receptors selectively, which results in receptor-mediated uptake and intracellular drug release. Moreover, biomolecular-induced drug delivery strategies can be tailored to exploit disease-specific biomarkers or microenvironments for precise drug targeting and release. For instance, nanocomposites functionalized with targeting ligands that recognize overexpressed receptors or antigens on cancer cells can achieve selective accumulation and retention within tumor tissues, resulting in decreased off-target effects and increased therapeutic effectiveness.

9.4.6 Light-Triggered Drug Delivery

The strong optical properties of nanoparticles make light-activated delivery of drugs a compelling therapeutic intervention strategy. This methodology relies on the incorporation of light-responsive materials into nanocomposite formulations, allowing for precise control over drug release through exposure to light of specific wavelengths. One of the key components of light-induced drug delivery is the use of photosensitive materials, such as photoresponsive polymers, organic dyes, or inorganic nanoparticles, within the nanocomposite matrix. When exposed to light, these materials alter chemically or physically, which causes the drug to release from the nanocomposite. For instance, when exposed to light, photoresponsive polymers may experience structural changes or photothermal conversion, which would release the medication that has been encapsulated.

In light-induced drug delivery systems, precise control over drug release is achieved by careful consideration of the light source and wavelength selection. Based on the unique needs of the drug delivery system, several light sources, such as visible, near-infrared (NIR), and ultraviolet (UV) light, can be used (Alvarez-Lorenzo, Bromberg, and Concheiro 2009). Additionally,

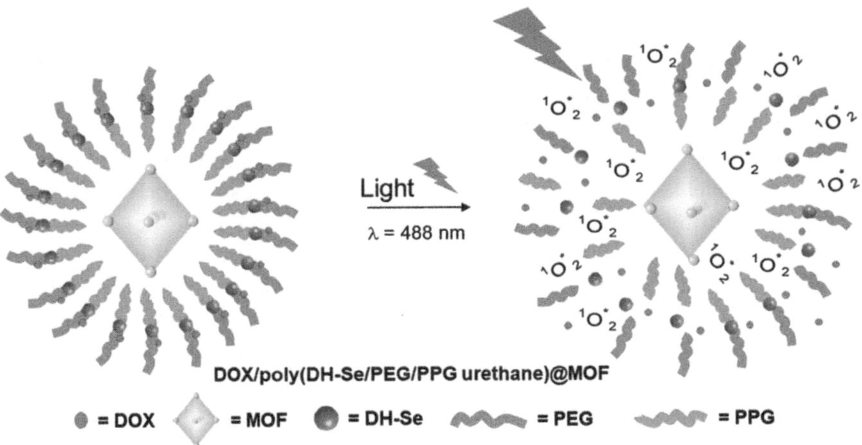

Figure 9.8 An illustration showing how the DOX/poly(DH-Se/PEG/PPG urethane) @ MOF nanocomposite releases drugs in vitro when exposed to light (reported with permission (Luo et al. 2019), ©Wiley Online Library).

the wavelength of light can be tailored to match the absorption spectrum of the photosensitive materials, allowing for selective activation and drug release at desired locations.

By combining the advantages of photosensitive porphyrin zirconium metal–organic frameworks as the core and redox-responsive selenium (Se) substituted polymer as the shell, Luo et al. created light-responsive drug delivery nanocomposites (Luo et al. 2019). Redox-cleavable di-(1-hydroxylundecyl)selenide (DH-Se) was polymerized in combination with biocompatible poly(ethylene glycol) (PEG) and poly(propylene glycol) (PPG) to create poly(DH-Se/PEG/PPG urethane). This polymer is then utilized to coat the porous porphyrin zirconium MOF formulation capable of generating reactive oxygen species (ROS), resulting in the formation of poly(DH-Se/PEG/PPG urethane) @MOF shell–core nanocomposites using an emulsion approach. Figure 9.8 illustrates how the light-triggered ROS generation by the MOF upon laser light irradiation allows the nanoparticles to assist a synergistic combination of photodynamic treatment and chemotherapy.

9.5 CONCLUSION

In conclusion, nanocomposites have emerged as versatile tools in both cytotoxicity assessment and drug delivery applications. In the realm of cytotoxicity assessment, nanocomposites offer precise platforms for evaluating the safety and biocompatibility of various materials. Through techniques such as cell viability assays, morphological analysis, apoptosis, necrosis assays, and inflammatory response assays, nanocomposites enable researchers to assess cytotoxicity accurately and efficiently. Moreover, advancements in nanocomposite design allow for the development of more biocompatible materials, mitigating concerns regarding nanotoxicity and enhancing the safety profile of nanomaterials for applications in biomedical area.

Nanocomposites show great promise for targeted and controlled or regulated drug release in drug delivery purposes. By harnessing the unique properties of nanoparticles, the multiple nanocomposites have developed that enable precise drug delivery to specific tissues or cells. Furthermore, strategies such as hydrophobicity-induced, pH-induced, temperature-induced, biomolecular-induced, and light-induced drug release provide with versatile tools to achieve spatiotemporal control over drug delivery. These advancements in nanocomposite-based drug delivery hold promise for enhancing drug efficacy, minimizing side effects, and overcoming challenges associated with drug resistance and barriers to drug penetration.

Overall, the integration of nanocomposites in cytotoxicity assessment and drug delivery represents a paradigm shift in biomedical research and clinical practice. By leveraging the unique properties of nanomaterials, researchers can address longstanding challenges and unlock new opportunities in drug development, disease diagnosis, and therapy. Nevertheless, more investigation is necessary to guarantee the safety and effectiveness of nanomaterials for therapeutic translation, improve biocompatibility, and optimize nanocomposite composition. With continued advancements in nanotechnology and interdisciplinary collaborations, nanocomposites are poised to revolutionize healthcare and pave the way for personalized medicine in the future.

REFERENCES

Afsharnezhad, Sima, Mehrdad Kashefi, Javad Behravan, Melika Ehtesham Gharaee, Mojtaba Meshkat, Khadijeh Shahrokh Abadi, and Masoud Homayoni Tabrizi. 2014. "Investigation of Nano-SiO2 Impact on Mechanical and Biocompatibility Properties of Cyanoacryalate Based Nanocomposites for Dental Application." *International Journal of Adhesion and Adhesives* 54 (October). Elsevier: 177–183. doi:10.1016/J.IJADHADH.2014.06.004.

Alvarez-Lorenzo, Carmen, Lev Bromberg, and Angel Concheiro. 2009. "Light-Sensitive Intelligent Drug Delivery Systems†." *Photochemistry and Photobiology* 85 (4). John Wiley & Sons, Ltd: 848–860. doi:10.1111/J.1751-1097.2008.00530.X.

Buck, Suzanne B., Jolene Bradford, Kyle R. Gee, Brian J. Agnew, Scott T. Clarke, and Adrian Salic. 2008. "Detection of S-Phase Cell Cycle Progression Using 5-Ethynyl-2'- Deoxyuridine Incorporation with Click Chemistry, an Alternative to Using 5-Bromo-2'-Deoxyuridine Antibodies." *BioTechniques* 44 (7). Future Science Ltd London, UK : 927–929. doi:10.2144/000112812/ASSET/IMAGES/LARGE/FIGURE2.JPEG.

Chen, Junjie, Longfei Yan, Wenya Song, and Deguang Xu. 2018. "Interfacial Characteristics of Carbon Nanotube-Polymer Composites: A Review." *Composites Part A: Applied Science and Manufacturing* 114 (November). Elsevier: 149–169. doi:10.1016/J.COMPOSITESA.2018.08.021.

Cui, Wei, Junbai Li, and Gero Decher. 2016. "Self-Assembled Smart Nanocarriers for Targeted Drug Delivery." *Advanced Materials* 28 (6). John Wiley & Sons, Ltd: 1302–1311. doi:10.1002/ADMA.201502479.

Ding, Li, Qi Wang, Ming Shen, Ying Sun, Xiangyu Zhang, Can Huang, Jianhua Chen, Rongxin Li, and Yourong Duan. 2017. "Thermoresponsive Nanocomposite Gel for Local Drug Delivery to Suppress the Growth of Glioma by Inducing Autophagy." *Autophagy* 13 (7). Taylor & Francis: 1176–1190. doi:10.1080/15548627.2017.1320634.

Doane, Tennyson, and Clemens Burda. 2013. "Nanoparticle Mediated Non-Covalent Drug Delivery." *Advanced Drug Delivery Reviews* 65 (5). Elsevier: 607–621. doi:10.1016/J.ADDR.2012.05.012.

Dumont, Vitor C., Herman S. Mansur, Alexandra A.P. Mansur, Sandhra M. Carvalho, Nádia S.V. Capanema, and Breno R. Barrioni. 2016. "Glycol Chitosan/Nanohydroxyapatite Biocomposites for Potential Bone Tissue Engineering and Regenerative Medicine." *International Journal of Biological Macromolecules* 93 (December). Elsevier: 1465–1478. doi:10.1016/J.IJBIOMAC.2016.04.030.

Feldman, Dorel. 2016. "Polymer Nanocomposites in Medicine." *Journal of Macromolecular Science, Part A* 53 (1). Taylor & Francis: 55–62. doi:10.1080/10601325.2016.1110459.

Fu, Shaoyun, Zheng Sun, Pei Huang, Yuanqing Li, and Ning Hu. 2019. "Some Basic Aspects of Polymer Nanocomposites: A Critical Review." *Nano Materials Science* 1 (1). Elsevier: 2–30. doi:10.1016/J.NANOMS.2019.02.006.

Goudarzi, Mojgan, Masoud Salavati-Niasari, and Mahnaz Amiri. 2019. "Effective Induction of Death in Breast Cancer Cells with Magnetite NiCo2O4/NiO Nanocomposite." *Composites Part B: Engineering* 166 (June). Elsevier: 457–463. doi:10.1016/J.COMPOSITESB.2019.02.017.

Hasanzadeh, Mohammad, Nasrin Shadjou, and Miguel de la Guardia. 2017. "Early Stage Diagnosis of Programmed Cell Death (Apoptosis) Using Electroanalysis: Nanomaterial and Methods Overview." *TrAC Trends in Analytical Chemistry* 93 (August). Elsevier: 199–211. doi:10.1016/J.TRAC.2017.06.007.

Hassan, Tufail, Abdul Salam, Amina Khan, Saif Ullah Khan, Halima Khanzada, Muhammad Wasim, Muhammad Qamar Khan, and Ick Soo Kim. 2021. "Functional Nanocomposites and Their Potential Applications: A Review." *Journal of Polymer Research* 28 (2). Springer: 1–22. doi:10.1007/S10965-021-02408-1.

Hu, Kesong, Dhaval D. Kulkarni, Ikjun Choi, and Vladimir V. Tsukruk. 2014. "Graphene-Polymer Nanocomposites for Structural and Functional Applications." *Progress in Polymer Science* 39 (11). Pergamon: 1934–1972. doi:10.1016/J.PROGPOLYMSCI.2014.03.001.

Hu, Z., G. Tong, D. Lin, C. Chen, H. Guo, J. Xu, and L. Zhou. 2016. "Graphene-Reinforced Metal Matrix Nanocomposites – a Review." *Materials Science and Technology* 32 (9). Taylor & Francis: 930–953. doi:10.1080/02670836.2015.1104018.

Ianchis, Raluca, Claudia M. Ninciuleanu, Ioana C. Gifu, Elvira Alexandrescu, Raluca Somoghi, Augusta R. Gabor, Silviu Preda, et al. 2017. "Novel Hydrogel-Advanced Modified Clay Nanocomposites as Possible Vehicles for Drug Delivery and Controlled Release." *Nanomaterials* 7 (12). Multidisciplinary Digital Publishing Institute: 443. doi:10.3390/NANO7120443.

Kang, Taegyu, Gi Doo Cha, Ok Kyu Park, Hye Rim Cho, Minjeong Kim, Jongha Lee, Dokyoon Kim, et al. 2023. "Penetrative and Sustained Drug Delivery Using Injectable Hydrogel Nanocomposites for Postsurgical Brain Tumor Treatment." *ACS Nano* 17 (6). American Chemical Society: 5435–5447. doi:10.1021/AC SNANO.2C10094/ASSET/IMAGES/LARGE/NN2C10094_0006.JPEG.

Kotal, Moumita, and Anil K. Bhowmick. 2015. "Polymer Nanocomposites from Modified Clays: Recent Advances and Challenges." *Progress in Polymer Science* 51 (December). Pergamon: 127–187. doi:10.1016/J. PROGPOLYMSCI.2015.10.001.

Koyanagi, Madoka, So Kawakabe, and Yutaka Arimura. 2016. "A Comparative Study of Colorimetric Cell Proliferation Assays in Immune Cells." *Cytotechnology* 68 (4). Springer Netherlands: 1489–1498. doi:10.1007/ S10616-015-9909-2/FIGURES/5.

Kuku, Gamze, Melike Saricam, Farida Akhatova, Anna Danilushkina, Rawil Fakhrullin, and Mustafa Culha. 2016. "Surface-Enhanced Raman Scattering to Evaluate Nanomaterial Cytotoxicity on Living Cells." *Analytical Chemistry* 88 (19). American Chemical Society: 9813–9820. doi:10.1021/ACS.ANA LCHEM.6B02917/ASSET/IMAGES/LARGE/AC-2016-02917C_0004.JPEG.

Kulkarni, Shrikaant. 2021. "Bionanocomposites for Biomedical Applications." *Applications of Biodegradable and Bio-Based Polymers for Human Health and a Cleaner Environment* (December). Apple Academic Press: 313–333. doi:10.1201/9781003146360-15.

Kumar, Hemant, Jitender Kumar, Balaram Pani, and Pramod Kumar. 2022. "Multifunctional Folic Acid-Coated and Doxorubicin Encapsulated Mesoporous Silica Nanocomposites (FA/DOX@Silica) for Cancer Therapeutics, Bioimaging and Invitro Studies." *ChemistrySelect* 7 (44). John Wiley & Sons, Ltd: e202203113. doi:10.1002/SLCT.202203113.

Kumar, Hemant, Balaram Pani, Jitender Kumar, and Pramod Kumar. 2022. "In Vitro and Bioimaging Studies of Mesoporous Silica Nanocomposites Encapsulated Iron-Oxide and Loaded Doxorubicin Drug (DOX/IO@Silica) as Magnetically Guided Drug Delivery System." *Current Pharmaceutical Biotechnology* 24 (10). Bentham Science Publishers: 1297–1306. doi:10.2174 /1389201023666220428084920.

Kumar, Jitender, and Indrajit Roy. 2024. "Upconverting Nanophosphors for Various Sensing Applications." *Talanta Open* 9 (August). Elsevier: 100302. doi:10.1016/J.TALO.2024.100302.

Lewinski, Nastassja, Vicki Colvin, and Rebekah Drezek. 2008. "Cytotoxicity of Nanoparticles." *Small* 4 (1). John Wiley & Sons, Ltd: 26–49. doi:10.1002/ SMLL.200700595.

Li, Mo, Xiangcun Li, Xinhong Qi, Fan Luo, and Gaohong He. 2015. "Shape-Controlled Synthesis of Magnetic Iron Oxide@SiO2-Au@C Particles with Core-Shell Nanostructures." *Langmuir* 31 (18). American Chemical Society: 5190–5197. doi:10.1021/ACS.LANGMUIR.5B00800/SUPPL_FILE/LA5B0 0800_SI_001.PDF.

Liu, Ying Ling, and Wei Hong Chen. 2007. "Modification of Multiwall Carbon Nanotubes with Initiators and Macroinitiators of Atom Transfer Radical Polymerization." *Macromolecules* 40 (25). American Chemical Society: 8881–8886. doi:10.1021/MA071700S/SUPPL_FILE/MA071700S-FILE00 3.PDF.

Luo, Zheng, Lu Jiang, Shaoxiong Yang, Zibiao Li, Wee Mia Wilson Soh, Liyan Zheng, Xian Jun Loh, and Yun Long Wu. 2019. "Light-Induced Redox-Responsive Smart Drug Delivery System by Using Selenium-Containing Polymer@MOF Shell/Core Nanocomposite." *Advanced Healthcare Materials* 8 (15). John Wiley & Sons, Ltd: 1900406. doi:10.1002/ADHM.201900406.

Maisanaba, Sara, Silvia Pichardo, María Puerto, Daniel Gutiérrez-Praena, Ana M. Cameán, and Angeles Jos. 2015. "Toxicological Evaluation of Clay Minerals and Derived Nanocomposites: A Review." *Environmental Research* 138 (April). Academic Press: 233–254. doi:10.1016/J.ENVRES.2014.12.024.

Mera, Gabriela, Markus Gallei, Samuel Bernard, and Emanuel Ionescu. 2015. "Ceramic Nanocomposites from Tailor-Made Preceramic Polymers." *Nanomaterials* 5 (2). Multidisciplinary Digital Publishing Institute: 468–540. doi:10.3390/NANO5020468.

Mohan, Tarun, Jitender Kumar, and Indrajit Roy. 2023. "Iron Selenide Nanorods for Light-Activated Anticancer and Catalytic Applications." *New Journal of Chemistry* 47 (5). The Royal Society of Chemistry: 2527–2535. doi:10.1039/ D2NJ05094C.

Oh, Seok Jeong, Hwa Kim, Yingqiu Liu, Hyo Kyung Han, Kyenghee Kwon, Kyung Hwa Chang, Kwangsik Park, et al. 2014. "Incompatibility of Silver Nanoparticles with Lactate Dehydrogenase Leakage Assay for Cellular Viability Test Is Attributed to Protein Binding and Reactive Oxygen Species Generation." *Toxicology Letters* 225 (3). Elsevier: 422–432. doi:10.1016/J. TOXLET.2014.01.015.

Omanović-Mikličanin, Enisa, Almir Badnjević, Anera Kazlagić, and Muhamed Hajlovac. 2020. "Nanocomposites: A Brief Review." *Health and Technology* 10 (1). Springer: 51–59. doi:10.1007/S12553-019-00380-X/FIGURES/3.

Park, Wooram, Jeane Chen, Soojeong Cho, Sin Jung Park, Andrew C. Larson, Kun Na, and Dong Hyun Kim. 2016. "Acidic PH-Triggered Drug-Eluting Nanocomposites for Magnetic Resonance Imaging-Monitored Intra-Arterial Drug Delivery to Hepatocellular Carcinoma." *ACS Applied Materials and Interfaces* 8 (20). American Chemical Society: 12711–12719. doi:10.10 21/ACSAMI.6B03505/ASSET/IMAGES/LARGE/AM-2016-03505Q_000 6.JPEG.

Ravichandran, Krishnasamy, Prabhakaran Kala Praseetha, Thirumurugan Arun, and Suyamprakam Gobalakrishnan. 2018. "Synthesis of Nanocomposites." *Synthesis of Inorganic Nanomaterials: Advances and Key Technologies* (January). Woodhead Publishing: 141–168. doi:10.1016/ B978-0-08-101975-7.00006-3.

Sanchez, Clément, Bénédicte Lebeau, Frédéric Chaput, and Jean Pierre Boilot. 2003. "Optical Properties of Functional Hybrid Organic–Inorganic Nanocomposites." *Advanced Materials* 15 (23). John Wiley & Sons, Ltd: 1969–1994. doi:10.1002/ADMA.200300389.

Sofi, Hasham S., Roqia Ashraf, Abdul Hanan Khan, Mushtaq A. Beigh, Shafaquat Majeed, and Faheem A. Sheikh. 2019. "Reconstructing Nanofibers from Natural Polymers Using Surface Functionalization Approaches for Applications in Tissue Engineering, Drug Delivery and Biosensing Devices." *Materials Science and Engineering: C* 94 (January). Elsevier: 1102–1124. doi:10.1016/J.MSEC.2018.10.069.

Sun, Xianxian, Chuanjin Huang, Lidong Wang, Lei Liang, Yuanjing Cheng, Weidong Fei, Yibin Li, et al. 2021. "Recent Progress in Graphene/Polymer Nanocomposites." *Advanced Materials* 33 (6). John Wiley & Sons, Ltd: 2001105. doi:10.1002/ADMA.202001105.

Wiemann, Martin, Antje Vennemann, Ursula G. Sauer, Karin Wiench, Lan Ma-Hock, and Robert Landsiedel. 2016. "An in Vitro Alveolar Macrophage Assay for Predicting the Short-Term Inhalation Toxicity of Nanomaterials." *Journal of Nanobiotechnology* 14 (1). BioMed Central: 1–27. doi:10.1186/S12951-016-0164-2.

Yoo, Sung Chan, Dongju Lee, Seong Woo Ryu, Byungchul Kang, Ho Jin Ryu, and Soon Hyung Hong. 2023. "Recent Progress in Low-Dimensional Nanomaterials Filled Multifunctional Metal Matrix Nanocomposites." *Progress in Materials Science* 132 (February). Pergamon: 101034. doi:10.1016/J.PMATSCI.2022.101034.

Zhao, Feng, Ying Zhao, Ying Liu, Xueling Chang, Chunying Chen, and Yuliang Zhao. 2011. "Cellular Uptake, Intracellular Trafficking, and Cytotoxicity of Nanomaterials." *Small* 7 (10). John Wiley & Sons, Ltd: 1322–1337. doi:10.1002/SMLL.201100001.

Zhu, Ying Jie, and Feng Chen. 2015. "PH-Responsive Drug-Delivery Systems." *Chemistry – An Asian Journal* 10 (2). John Wiley & Sons, Ltd: 284–305. doi:10.1002/ASIA.201402715.

Chapter 10

Polymer-based Bionanocomposites

Smart Adsorbents for Detection and Removal of Metal Contaminants from Water

*Pooja Kumari, Tabassum Nike,
Deepika Kaushal, Vivek Sheel Jaswal,
Vinay Chauhan, and Manish Kumar*

10.1 INTRODUCTION

Hazardous metal contamination is one, among various important environmental issues, that affect humans as well as other forms of life worldwide due to the rapid population growth, urbanization and continuously growing industrialization (Zhao et al., 2018). Humans are constantly exposed to a wide range of toxins present in environment like heavy metal ions. The health of humans is adversely damaged by these heavy metals (Zhang & Fang, 2010). Metal ions like mercury(II), lead(II), Cadmium(II), and Chromium(II) have been identified as environmental pollutants because a variety of these metal ions are harmful even in ppm concentrations (Muthivhi et al., 2018). Many chemical industries like fertilizer, leather, textile, cosmetics, pharmaceuticals, and many others produce large amounts of wastewater that contains trace amounts of various contaminants like dyes, detergents, pesticides, hydrocarbons, and heavy metals. Out of these contaminants heavy metal ions do not break down and have a propensity to accumulate in internal systems of living creatures, which leads to numerous diseases and ailments (Chakraborty et al., 2021)(Orta et al., 2020). Agrochemicals used in agriculture, such as fertilizers and plant nutrients, can considerably increase the amounts of these metal ions in soil and water resources. These heavy metals could build up in significant quantities in the various soil layers, and with time these migrate to water sources (surface and groundwater), which have a negative impact on human health. Several harmful health effects are caused by Heavy metals (especially As and Cd) when enter the body systems, including hypersensitivity, and hyperpigmentation, and these are also carcinogenic (Wongsasuluk et al., 2014) (Badsha et al., 2021). The toxic effect of the metals is attributed to their strong binding

DOI: 10.1201/9781003470311-10

affinities for the thiol group of proteins (Gumpu et al., 2015; Turdean, 2011) (Tag et al., 2007). Heavy metals including Hg, As, Pb, Cr, Ni, and Cd are highly dangerous in terms of toxicity and carcinogenic properties, even at a ppm level. Heavy metals accumulate in the system, increasing toxicity and impacting many physiological systems such as the central nervous system, liver, kidney, skin, bone, and teeth (Aragay et al., 2011; Duffus, 2002; Li et al., 2013). It was investigated that very low concentrations upto 10 µM of nickel (Ni) can cause oxidative stress, DNA strand breakage, and apoptosis when its effects on normal rat kidney cells were studied (Badsha et al., 2021; Wongsasuluk et al., 2014). Thus, it is crucial to reliably, quickly, and quantitatively measure these harmful metals in water sources using in situ trace detection methods and then remove the same by suitable techniques (Chakraborty et al., 2021) (Zhang & Fang, 2010).

There have been a variety of approaches for removing metal ions from water, like ion exchange, coagulation, oxidation/precipitation, and membrane separations. Although these methods are easy, they have several drawbacks, including a large amount of hazardous sludge, delayed metal precipitation, poor sedimentation, and agglomeration of metal residues, all of which require additional treatment before release into the surroundings. Fouling and clogging of membranes, high costs, and more complex procedures are a few downsides of membrane technology (Asere et al., 2019; Nasrollahzadeh et al., 2021; Orta et al., 2020)(Özkahraman et al., 2018; Singh et al., 2015).

Because of easy procedures involved, inexpensive and easily available adsorbents, adsorption is considered among the most effective and simple methods for treating metal-polluted water. Among various adsorbents natural polymers based composites are ideal candidates for usage as potential adsorbents due to their suitable structural features, modifiable functional groups present on surface which can be modified according to required functional properties, economical and easy regeneration, and environment-friendly and biodegradable nature. The low selectivity and adsorption capacity, high swelling abilities and poor mechanical strength and stability of pure polymers, needed to be improved for use in actual applications (Zhao et al., 2018). Fillers of various sizes are frequently used as reinforcement for polymers to make them more suitable for use. An innovative replacement for traditional fillers has been made possible by the use of nano-fillers to improve the stiffness/mechanical strength and other physical attributes of polymer based composites (Fu et al., 2019). By inserting metal nanoparticles into polymer matrices one can take the benefits of both nanoparticles and polymer. This method is one of the best ways to keep metal particles under surveillance and minimize the chances of their aggregation. As a result, polymer/metal nanocomposites that use polymer phases as stabilizers, templates, or protective agents exhibit a number of significantly improved properties (Nasrollahzadeh et al., 2021; Zare &

Sahani, 2016). Over the past years, a wide variety of bionanocomposites that are derived by use of natural biopolymers, including chitosan, cellulose, starch, alginate, sacran, zein, and gelatin, have been synthesized by various researchers and have been used in different fields (Orta et al., 2020).

10.2 MATERIALS AND METHODS

10.2.1 Materials

A wide variety of natural polymers are there which have been employed by various researchers in the preparations of different kind of polymer based nanocomposites used for metal ion detection and removal. Some major and commonly used polymers along with their important properties are described here.

10.2.1.1 Chitosan

Chitosan has drawn a lot of interest among the various renewable polymer-based materials due to its advantageous properties, including its strong antibacterial properties, biodegradability, biocompatibility, applications in sensing biomaterials, non-toxic nature, and uses for food packaging and texture correction (Azizi-Lalabadi & Jafari, 2021). It possesses exceptional chelating qualities and is loaded with remarkable reactivity due to the abundance of hydroxyl (-OH) and amino ($-NH_2$) functional groups in it which are quite reactive (Hu et al., 2020; Mahmoud et al., 2021; Shahraki et al., 2019; Kayalvizhi et al., 2022). It has been found that tailoring chitosan physically and chemically enhances its ability to adsorb metal ions. Its flexibility and chemically stable nature can be improved through chemical functionalization and surface modifications, which can also reduce its reactivity to acid media (Shahraki et al., 2019; Kayalvizhi et al., 2022).

10.2.1.2. Starch

One of the several major neutral polysaccharide polymers utilized in research is starch, a biodegradable agriculturally generated biopolymer. Materials made of starch alone are not particularly suited for applications as sorbents since they require regulated molecular dimensions as well as appropriate durability against wear, strength, and permeability. Starch has the ability to combine various metal particles. Starch can be chemically modified to improve its qualities significantly. This interaction ability can be increased by altering starch with relevant functional groups via the process of esterification, making cross-links with suitable reagents, and oxidation reactions to make changes. For a long time, a wide range of starch and its analogs have been made by the modifications of infunctional groups including amide, amino, and carboxyl by different researchers and have been used in water contaminant removal studies (Abdul-Raheim et al., 2016; Saberi et al., 2019).

10.2.1.3 Cellulose

Cellulose is among one of the highest predominant biopolymer on planet Earth. Cellulose contains several hydroxyl groups that, when combined with metal form chelate complexes and exhibit strong hydrogen bonding abilities, so can remove heavy metal ions or other particles from wastewater. As a result, cellulose and its derivatives are gaining popularity as practical components for wastewater treatment processes. However, pristine cellulose was not able to attain sufficient binding capability. All agricultural by-products containing cellulose can be used for adsorption. By physically or chemically altering cellulose, it can be employed as an adsorbent in a variety of applications. It is coupled with diverse organic-inorganic materials/nanomaterials for this purpose to generate hybrid composites with enhanced characteristics (Jamshaid et al., 2017; Liu et al., 2018).

10.2.1.4 Alginate

Alginate (G) is a polymer of biological origin isolated from brown seaweeds. This biopolymer is safe to use, biocompatible, environmentally friendly, and biodegradable. It is composed of guluronic and mannuronic acid units by specific connectivity pattern. Alginate can easily produce crosslinked gel matrices when present along with divalent cations, particularly Ca^{2+} ions. The Ca-crosslinked alginate matrices when used in synthesis of adsorbent, their consistency was like gels. These gel-like alginate composites are better than powder forms as their handling and working conditions are more convenient. The alginate-based combinations contain abundant carboxylic (-COOH) groups on their surfaces, which form strong complexes with the metal ions and hence are effective in their removal from the wastewater.

10.2.2 Methods

Polymer nanocomposites can be synthesized using melt intercalation, template synthesis (sol–gel technology), exfoliation adsorption (polymer or prepolymer intercalation), and in situ polymerization methods.

10.2.2.1 In Situ Polymerization Intercalation

In situ polymerization, as reported by Toyota researchers, played a pivotal role in catalyzing exponential growth in the field of nanocomposite research (Mittal, 2009). In situ polymerization occurs when stacked silicates expand upon exposure to a liquid monomer or solution containing a monomer,

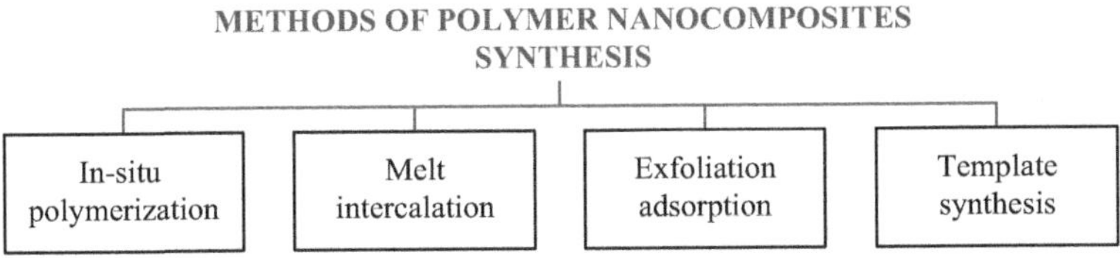

Figure 10.1 Method of polymer nanocomposite synthesis.

allowing polymer formation within the intercalated layers. Polymerization can be carried out by employing various methods such as heat, radiation, or the introduction of an appropriate initiator through diffusion. In addition, an inorganic initiator or catalyst can be introduced into the interlayer through cationic exchange before the stage of monomer swelling in order to start the reaction (Abedi & Abdouss, 2014). Through this mode of synthesis, thermoplastic as well as thermoset-based nanocomposites can be developed (Alexandre & Dubois, n.d.).

10.2.2.2 Melt Intercalation

Synthesizing polymer nanocomposites using melt intercalation is a method that does not require the use of any solvents, is good to the environment, and is cost-effective, which is more advantageous than in situ polymerization and solution intercalation. The process of melt intercalation includes annealing and combining a mixture of clay that is organophilic and polymer. During annealing, the polymer chains are inserted into the organophilic clay, resulting in the formation of intercalated nanocomposites based on polymer (Pavlidou & Papaspyrides, 2008). A vast number of polymers including polystyrene and styrene derivatives, polyamides 6, poly(styrene-b-butadiene) copolymer, PEO (polyethylene oxide), and polyethylene-poly(ethylene glycol) diblock copolymer have been inserted into organo-modified clays to synthesize melt intercalated nanocomposites (Shen et al., n.d.). Lee et al. synthesized polyethylene and clay nanocomposites through a melt-intercalation process using polyethylene-graft-malic anhydride (PP-g-MA) or polypropylene-graft-malic anhydride (PP-g-MA) as a compatibilizer and the swelling agent used was octadecylamine. Compared to pure polyethylene, with the incorporation of 7% clay into the material, there was a 49% enhancement in the tensile modulus and 15% improvement in tensile strength (Lee et al., 2005).

10.2.2.3 Exfoliation Adsorption

In the process of exfoliation adsorption, layered silicates which are stacked are separated. This is done by utilizing a solvent in which the polymer can dissolve the layers that are stacked on top of one another, and are separated into their distinct forms. After the organoclay has been dissolved in the solvent and allowed to swell, the polymer will be added to the solution and will begin to intercalate between the layers of clay. In the final step, the solvent is extracted, which commonly involves vaporization, frequently occurring in conditions of vacuum, or by precipitation. After that the separate layers begin to reassemble, which results in the formation of a nanocomposite structure and encapsulation of the polymer (Pavlidou & Papaspyrides, 2008). Exfoliation adsorption relies on the increase in entropy achieved through solvent desorption, this compensatory mechanism counterbalances the reduced entropy caused by the confinement of intercalated chains (Mittal, 2009).

10.2.2.4 Template Synthesis

The production of clay minerals through the use of an aqueous solution that contains both polymer and silicate building blocks is at the heart of the Sol-gel technique, which is also known as template synthesis. The polymer performs the function of a nucleation catalyst, hence promoting the growth of inorganic host crystals, which then leads to the formation of a nanocomposite through crystal growth. Primarily, it finds its primary application in producing double-layer hydroxide-based nanocomposites, with relatively limited development for generating layered silicates. The reason for this disparity lies in the elevated synthesis temperatures that can cause polymer degradation and lead to increased aggregation of the emerging inorganic crystals. Consequently, this method is not widely employed (Mittal, 2009; Pavlidou & Papaspyrides, 2008).

10.3 RESULTS AND DISCUSSION

10.3.1 Chitosan

10.3.1.1 Chitosan-based Bionanocomposites for Removal of Metal Contaminants from Water

By employing the Schiff base ligand to modify chitosan, Shahraki et al. created the magnetic chitosan-(2-iminothiophenol methyl) benzaldehyde Schiff base-based adsorbent (MCS-ITMB), which they proved to be a successful adsorbent for the removal of Pb(II) from water-based solutions. They also discovered that the adsorbents containing an aromatic ring are more beneficial to Pb^{+2} ion absorption. The removal efficacy of the MCS-ITMB in the removal of Pb^{+2} was investigated using optimized parameters. When applied to isotherm models, MCS-ITMB was found to have a total adsorption efficiency of 134.10 mg/g. MCS-ITMB demonstrated good reusability and was able to keep specific efficacy of removal after five adsorption-desorption cycles. The initial pH substantially influenced Pb^{+2} ion adsorption abilities. Initially adsorption percentage of the Pb^{+2} metal increases with variation of pH from 1.0 to 5.0, after that a rapid decline in metal ion adsorption when pH values further increased above 5.0 in pH studies. As the MCS-ITMB adsorbents contains several reactive groups which can be protonated within normal aqueous environment at lower values of pH (below 5), and thus the species have lower electron density which is a requisite for bonding with metal ions. The protonated forms of adsorbent exhibited electrostatic repulsion with the Pb^{+2} ion and resulting in less adsorption ability. When there was an increase in pH values, the adsorption ability for Pb^{2+} increased as the protonation decreased and interaction between metal ion and adsorbent increased. Adsorption isotherms experiments were carried out to calculate some constants which were further used to investigate various properties determining the surface morphologies and functionalities which help in the determination of affinities present on the surface of synthesized composites. When initial metal ion concentration was increased, there was a dramatic rise in adsorption capability also. At C_0 = 60 mg/L, the adsorption efficiency reached its maximum. Above C_0 = 60 mg/L concentration there was a decrease in adsorption efficiency and finally it became unchanged. Desorption in an acidic solution was done to test the reusability of the MCS-ITMB. Adsorption process was repeated after regenerating the adsorbent five times consecutively. The total adsorption efficiency of the adsorbent remained almost constant with a minimal decline in adsorption capacity at each cycle. So the adsorbent can be employed as a possibly interesting material to remove Pb^{2+}ions from polluted water repeatedly (Shahraki et al., 2019).

Using a simple sonochemical approach, Eldeeb et al. created a nanocomposite adsorbent which are magnetic in nature from carbon nanotubes and chitosan, followed by cross-linking when citric acid used as a cross-linker. The prepared materials were employed to check the removal effectiveness of Cu^{2+} ions from their water-based solution. The adsorbent takes nearly 20 minutes to reach optimum adsorption ability for Cu^{2+} ions. The optimal pH range was in between 5.8 and 6.0. The Langmuir isotherm model was applied and data results best suited to the model and good adsorption ability of 11.77 mg g^{-1}. The magnetic MWCNTs/Cs have a magnetization of 11.591 emu/g and showed an S-shaped hysteresis loop. The magnetic characteristic of nanocomposites makes the process of removal easier (Eldeeb et al., 2021).

Hu et al. combined chitosan and polyacrylic acid (PAA). Iron nanoparticles were integrated into CS-PAA to give them magnetic characteristics and called magnetic-CS-PAA (MCS-PAA) nanocomposites. It was discovered that the maximum adsorption capacity was 204.89 mg/g when there was a presence of Pb(II) in the solution of 100 mg/L and when the equilibrium period was 70 minutes. The presence of the -COOH, -NH$_2$, and -OH in synthesized nanocomposite plays the role of lead absorption (Hu et al., 2020).

Mohamed et al. synthesized two different nanocomposites TiO_2NP-chitosan and ZrO_2NP-chitosan with a microwave-assisted method for the creation of crosslinked $NTiO_2$-Ch@$NZrO_2$-Ch nanocomposites and used them in the trivalent Gd and Sm ion removal from aqueous solution containing the mentioned ions. The formed $NTiO_2$-Ch@$NZrO_2$-Ch composite materials demonstrated excellent sorption characteristics. Overall, the experimental results demonstrated that changes in the pH of the medium, initial metal ion concentration, contact time for the reaction, and amounts of the synthesized composite used per experiment all have a significant impact on adsorption ability. At pH 7, the maximal absorption capacities for trivalent Gd were 450 and Sm was 650 mol/g, utilizing 10 mg $NTiO_2$-Ch@$NZrO_2$-Ch composite material per 10mL of Gd (III) and Sm (III) ion solution (Mahmoud et al., 2021).

Kayalvizhi et al. explored the adsorption performance of activated Sawdust-Chitosan nanocomposite beads (SDNCB) powder to examine the extraction efficiency of some ions of heavy metals like Nickel and Copper from water-based media. Synthesized cellulose and chitosan beads have suitable surface area and functional groups responsible for the fast rate of sorption kinetics of Cu^{2+} and Ni^{2+} ions. For ion adsorption, the equilibrium period was reported to be 70 minutes and the optimal pH was 5 and 6 respectively. The appearance of a negative G value confirms the spontaneity of ion adsorption process. The observed enthalpy (H) and entropy (S) values showed that it was an exothermic process accompanied by an increase in entropy (Kayalvizhi et al., 2022).

10.3.1.2 Chitosan-based Bionanocomposites for Detection of Metal Contaminants from Water

Luo et al. synthesized a unique nanocomposite for the successful detection and elimination of chromium (VI) which is a chitosan-based fluorescent hydrogel with cellulose and titanate nanofibers enhanced with carbon dots. Adsorption equilibrium isotherm results showed Langmuir type of mechanism was followed and kinetics results showed that adsorption follows pseudo-second-order model. The maximum sorption capacity for chromium (VI) was 228.2 mg g^{-1}. Chromium (VI) was measured quantitatively using a linear range of 10-80 mg L^{-1}. The mechanism underlying the highly effective detection and adsorption of Chromium (VI) in this composite was also examined using FTIR and XPS techniques. These findings demonstrated that the porous structures of nanocomposites along with presence of carbon dots modified cellulose and titanate nanofibers may be primarily responsible for chromium (VI) great sorption and detection capabilities (Luo et al., 2021).

Using glutaric aldehyde as a cross-linker, Geng et al. manufactured 3D fluorescent chitosan hydrogel (3D-FCH) effectively. The hydrogels have a limit of detection of 0.9 nM. It was found that for an analytical linear range of up to 50 nM the resultant 3D-FCH displayed exceptional fluorescence properties and were sensitive and selective for determination of Hg^{+2} in aqueous media in this range (Geng et al., 2015).

For the concurrent fluorescence adsorption and to detect copper (II) cations and Chromium (VI) anion, Chen et al. synthesized unique self-assembled nitrogen-doped carbon dots (NCDs) with cellulose nanofibril (CNF) and chitosan (CS) based hydrogel (NCDs-CNF/CS gel). The second layer of the chitosan network was created via the replacement of solvent. The NCDs cross-linked CNF hydrogel network was created using a low-temperature eco-friendly hydrothermal technique. This composite had a higher selectivity and sensitivity of fluorescence response for Chromium (VI) with a linear range of 1-50mg/L and limit of detection (LOD) of 0.7093 mg/L. A broad linear range of fluorescence of Copper(II) was found to be 50-1000 mg/L and LOD of 40.339 mg/L. For Copper(II) and Chromium(VI), this composite had remarkable adsorption rates of 148.30 mg/g and 294.46 mg/g, respectively, (Xueqi Chen, 2022).

10.3.2 Starch

10.3.2.1 Starch-based Bionanocomposites for Removal of Metal Contaminants from Water

Abdul-Raheim et al. used potato peels for extraction of starch and processed it with acrylic acid to make modifications in their research studies. The modified starch polymer was used for the synthesis of Nanoparticles along with Fe_3O_4 and was named (modified potato starch-magnetic nanoparticles, MPS-MNPs). They were specifically utilized to remove Pb^{2+}, Ni^{2+}, and Cu^{2+} ions from contaminated water selectively. Adsorption equilibrium was achieved in 60 minutes, and maximum adsorption for Cu^{2+}, Pb^{2+}, and Ni^{2+} were 100, 70, and 100 mg^{-1} at 35°C, respectively. PS-MNPs specifically absorbed Ni^{2+} ions with an adsorption preference order of $Ni^{2+}>Cu^{2+}>Pb^{2+}$. pH 5.5 was best as at this pH the maximum adsorption efficiency results were obtained (Abdul-Raheim et al., 2016).

In their study, Baghbadorani et al. looked into the efficacy of starch-g-poly(acrylic acid) (St-g-PAA) superabsorbent hydrogels mixed with cellulose nanofibers (CNFs). The synthesized superabsorbent materials were employed for testing Cu^{2+} ion elimination efficiencies. It was discovered that the maximum monolayer adsorption capacities of the St-g-PAA hydrogels without reaction with CNF and the hydrogels reacted with CNFs, respectively, were 0.736 g/g and 0.957 g/g when reaction carried out in 0.6 g/L concentration of Cu^{2+} in solution having an acidic pH of 5. The adsorption data was not fitted in the Freundlich model accurately. In simple terms, the model's curves could not be fitted since they were not linear. The different adsorption parameters in the Freundlich model isotherm (n and k) for the hydrogels reacted with CNF were 2.796 and 0.896 (L/g). For the hydrogels not reacted with CNF the same parameters had values of 2.680 and 1.347 (L/g) respectively. However, n and k values for both were not sufficiently high to make data valid for the model. On the other hand, the R^2 values for both types of hydrogels was 0.9980 and 0.9831, correspondingly, reveal the agreement among the adsorption behavior of both when applied to the Langmuir adsorption model. In Langmuir isotherm the predicted monolayer adsorption efficiency and the constant value of the samples without reaction with CNF were determined to be 0.736 g/g and 13.710 L/g respectively. The same parameter values for samples reacted with CNF were calculated to be 0.957 g/g and 20.691 L/g respectively. As there is an abundance of anionic functional groups in the composites formed by reaction with CNF, they have greater interactions with the pollutant metal which indicates that composites were better in their removal (Bahadoran Baghbadorani et al., 2019).

Starch and sodium montmorillonite were combined to create starch/Na-MMT nanocomposites by Garca-Padilla et al. By using the intercalation process in an acetic acid solution, composites with varied starch and nano clay ratios (SN) selected as 5:1, 10:1, and 10:3 were created. These composites were further employed for metals Ni and Co removal studies. After calculating the removal efficiency (97.1%) and adsorptive favorability for Ni ions, it was determined that pH value 4.5, initial concentration of 100 ppm of metal, and SN ratio 10:1 were the favorable values of parameters. For cobalt ions, a pH value of 6, 140 ppm concentration of cobalt metal, and an SN ratio of 10:3 gave maximum removal yield (78.07%). (García-Padilla et al., 2020). Starch-based/AcA hydrogel (St-AcAH) and starch-poly (acrylic acid) nanocomposites hydrogel with Fe_3O_4 (Fe_3O_4@ St-AcANCH) was devised and created by Saberi et al. using a free radical, chemical crosslinking approach with the aim of removing harmful dyes waste and harmful metals which are magnetic in nature due to incorporation of Fe_3O_4. With respect to copper, lead, Methylene Violet (MV), and Congo Red (CR) solution, the synthesized nanocomposites hydrogel exhibits excellent absorption percentages by a natural physisorption process that exhibits strong consistency with Langmuir isotherm and pseudo-second-order models. According to research, nanocomposite hydrogel so formed was a powerful adsorbent for eliminating metals and dyes from solution, opening up new opportunities for water and environmental concerns. Following 7 successive rounds of adsorption–desorption, St-AcAH, and Fe_3O_4@StAcANCH both retained almost 66.0% and 89.1% of their initial adsorption capacities, respectively (Saberi et al., 2019).

10.3.2.2 Starch-based Bionanocomposites for Detection of Metal Contaminants from Water

Balasurya et al. synthesize and characterize Fe@Ag-starch nanocomposite by a variety of characterization methods, where XRD patterns confirm that the fabricated particle was crystalline and pure in composition. Fe@Ag-starch nanocomposite conjugated with phenylalanine was used to investigate mercury detection. The outcomes demonstrate that the detection was accurate and focused on Hg^{+2} ions. For the purpose of detecting Hg^{+2}, it was determined that the current probe has a limit of detection of 1.84 nM. They also validate the impact of different metal ions on the detection efficiency of Hg^{+2} and showed that they had no effect on the Fe@Ag-starch phenylalanine conjugate's ability to detect Hg^{+2} ions. At 40°C, pH=5, and 0.1% saline content, the detection of Hg^{+2} ions was successful. As a result, the produced probe can also be utilized to detect Hg^{+2} ions from a variety of environmental samples (Balasurya et al., 2021).

10.3.3 Cellulose

10.3.3.1 Cellulose-based Bionanocomposites for Removal of Metal Contaminants from Water

Liu et al. offer a sustainable and inexpensive method for creating a composite made of polydopamine (PDA), cellulose fibers (CF), and titanium dioxide nanoparticles (TiO_2 NPs) called TiO_2/PDA/CF in which PDA form a protective layering. The PDA layer inspired by mussels, stuck to CF stably, and TiO_2 NPs were immobilized on the surface of the layer so formed which were formed by $TiOSO_4$ hydrolysis. The PDA layer contributed to the enhancement of composite's stability and superior reutilization properties. Additionally, the adsorption capabilities of lead and methylene blue which were calculated as 20 mg/g for Pb^{2+} and 15 mg/g for methylene blue were significantly improved by the TiO_2/PDA functional layer than by the use of only cellulose fiber. The adsorption capacity of the TiO_2/PDA/CF was greater than TiO_2/CF at equilibrium (qe). The negative charges of cellulose and PDA are widely known to exist over a large pH range, and the TiO_2 NPs likewise exhibit an isoelectric point at pH 6.2. Because of the protonation of the functional groups on the surface of adsorbents in low pH solution and the intense electrostatic repulsion created between protonated functional groups on absorbents and positively charged metal ions, (Pb^{2+}) has low adsorption capabilities in low pH or acidic conditions (Liu et al., 2018).

Making composite membranes that have excellent adsorption capacities for water treatment is an alternative way to use biopolymers. In the study, Saber-Samandari et al. synthesized a membrane by grafting between carboxymethyl cellulose and poly(acrylic acid) with the inclusion of

Table 10.1 List of nanocomposites and the corresponding metal ions they remove

Sr. No.	Type of nanocomposites	Metal ion removal	References
1.	Chitosan-(2-iminothiophenol methyl) benzaldehyde Schiff base-based adsorbent (MCS-ITMB)	Pb^{+2}	Shahraki et al., 2019
2.	Carbon nanotubes with chitosan	Cu(II)	Eldeeb et al., 2021
3.	Magnetic-CS-PAA (Chitosan and polyacrylic acid)	Pb(II)	Hu et al., 2020
4.	$NTiO_2$-Ch@$NZrO_2$-Ch	Gd and Sm ion	Mahmoud et al., 2021
5.	Sawdust-Chitosan nanocomposite beads (SDNCB)	Nickel and Copper	Kayalvizhi et al., 2022
6.	Modified potato starch-magnetic nanoparticles, MPS-MNPs)	Pb^{2+}, Cu^{2+}, and Ni^{2+}	Abdul-Raheim et al., 2016
7.	Starch-g-poly(acrylic acid) (St-g-PAA) with cellulose nanofibers (CNFs).	Cu^{2+}	Bahadoran Baghbadorani et al., 2019
8.	Starch and sodium montmorillonite (starch/Na-MMT) nanocomposites	Ni and Co	García-Padilla et al., 2020
9.	Starch-based/AcA hydrogel (St-AcAH) and Starch-poly(acrylic acid) nanocomposites hydrogel with Fe_3O_4 (Fe_3O_4@St-AcANCH)	Copper, lead, Methylene Violet (MV), and Congo Red (CR) solution,	Saberi et al., 2019
10.	Polydopamine (PDA), cellulose fibers (CF), and titanium dioxide nanoparticles (TiO_2 NPs) (TiO_2/PDA/CF) nanocomposite	lead and methylene blue	Liu et al., 2018
11.	carboxymethyl cellulose and poly(acrylic acid) with silica gel	cadmium (Cd (II)) and crystal violet (CV) dye	Saber-Samandari et al., 2016
12.	cobalt ferrite nanoparticles (CF), titanate nanotubes (T), and alginate (G) nanocomposite (CF/G and T/G)	copper, iron, and Arsenic ions Cu^{2+}, Fe^{3+}, and As^{3+}	Esmat et al., 2017
13.	Multi-walled carbon nanotubes with amide groups (CNT-$CONH_2$)	Co (II) ions	Karkeh-abadi et al., 2016
14	alginate beads with Ni(II) imprinting and non-imprinted alginate beads	Ni(II) ion	Özkahraman et al., 2018

an inorganic filler (silica gel) to create a back to strengthen the membrane. Subsequently, various concentrations of bentonite were added as a multipurpose crosslinker to the above-mentioned cellulose-grafted networks to create nanocomposite membranes. The newly created nanocomposite membranes were used as base material to remove the ions of cadmium (Cd (II)) and crystal violet (CV) dye efficiently (Saber-Samandari et al., 2016).

10.3.3.2 Cellulose-based Bionanocomposites for Detection of Metal Contaminants from Water

Luo et al. employed a crosslinking technique to effectively produce a fluorescent magnetic hydrogel with amino-functionalized Fe_3O_4 nanoparticles (AF-Fe_3O_4NPs) and cellulose nanoparticles (CNFs) modified with carbon dots (CDs). The selectivity and detection sensitivity of the fluorescence sensor for Chromium (VI) were investigated. 20-800 mg/L range was used to obtain the quantitative detection of chromium(VI). Meanwhile, to analyze the highly effective detection and adsorption of FMCH for chromium(VI) FTIR and XPS techniques were used. These findings demonstrated that chromium(VI)'s outstanding sorption and detecting properties which may be primarily because of porous structures that offered a large number of active sites and also contain ion transport channels in between pores. The additional AF-Fe_3O_4 and CNFs modified with CDs had enhanced chromium(VI)'s sorption capacity and provided a quick visual reaction to chromium(VI). It demonstrates how the FMCH may be effectively utilized to detect and remove chromium(VI) from wastewater (Yong Luo, 2023).

Oyuz et al. synthesized inexpensive ecologically friendly material for Fe(III) ions so that these ions can be removed and detected from polluted streams. For this, basic cellulose in a powdered state was initially produced by immobilizing hexamethylene diisocyanate. After being activated, cellulose was changed with a bodipy (fluorinated boron-dipyrromethene) for practical spectroscopic tests to efficiently detect and eliminate Fe(III) ions from the contaminated medium. For detecting Fe(III) ions under both long-wave light and daytime, the Bodipy-based cellulose demonstrated outstanding performance (Oguz et al., 2020).

By utilizing cellulose/CBIMMT modified-ligand nanocomposite, an extremely small quantity of Bi(III) ions was determined in realistic water samples by Asadi-Ojaee et al. 4-(40-chlorobenzylideneimino)-3-methyl-5-mercapto-1,2,4-triazole (CBIMMT) employed to produce a ligand which is then immobilized on nanocellulose and then used to develop the designed composites. With a limit of detection of 2.68 ng mL^{-1}, the as-prepared calibration graph displays a uniform curve of bismuth (III) ions for a concentration range of 10–500 ng mL^{-1}. 1.5% was the value of the calculated RSD. The as-synthesized nanocomposites were used as sensing materials for the detection of Bi(III) ions present in the original water samples (Asadi-Ojaee et al., 2019).

10.3.4 Alginate

10.3.4.1 Alginate-based Bionanocomposites for Removal of Metal Contaminants from Water

Esmat et al. first synthesized cobalt ferrite nanoparticles (CF), titanate nanotubes (T), and alginate (G), and then used these to synthesize their nanocomposite materials (CF/G and T/G) by using CF, T as nanofillers and employed for successful elimination of copper, iron, and Arsenic ions. Cu^{2+}, Fe^{3+}, and As^{3+} removal efficiencies were found to be quite good. The construction of composites makes composites easier to manage than single counterparts (Esmat et al., 2017).

Multi-walled carbon nanotubes with amide groups ($CNT-CONH_2$) were imprinted in a composite made of sodium alginate incorporating hydroxyapatite by Karkeh-abadi et al. and finally led to nanocomposite beads synthesis. A major issue with sodium alginate and its derived compounds is their lack of strength and elasticity due to their high water-retention abilities. Hydroxyapatite was found to be uniformly distributed in the matrix of polymers with lower strength like alginate to make polymer mechanical characteristics better. The nanocomposite beads were produced and employed as an adsorbent for Cobalt ions adsorption from their solution. In the optimum reaction parameters, the maximum Co (II) ion binding efficiency of the produced nanocomposite beads was 347.8 mg^{-1}. Adsorption of divalent cobalt ions in an environment of other competing foreign ions including Fe(III), Zn(II), Ni(II), Pb(II), Cu(II), Ca(II), and Hg(II) etc. has been performed. Because of competition with Cobalt ions to bind at the top of the adsorbent, the adsorbents can only consume nearly half their total binding abilitiesfor Co(II) ions. The results clearly indicate that the mechanism of Co absorption was not selective, and thus the synthesized composite can be employed in the removal of a variety of ionic pollutants (different ions) from wastewater (Karkeh-abadi et al., 2016).

The authors Özkahramanet al. used a very different way of developing Ni(II) ion selectivity. They prepared two different types of alginate beads one with Ni(II) imprinting (first synthesis with Ni and then its Desorption) and other simple non-imprinted alginate beads (synthesis without Ni) and employed in the adsorption experiments of the nickel ions. The maximum and selective adsorption capacity of Ni(II) imprinted alginate beads (IIP) was 6.00 mmol g^{-1}. By virtue of the imprinted pits that formed in the IIP alginate bead which resembles divalent nickel ions in both form and size, the Nickel imprinted bead showed a high ability to selectively adsorb Ni(II) when present along with Cu(II), Co(II), and Zn(II) ions. Due to the lack of specific binding pits, NIP alginate beads exhibited almost similar binding affinities for all other metals except Nickel (Özkahraman et al., 2018).

10.3.4.2 Alginate-based Bionanocomposites for Detection of Metal Contaminants from Water

Faghiri et al. fabricated a novel hybrid nano-sensor of silver nanoparticles incorporated sodium alginate composites (SA-Ag NPs) with a solvent casting approach and further employed the same for the detection of heavy metal Hg^{+2} ions in sample solutions calorimetrically and visually. The viability of synthesized Sodium alginate and silver nanoparticle nano-sensors was verified for preservation over time. According to the optimization results, this nanosensor was extremely effective for detecting Hg^{+2} ions at pH 6 with 7 minutes response time, and 5.29nM limit of detection. Within the range of concentrations of 0.025-50nM, an acceptable linear connection with the LSPR (localized surface plasmon resonance) absorbance and the concentration of Hg^{+2} ions was found. The created nanosensor also had an exceptionally high selectivity for the Hg^{+2} ion when compared to the other ions used in the experiment, and it was effectively used to determine the presence of Hg^{+2} in different samples collected from various environmental segments. Consequently, Sodium alginate and silver nanoparticles can be utilized in various fields as have broad areas of potential applications and great marketing value (Faghiri & Gorbani, 2019).

10.4 CONCLUSION

From the above discussion it can be concluded that tremendous research has already been done in the field of metal ion removal by natural polymer-based nanocomposites, but not in the field of metal detection by the same when both are compared. Almost every natural polymer has been utilized to large or small extent in this field because of their non-toxic biocompatible nature and also due to easy availability and less cost, but we had discussed only few in detail as the literature is very vast. So far, we have discussed that the natural polymers have good adsorbing abilities but still have some limitations like low mechanical strength which are enhanced by creating their nanocomposites which combine the advantages of both. The polymer nanocomposites thus formed are found to be reusable up to 5–6 times as reported in most of cases. Despite these advantages there are still some facts on which further research is needed. Firstly, the use of nanocomposites in metal detection is less that should be on the focus in future research. Also, their reusability properties should be more so that the polymer nanocomposites can

Table 10.2   List of nanocomposites and the corresponding metal ions they detect

Sr. No.	Type of nanocomposites	Metal ion detected	References
1.	Chitosan-based fluorescent hydrogel with cellulose and titanate nanofibers enhanced with carbon dots	Chromium (VI)	Luo et al., 2021
2.	3D fluorescent chitosan hydrogel (3D-FCH)	Hg^{+2}	Geng et al., 2015
3.	Nitrogen-doped carbon dots (NCDs) with cellulose nanofibril (CNF) and chitosan (CS) based hydrogel (NCDs-CNF/CS gel).	Copper (II) cations and Chromium (VI) anion	Xueqi Chen, 2022
4.	Fe@Ag-starch	Hg^{+2}	Balasurya et al., 2021
5.	Fluorescent magnetic hydrogel with amino-functionalized Fe_3O_4 nanoparticles (AF-Fe_3O_4NPs) and cellulose nanoparticles (CNFs) modified with carbon dots (CDs).	Chromium (VI)	(Yong Luo, 2023)
6.	Bodipy (Fluorinated Boron-Dipyrromethene)	Fe (III)	Oguz et al., 2020
7.	Cellulose/CBIMMT (4-(40-chlorobenzylideneimino)-3-methyl-5-mercapto-1, 2, 4-triazole) nanocomposite	Bi (III)	Asadi-Ojaee et al., 2019
8.	Silver nanoparticles with sodium alginate (SA-Ag NPs)	Hg^{+2}	(Faghiri & Gorbani, 2019

be utilized in practical applications. So further research is required in the reusability studies. One more issue which is of importance is that in actual practices the metal contaminants are not present as isolated system, but there is various other pollutant in the polluted water, which can interfere, so further studies to resolve these practical problems is needed. From whole studies we can say that polymer-based nanocomposites are among best metal ion removal materials, and can be utilized in actual practices with some deep research in abovementioned issues.

REFERENCES

Abdul-Raheim, A. R. M., El-Saeed Shimaa, M., Farag, R. K., & Abdel-Raouf Manar, E. (2016). Low cost biosorbents based on modified starch iron oxide nanocomposites for selective removal of some heavy metals from aqueous solutions. *Advanced Materials Letters*, 7(5), 402–409. https://doi.org/10.5185/amlett.2016.6061

Abedi, S., & Abdouss, M. (2014). A review of clay-supported Ziegler-Natta catalysts for production of polyolefin/clay nanocomposites through in situ polymerization. In *Applied Catalysis A: General* (Vol. 475, pp. 386–409). https://doi.org/10.1016/j.apcata.2014.01.028

Alexandre, M., & Dubois, P. (n.d.). *Polymer-layered Silicate Nanocomposites: Preparation, Properties and Uses of a New Class of Materials, Materials Science and Engineering: R: Reports,* 28 (1-2), pp. 1–63.

Aragay, G., Pons, J., & Merkoçi, A. (2011). Recent trends in macro-, micro-, and nanomaterial-based tools and strategies for heavy-metal detection. In *Chemical Reviews* (Vol. 111, Issue 5, pp. 3433–3458). https://doi.org/10.1021/cr100383r

Asadi-Ojaee, S. S., Mirabi, A., Rad, A. S., Movaghgharnezhad, S., & Hallajian, S. (2019). Removal of Bismuth (III) ions from water solution using a cellulose-based nanocomposite: A detailed study by DFT and experimental insights. *Journal of Molecular Liquids,* 295. https://doi.org/10.1016/j.molliq.2019.111723

Asere, T. G., Stevens, C. V., & Du Laing, G. (2019). Use of (modified) natural adsorbents for arsenic remediation: A review. In *Science of the Total Environment* (Vol. 676, pp. 706–720). Elsevier B.V. https://doi.org/10.1016/j.scitotenv.2019.04.237

Azizi-Lalabadi, M., & Jafari, S. M. (2021). Bio-nanocomposites of graphene with biopolymers; fabrication, properties, and applications. In *Advances in Colloid and Interface Science* (Vol. 292). Elsevier B.V. https://doi.org/10.1016/j.cis.2021.102416

Badsha, M. A. H., Khan, M., Wu, B., Kumar, A., & Lo, I. M. C. (2021). Role of surface functional groups of hydrogels in metal adsorption: From performance to mechanism. In *Journal of Hazardous Materials* (Vol. 408). Elsevier B.V. https://doi.org/10.1016/j.jhazmat.2020.124463

Bahadoran Baghbadorani, N., Behzad, T., Etesami, N., & Heidarian, P. (2019). Removal of Cu2+ ions by cellulose nanofibers-assisted starch-g-poly(acrylic acid) superadsorbent hydrogels. *Composites Part B: Engineering,* 176. https://doi.org/10.1016/j.compositesb.2019.107084

Balasurya, S., Syed, A., Swedha, M., Harini, G., Elgorban, A. M., Zaghloul, N. S. S., Das, A., & Khan, S. S. (2021). A novel SPR based Fe@Ag core–shell nanosphere entrapped on starch matrix an optical probe for sensing of mercury(II) ion: A nanomolar detection, wide pH range and real water sample application. *Spectrochimica Acta - Part A: Molecular and Biomolecular Spectroscopy,* 263. https://doi.org/10.1016/j.saa.2021.120204

Chakraborty, G., Katiyar, V., & Pugazhenthi, G. (2021). Improvisation of polylactic acid (PLA)/exfoliated graphene (GR) nanocomposite for detection of metal ions (Cu2+). *Composites Science and Technology,* 213. https://doi.org/10.1016/j.compscitech.2021.108877

Duffus, J. H. (2002). "Heavy metals"-A meaningless term? (IUPAC technical report). In John H. Duffus (Ed.), *Pure and Applied Chemistry* (pp. 793–807), (Vol. 74, Issue 5). W. A. Temple.

Eldeeb, T. M., El Nemr, A., Khedr, M. H., & El-Dek, S. I. (2021). Efficient removal of Cu(II) from water solution using magnetic chitosan nanocomposite. *Nanotechnology for Environmental Engineering,* 6(2). https://doi.org/10.1007/s41204-021-00129-w

Esmat, M., Farghali, A. A., Khedr, M. H., & El-Sherbiny, I. M. (2017). Alginate-based nanocomposites for efficient removal of heavy metal ions. *International Journal of Biological Macromolecules, 102,* 272–283. https://doi.org/10.1016/j.ijbiomac.2017.04.021

Faghiri, F., & Ghorbani, F. (2019). Colorimetric and naked eye detection of trace Hg2+ ions in the environmental water samples based on plasmonic response of sodium alginate impregnated by silver nanoparticles. *Journal of Hazardous Materials, 374,* 329–340. https://doi.org/10.1016/j.jhazmat.2019.04.052

Fu, S., Sun, Z., Huang, P., Li, Y., & Hu, N. (2019). Some basic aspects of polymer nanocomposites: A critical review. *Nano Materials Science, 1*(1), 2–30. https://doi.org/10.1016/j.nanoms.2019.02.006

García-Padilla, Á., Moreno-Sader, K. A., Realpe, Á., Acevedo-Morantes, M., & Soares, J. B. P. (2020). Evaluation of adsorption capacities of nanocomposites prepared from bean starch and montmorillonite. *Sustainable Chemistry and Pharmacy, 17.* https://doi.org/10.1016/j.scp.2020.100292

Geng, Z., Zhang, H., Xiong, Q., Zhang, Y., Zhao, H., & Wang, G. (2015). A fluorescent chitosan hydrogel detection platform for the sensitive and selective determination of trace mercury(II) in water. *Journal of Materials Chemistry A, 3*(38), 19455–19460. https://doi.org/10.1039/c5ta05610a

Gumpu, M. B., Sethuraman, S., Krishnan, U. M., & Rayappan, J. B. B. (2015). A review on detection of heavy metal ions in water - An electrochemical approach. In *Sensors and Actuators, B: Chemical* (Vol. 213, pp. 515–533). Elsevier B.V. https://doi.org/10.1016/j.snb.2015.02.122

Hu, D., Lian, Z., Xian, H., Jiang, R., Wang, N., Weng, Y., Peng, X., Wang, S., & Ouyang, X. –K. (2020). Adsorption of Pb(II) from aqueous solution by polyacrylic acid grafted magnetic chitosan nanocomposite. *International Journal of Biological Macromolecules, 154,* 1537–1547. https://doi.org/10.1016/j.ijbiomac.2019.11.038

Jamshaid, A., Hamid, A., Muhammad, N., Naseer, A., Ghauri, M., Iqbal, J., Rafiq, S., & Shah, N. S. (2017). Cellulose-based materials for the removal of heavy metals from wastewater – an overview. In *ChemBioEng Reviews* (Vol. 4, Issue 4, pp. 240–256). Wiley-Blackwell. https://doi.org/10.1002/cben.201700002

Karkeh-abadi, F., Saber-Samandari, S., & Saber-Samandari, S. (2016). The impact of functionalized CNT in the network of sodium alginate-based nanocomposite beads on the removal of Co(II) ions from aqueous solutions. *Journal of Hazardous Materials, 312,* 224–233. https://doi.org/10.1016/j.jhazmat.2016.03.074

Kayalvizhi, K., Alhaji, N. M. I., Saravanakkumar, D., Mohamed, S. B., Kaviyarasu, K., Ayeshamariam, A., Al-Mohaimeed, A. M., AbdelGawwad, M. R., & Elshikh, M. S. (2022). Adsorption of copper and nickel by using sawdust chitosan nanocomposite beads – A kinetic and thermodynamic study. *Environmental Research, 203.* https://doi.org/10.1016/j.envres.2021.111814

Lee, J. H., Jung, D., Hong, C. E., Rhee, K. Y., & Advani, S. G. (2005). Properties of polyethylene-layered silicate nanocomposites prepared by melt intercalation with a PP-g-MA compatibilizer. *Composites Science and Technology, 65*(13), 1996–2002. https://doi.org/10.1016/j.compscitech.2005.03.015

Li, M., Gou, H., Al-Ogaidi, I., & Wu, N. (2013). Nanostructured sensors for detection of heavy metals: A review. *ACS Sustainable Chemistry and Engineering, 1*(7), 713–723. https://doi.org/10.1021/sc400019a

Liu, R., Dai, L., & Si, C. L. (2018). Mussel-inspired cellulose-based nanocomposite fibers for adsorption and photocatalytic degradation. *ACS Sustainable Chemistry and Engineering, 6*(11), 15756–15763. https://doi.org/10.1021/acssuschemeng.8b04320

Luo, Q., Huang, X., Luo, Y., Yuan, H., Ren, T., Li, X., Xu, D., Guo, X., & Wu, Y. (2021). Fluorescent chitosan-based hydrogel incorporating titanate and cellulose nanofibers modified with carbon dots for adsorption and detection of Cr(VI). *Chemical Engineering Journal, 407*. https://doi.org/10.1016/j.cej.2020.127050

Mahmoud, M. E., Nabil, G. M., & Elweshahy, S. M. T. (2021). Novel NTiO2-chitosan@NZrO2-chitosan nanocomposite for effective adsorptive uptake of trivalent gadolinium and samarium ions from water. *Powder Technology, 378*, 246–254. https://doi.org/10.1016/j.powtec.2020.09.058

Mittal, V. (2009). Polymer layered silicate nanocomposites: A review. *Materials, 2*(3), 992–1057. https://doi.org/10.3390/ma2030992

Muthivhi, R., Parani, S., May, B., & Oluwafemi, O. S. (2018). Green synthesis of gelatin-noble metal polymer nanocomposites for sensing of Hg2+ ions in aqueous media. *Nano-Structures and Nano-Objects, 13*, 132–138. https://doi.org/10.1016/j.nanoso.2017.12.008

Nasrollahzadeh, M., Sajjadi, M., Iravani, S., & Varma, R. S. (2021). Starch, cellulose, pectin, gum, alginate, chitin and chitosan derived (nano)materials for sustainable water treatment: A review. In *Carbohydrate Polymers* (Vol. 251). Elsevier Ltd. https://doi.org/10.1016/j.carbpol.2020.116986

Oguz, M., Kursunlu, A. N., & Yilmaz, M. (2020). Low-cost and environmentally sensitive fluorescent cellulose paper for naked-eye detection of Fe(III) in aqueous media. *Dyes and Pigments, 173*. https://doi.org/10.1016/j.dyepig.2019.107974

Orta, M. del M., Martín, J., Santos, J. L., Aparicio, I., Medina-Carrasco, S., & Alonso, E. (2020). Biopolymer-clay nanocomposites as novel and ecofriendly adsorbents for environmental remediation. In *Applied Clay Science* (Vol. 198). Elsevier Ltd. https://doi.org/10.1016/j.clay.2020.105838

Özkahraman, B., Özbaş, Z., & Bal Öztürk, A. (2018). Synthesis of Ion-imprinted alginate based beads: selective adsorption behavior of Nickel (II) Ions. *Journal of Polymers and the Environment, 26*(11), 4303–4310. https://doi.org/10.1007/s10924-018-1292-6

Pavlidou, S., & Papaspyrides, C. D. (2008). A review on polymer-layered silicate nanocomposites. In *Progress in Polymer Science (Oxford)* (Vol. 33, Issue 12, pp. 1119–1198). https://doi.org/10.1016/j.progpolymsci.2008.07.008

Saberi, A., Alipour, E., & Sadeghi, M. (2019). Superabsorbent magnetic Fe3O4-based starch-poly (acrylic acid) nanocomposite hydrogel for efficient removal of dyes and heavy metal ions from water. *Journal of Polymer Research, 26*(12). https://doi.org/10.1007/s10965-019-1917-z

Saber-Samandari, S., Saber-Samandari, S., Heydaripour, S., & Abdouss, M. (2016). Novel carboxymethyl cellulose based nanocomposite membrane: Synthesis, characterization and application in water treatment. *Journal of Environmental Management, 166*, 457–465. https://doi.org/10.1016/j.jenvman.2015.10.045

Shahraki, S., Delarami, H. S., & Khosravi, F. (2019). Synthesis and characterization of an adsorptive Schiff base-chitosan nanocomposite for removal of Pb(II) ion from aqueous media. *International Journal of Biological Macromolecules, 139*, 577–586. https://doi.org/10.1016/j.ijbiomac.2019.07.223

Shen, Z., Simon, G. P., & Cheng, Y.-B. (n.d.). Comparison of solution intercalation and melt intercalation of polymer±clay nanocomposites. www.elsevier.com/locate/polymer

Singh, R., Singh, S., Parihar, P., Singh, V. P., & Prasad, S. M. (2015). Arsenic contamination, consequences and remediation techniques: A review. In *Ecotoxicology and Environmental Safety* (Vol. 112, pp. 247–270). Academic Press. https://doi.org/10.1016/j.ecoenv.2014.10.009

Tag, K., Riedel, K., Bauer, H. J., Hanke, G., Baronian, K. H. R., & Kunze, G. (2007). Amperometric detection of Cu2+ by yeast biosensors using flow injection analysis (FIA). *Sensors and Actuators, B: Chemical, 122*(2), 403–409. https://doi.org/10.1016/j.snb.2006.06.007

Turdean, G. L. (2011). Design and development of biosensors for the detection of heavy metal toxicity. *International Journal of Electrochemistry, 2011*, 1–15. https://doi.org/10.4061/2011/343125

Wongsasuluk, P., Chotpantarat, S., Siriwong, W., & Robson, M. (2014). Heavy metal contamination and human health risk assessment in drinking water from shallow groundwater wells in an agricultural area in Ubon Ratchathani province, Thailand. *Environmental Geochemistry and Health, 36*(1), 169–182. https://doi.org/10.1007/s10653-013-9537-8

Xueqi Chen, Z. S. (2022). Fluorescent carbon dots crosslinked cellulose Nanofibril/Chitosan interpenetrating hydrogel system for sensitive detection and efficient adsorption of Cu(II) and Cr(VI). *Chemical Engineering Journal, 430*. https://doi.org/10.1016/j.cej.2021.133154

Yong Luo, Z. H. (2023). Fluorescent magnetic chitosan-based hydrogel incorporating Amino-Functionlized Fe3O4 and cellulose nanofibres modified with carbon dots for adsorption and detection of Cr(VI). *Colloids and Surfaces A: Physicochemical and Engineering Aspects, 658*. https://doi.org/10.1016/j.colsurfa.2022.130673

Zare, Y., & Shabani, I. (2016). Polymer/metal nanocomposites for biomedical applications. In *Materials Science and Engineering* C (Vol. 60, pp. 195–203). Elsevier Ltd. https://doi.org/10.1016/j.msec.2015.11.023

Zhang, L., & Fang, M. (2010). Nanomaterials in pollution trace detection and environmental improvement. In *Nano Today* (Vol. 5, Issue 2, pp. 128–142). https://doi.org/10.1016/j.nantod.2010.03.002

Zhao, G., Huang, X., Tang, Z., Huang, Q., Niu, F., & Wang, X. (2018). Polymer-based nanocomposites for heavy metal ions removal from aqueous solution: A review. In *Polymer Chemistry* (Vol. 9, Issue 26, pp. 3562–3582). Royal Society of Chemistry. https://doi.org/10.1039/c8py00484f

Chapter 11

Biomimetic Nanocomposites for Orthopedic Applications

Milad Heidari, Sivasakthivel Thangavel, and Ashwani Kumar

11.1 INTRODUCTION

Orthopedic applications, that deal with musculoskeletal issues, require materials that go beyond the limitations of traditional options like metals and polymers. The need for innovative materials arises from challenges related to biocompatibility, mechanical properties, and long-term performance. Unlike conventional materials, innovative materials prioritize seamless integration with the biological environment, ensuring better biocompatibility and minimizing complications such as inflammation and rejection. These materials are designed to exhibit mechanical properties that resemble natural tissues, providing the necessary strength, flexibility, and durability within the musculoskeletal system. They also often possess regenerative capabilities, promoting tissue growth and supporting natural healing processes [1–3].

Innovative materials aim to overcome issues associated with traditional implants, including infection, wear, and implant loosening, thereby enhancing the overall success and longevity of orthopedic interventions. The field of orthopedics is evolving towards patient-specific solutions, and advanced materials allow for the development of custom-designed implants tailored to individual anatomy and specific orthopedic conditions. Ultimately, the pursuit of innovative materials is crucial in advancing orthopedic treatments, improving patient outcomes, and restoring health and functionality in the musculoskeletal system. The importance of biomimicry in designing nanocomposites for orthopedics lies in the ability to take inspiration from the intricate designs and adaptive mechanisms found in nature. Biomimicry involves emulating biological structures and processes to create materials that closely mimic the properties and behaviors of natural tissues. In the realm of orthopedics, where the goal is to seamlessly integrate implants with the human body, biomimetic nanocomposites offer unique advantages.

DOI: 10.1201/9781003470311-11

The optimization of mechanical strength, flexibility, and biocompatibility in materials is a skill that nature has perfected. By imitating these qualities, biomimetic nanocomposites can closely resemble bones, cartilage, and other musculoskeletal components. This similarity improves compatibility with the body, reducing the risk of negative reactions and enhancing the success of orthopedic procedures. Additionally, biomimetic design principles aid in the development of nanocomposites that interact actively with the biological environment, promoting regenerative processes. By replicating the hierarchical structures found in natural tissues, cell adhesion, proliferation, and differentiation can be improved. This biomimetic approach fosters tissue growth and regeneration, which are crucial factors in orthopedic applications focused on repairing or replacing damaged musculoskeletal structures [4, 5].

Orthopedic materials today confront a formidable task in addressing the many facets of mechanical integrity, biocompatibility, and long-term performance. Conventional materials used in orthopaedic applications frequently don't mesh well with the intricate biological environment, leading to problems like rejection, inflammation, and reduced functionality. The gap that currently exists highlights the critical need for novel materials that can get past these constraints and provide better durability and biocompatibility. Biomimetic nanocomposites present a promising approach by striving to mimic the complex architecture and characteristics of biological tissues. This chapter looks at how biomimetic nanocomposites can transform orthopedic materials and improve patient care to investigate and close this important gap.

11.2 FUNDAMENTALS OF BIOMIMETIC NANOCOMPOSITES

Biomimetic materials are inspired by nature and are designed with specific properties in mind by mimicking the structures, functions, and processes found in biological systems. These materials mimic the efficiency and resilience of nature by imitating its molecular makeup and hierarchical organization. Biomimetic materials aim to improve biocompatibility, durability, and functionality by mimicking the complexity of living organisms. These materials tackle difficult problems in a variety of fields by utilizing the design principles found in nature, providing answers that closely resemble the adaptability and efficiency found in biological entities. Biomimetic materials are essential in orthopedics because they can be used to create nanocomposites that are specifically designed to resemble the mechanical properties of bones and tissues [6, 7].

11.2.1 Overview of Nanocomposites and their Relevance to Orthopedics

The overview of nanocomposites and how they relate to orthopedics reveals a paradigm shift in material science that could greatly improve the care of musculoskeletal conditions. A class of materials known as nanocomposites is created when nanoscale reinforcements – typically nanoparticles or nanofibers – are incorporated into a matrix to improve the material's mechanical, biological, and thermal properties. The application of nanocomposites presents a novel strategy in orthopedics to overcome the drawbacks of traditional materials. These cutting-edge materials meet the complex needs of the musculoskeletal system by providing enhanced strength, flexibility, and biocompatibility. Materials can be engineered with specific properties using nanocomposites, enabling customization for particular orthopedic applications. Finer control over material characteristics is made possible by the nanoscale components, guaranteeing a closer match to the mechanical properties of bones and tissues

Relevance to orthopedics extends beyond mechanical performance. Nanocomposites can mimic the hierarchical structures found in natural tissues, fostering improved cell adhesion, proliferation, and tissue regeneration. This biomimetic approach is particularly significant in orthopedic applications where the seamless integration of implants with biological systems is paramount for successful outcomes. Moreover, nanocomposites show promise in drug delivery systems, enabling targeted and controlled release of therapeutic agents for localized treatment of orthopedic conditions, such as osteoarthritis or bone infections. The nanoscale architecture facilitates interactions at the cellular level, opening avenues for innovative treatments and accelerated healing processes [8, 9].

Notwithstanding these encouraging developments, issues with scalability, affordability, and long-term safety still exist. This chapter will examine recent developments and how nanocomposites might be able to help with these problems, highlighting how they could influence orthopedic materials in the future. This chapter seeks to shed light on the rapidly changing field of nanocomposites and their critical role in transforming orthopedic interventions through a thorough analysis.

11.2.2 Key Properties of Biomimetic Nanocomposites

Key properties of biomimetic nanocomposites include enhanced biocompatibility, replicating natural tissue structures, and promoting regenerative responses. These materials exhibit superior mechanical strength, mimicking the resilience of biological counterparts. Tailored at the nanoscale, they enable precise control over properties, fostering optimal integration with the musculoskeletal system for advanced orthopedic applications (Table 11.1).

Table 11.1   Properties of biomimetic nanocomposites.

Key properties of biomimetic nanocomposites
Enhanced Biocompatibility
Replication of Natural Tissue Structures
Promotion of Regenerative Responses
Superior Mechanical Strength
Nanoscale Tailoring for Precise Control
Optimal Integration with Musculoskeletal System
Advanced Orthopedic Application Capabilities

11.3 BIOMIMETIC DESIGN PRINCIPLES

Based on the idea of biomimicry, biomimetic design principles offer a convincing strategy for directing the creation of novel materials for orthopedic applications. By mimicking nature's creative responses to difficult problems, biomimicry aims to develop materials with the same adaptability, resilience, and efficiency as biological systems.

These design principles apply to biomimetic nanocomposites for orthopedics and include the examination and integration of natural structures and processes. From the self-healing properties of certain organisms to the hierarchical organization of bone microstructures, nature is a rich source of inspiration. The identification and comprehension of these biological blueprints is covered in the discussion of biomimetic design principles. Through the application of natural systems' innate wisdom, scientists seek to mimic the anatomical and functional properties that make natural tissues resilient and flexible. Analyzing biological materials' molecular makeup, spatial organization, and dynamic responses is required [10, 11].

Moreover, the engineering of nanocomposites to closely resemble the behavior of living tissues is guided by the principles of biomimetic design. This entails modifying surface features, mechanical attributes, and biocompatibility to match the particular requirements of orthopedic applications. By taking cues from natural processes, these principles help to develop materials that work in harmony with the human body to enhance patient outcomes and extend the life of orthopedic interventions. Table 11.2 illustrates how biomimetic nanocomposites can be designed using natural materials as a model, leading to advancements in orthopedic biomaterials.

Applying biomimetic design principles to nanocomposite design represents a cutting-edge approach, seamlessly integrating biological inspiration into the meticulous engineering of advanced materials. The process begins with an in-depth analysis of the hierarchical structures, molecular compositions, and dynamic functionalities inherent in natural materials, such as bone or cartilage. This comprehensive understanding serves as the

Table 11.2 Examples of natural materials inspiring design [12–17]

Natural materials	Inspiring design in biomimetic nanocomposites
Bone Structure	• Hierarchical Composition: Emulating the arrangement of collagen and hydroxyapatite at the nanoscale for enhanced mechanical strength.
Cartilage	• Viscoelastic Properties: Replicating the dynamic response of natural cartilage with collagen and proteoglycans for flexibility and compressive strength.
Spider Silk	• High Tensile Strength and Flexibility: Mimicking the molecular structure to create nanocomposites with superior mechanical properties.
Sea Shells	• Self-Healing Capabilities: Integrating self-healing mechanisms inspired by sea shells for enhanced durability and longevity.
Gecko Feet	• Adhesive Capabilities: Drawing from microscopic structures on gecko feet to improve adhesion in nanocomposites for stable implant integration.
Coral Skeletons	• Porosity and Strength: Emulating the porous yet strong structure of coral skeletons for improved material porosity and tissue integration.

foundation for selecting and arranging nanoscale components within the composite matrix.

A crucial facet of the design of biomimetic nanocomposite materials is the emulation of the complex architecture present in biological tissues. For example, improving the mechanical strength of the composite by nanoscalely imitating the collagenous architecture of bone lays the groundwork for biomechanically robust orthopedic materials. Natural materials are arranged hierarchically, which provides a model for the synthesis of nanocomposites with customized characteristics to meet particular needs in orthopedic applications. Furthermore, biomimetic nanocomposites incorporate the self-assembling and self-organizing processes found in nature. This entails the self-organization of nanoscale constituents to resemble the exact structures present in biological tissues. Molecular self-assembly improves the nanocomposite's structural integrity and makes it easier to create materials that closely resemble the structure and capabilities of natural tissues [18, 19].

To mimic the adaptability and responsiveness of biological systems, stimuli-responsive elements are also explored in biomimetic nanocomposite design. These nanocomposites respond dynamically to their environment by integrating components that change in response to mechanical loads or temperature fluctuations. For example, nanocomposites that draw inspiration from the viscoelasticity of cartilage exhibit mechanical stress adaptation, offering natural tissues-like flexibility and responsiveness.

11.4 CHARACTERIZATION OF BIOMIMETIC NANOCOMPOSITES

Characterizing biomimetic nanocomposites is a critical aspect of their development, ensuring a comprehensive understanding of their structural, mechanical, and biological properties. This multifaceted characterization is imperative for assessing the performance and applicability of these innovative materials in orthopedic applications.

11.4.1 Structural Characterization

Techniques including transmission electron microscopy (TEM) and scanning electron microscopy (SEM) are used to analyze the structural characteristics of biomimetic nanocomposites. By enabling high-resolution imaging, these techniques guarantee the replication of biomimetic design principles and enable researchers to see the nanoscale architecture. Furthermore, information about crystallographic structures can be obtained by X-ray diffraction (XRD), which validates the biomimetic composite's alignment with natural materials such as cartilage or bone.

11.4.2 Mechanical Characterization

Biomimetic nanocomposites' ability to function well in orthopedic applications depends on their mechanical characteristics. To assess qualities like strength, elasticity, and hardness, techniques like nanoindentation, compression testing, and tensile testing are used. By emulating the mechanical properties of natural tissues, like bone, the nanocomposites are guaranteed to be able to tolerate physiological loads and offer the required support to the musculoskeletal system.

11.4.3 Biological Characterization

Assessing the biological performance of biomimetic nanocomposites involves studying their interaction with living tissues. Cell culture experiments evaluate biocompatibility, cell adhesion, and proliferation on the surface of the nanocomposite. Additionally, in vitro and in vivo studies explore the material's impact on tissue regeneration and integration. Techniques like immunohistochemistry and gene expression analysis provide insights into the cellular response, ensuring that the nanocomposites foster a favorable environment for tissue growth.

11.4.4 Chemical Characterization

Validating the biomimetic nature of biomimetic nanocomposites requires an understanding of their chemical composition. Nuclear magnetic resonance

(NMR) spectroscopy and Fourier-transform infrared spectroscopy (FTIR) can clarify molecular structures and verify the existence of particular biomimetic components. Chemical analysis guarantees that the intended biomimetic properties are met by the nanocomposite formulation.

11.4.5 Dynamic Characterization

Dynamic behavior, such as responsiveness to environmental stimuli, is a key consideration. Dynamic mechanical analysis (DMA) assesses the viscoelastic properties of the nanocomposite, providing insights into its ability to adapt to changing mechanical conditions. This dynamic characterization is crucial for applications where the material needs to respond to physiological stresses within the body. It is impossible to exaggerate the significance of careful characterization when evaluating the effectiveness of biomimetic nanocomposites, especially when considering orthopedic applications. Thorough characterization is essential to verifying the functionality, safety, and effectiveness of these cutting-edge materials and facilitating their seamless integration into intricate biological settings [20, 21].

Extensive characterization guarantees biomimetic nanocomposites' dependability and consistency. Researchers can create a baseline for performance metrics and make precise comparisons between various formulations and iterations by using standardized testing protocols and techniques. This makes research findings more credible and makes successful biomimetic designs easier to replicate.

To guarantee that biomimetic nanocomposites fulfill the high standards required for orthopedic applications, characterization is essential to quality control. To ensure the predictability and dependability of performance over time, material properties must be consistent. Strict characterization procedures are a tool for quality control that reduces the possibility of process variability in manufacturing. Extensive characterization enables scientists to customize biomimetic nanocomposites for particular orthopedic uses. Comprehending the material's mechanical, biological, and structural characteristics allows for the customization of its composition to specifically address the needs of orthopedic interventions such as joint replacements or bone regeneration. The optimal performance in various clinical scenarios is ensured by this customization [22, 23].

Characterization provides valuable insights into the limitations of biomimetic nanocomposites. By identifying weaknesses or potential areas for improvement, researchers can refine formulations and optimize material properties. This iterative process, guided by thorough characterization, is essential for advancing the field, and pushing the boundaries of biomimetic design to achieve enhanced performance.

11.5 APPLICATIONS IN ORTHOPEDICS

Table 11.3 & Figure 11.1 outlines various orthopedic applications and highlights the role of biomimetic nanocomposites in each context.

Inspired by the principles of design found in nature, biomimetic nanocomposites have the potential to offer numerous benefits over conventional materials, thereby ushering in a new era of sustainability and innovation. Their superior mechanical properties constitute one of their main advantages. Biomimetic nanocomposites can achieve remarkable strength, toughness, and flexibility by mimicking the structural details present in natural materials like bone or nacre. This makes it possible to create materials with

Table 11.3 Overview of specific orthopedic applications [24–30]

Orthopedic application	Description
Bone Regeneration	Biomimetic nanocomposites play a crucial role in bone regeneration, providing a scaffold for cell adhesion, proliferation, and differentiation. Controlled release of growth factors enhances regenerative potential, mimicking natural extracellular matrix for tissue growth. The nanocomposites, replicating hierarchical bone structures, offer improved mechanical support and biocompatibility for bone defect repairs.
Joint Replacements	In joint replacements, biomimetic nanocomposites focus on replicating natural joint mechanics. These materials offer superior wear resistance, reducing implant deterioration. Lubricious properties mimic synovial fluid, minimizing friction and wear on articulating surfaces. Tailored surface properties promote osseointegration, ensuring stable and enduring joint replacements. The biomimetic approach aims to provide implants closely emulating native joints in function and longevity.
Cartilage Repair	Biomimetic nanocomposites are utilized in cartilage repair by mimicking the viscoelastic properties of natural cartilage. These materials provide a conducive environment for chondrocyte growth and regeneration. They aim to restore the biomechanical properties of damaged cartilage and offer a promising solution for treating osteoarthritis and other cartilage-related conditions.
Spinal Fusion	For spinal fusion applications, biomimetic nanocomposites contribute to improved fusion outcomes. Mimicking the structural properties of vertebral bone, these materials provide a supportive matrix for spinal fusion, enhancing stability and reducing complications. Controlled release of bioactive agents aids in promoting bone growth and fusion in spinal surgeries.
Soft Tissue Repair	Biomimetic nanocomposites are explored in soft tissue repair, replicating the tensile strength and flexibility of natural tissues. These materials aim to provide robust and resilient solutions for repairing ligaments, tendons, and other soft tissues. The biomimetic design enhances compatibility and reduces the risk of adverse reactions, promoting successful soft tissue repair.

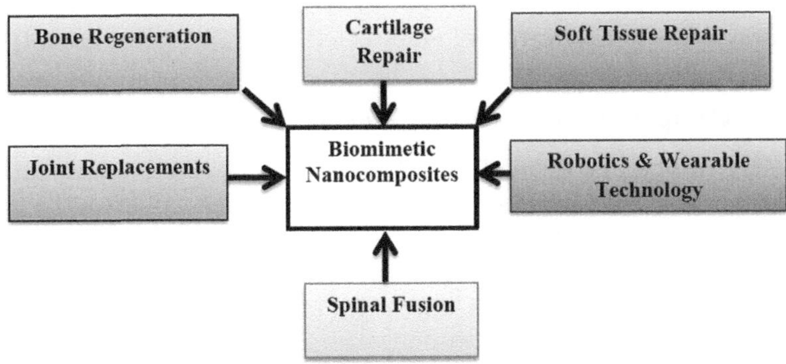

Figure 11.1 Different applications of biomimetic nanocomposites.

improved performance qualities that are appropriate for a variety of uses, including biomedical devices and structural engineering. The biomimetic nanocomposites' low weight is another important benefit. These composites have a high strength-to-weight ratio because they mimic the micro and nanostructures found in strong, lightweight natural materials like plant fibers or bird feathers. This feature helps to increase fuel efficiency and overall sustainability and is especially useful in sectors like aerospace and automotive manufacturing where weight reduction is crucial [31, 32].

Additionally, biomimetic nanocomposites show exceptional flexibility and reactivity to outside stimuli. These materials can be designed to react to variables like temperature, pressure, or moisture by taking inspiration from the way that nature can change with its surroundings. This creates opportunities for the creation of smart materials that can self-heal, have shape memory effects, and dynamically alter their structure. These developments could lead to advancements in robotics, wearable technology, and medical devices. Moreover, sustainable and bioderived materials are frequently used in the creation of biomimetic nanocomposites. This is in contrast to many conventional materials, which are produced using energy-intensive processes and non-renewable resources. By utilizing bio-inspired strategies, materials with a smaller environmental impact can be produced, which is in line with the increasing emphasis on eco-friendly and circular economy practices worldwide [33].

11.6 CHALLENGES AND FUTURE DIRECTIONS

11.6.1 Current Challenges in the Development of Nanocomposites

Determining the present obstacles in the creation and application of biomimetic nanocomposites is essential to the advancement of this cutting-edge area of materials science. Although biomimetic nanocomposites are very promising, several issues need to be resolved before they can be fully utilized in real-world applications [34, 35].

11.6.1.1 Complex Manufacturing Processes

Complicated Manufacturing Procedures: The creation of biomimetic nanocomposites frequently entails complex procedures that call for accuracy and nanoscale control. These procedures could be pricey, time-consuming, and complex. The creation of affordable and scalable manufacturing techniques is still a major obstacle to their broad adoption [36, 37].

11.6.1.2 Standardization and Characterization

Standardization and Characterization: In order to guarantee consistent quality and performance, it is essential to establish standardized testing and characterization procedures for biomimetic nanocomposites. The variability of manufacturing processes combined with the absence of widely recognized testing protocols makes cross-industry comparison of results difficult.

11.6.1.3 Durability and Long-Term Performance

Evaluating the biomimetic nanocomposites' long-term performance and durability is a significant task. For these materials to remain safe and reliable over time, many factors need to be thoroughly investigated, including fatigue, aging effects, and exposure to the environment. This is especially important for applications where maintaining structural integrity is critical.

11.6.1.4 Integration with Existing Materials and Technologies

Integration with Current Materials and Technologies: It can be difficult to integrate biomimetic nanocomposites with current materials and technologies. Compatibility problems can impact the overall performance of the system, particularly when combining biomimetic materials with conventional materials. Resolving bonding, interface strength, and general material compatibility problems is necessary to achieve seamless integration.

11.6.1.5 Regulatory Compliance and Safety Concerns

The development of biomimetic nanocomposites introduces new materials with unique properties, raising concerns about their potential environmental and health impacts. Ensuring compliance with regulatory standards and conducting thorough risk assessments are imperative. Addressing safety concerns is essential for gaining regulatory approval and fostering public acceptance.

11.6.1.6 Cost Barriers

Cost Barriers: One major obstacle to the widespread adoption of biomimetic nanocomposites is the cost of production, particularly for those containing specialized or rare biomimetic components. To ensure that these materials are economically viable for a range of applications, research endeavors ought to concentrate on devising economical sourcing and production strategies.

11.6.2 Ongoing Research to Address These Challenges

Research efforts are currently underway to tackle the various aspects linked to the creation and application of biomimetic nanocomposites. To ensure regulatory compliance, overcome manufacturing complexities, improve standardization, ensure durability, facilitate integration, and address cost barriers, researchers are focusing their efforts on innovative solutions

11.6.2.1 Manufacturing Innovation

New manufacturing techniques that strike a balance between accuracy and scalability are being investigated by research initiatives. Growing interest is being paid to advances in nanofabrication technologies, like molecular self-assembly and 3D printing, to improve reproducibility and optimize production procedures for biomimetic nanocomposites [38–40].

11.6.2.2 Standardization and Characterization Methods

The scientific community is working hard to create protocols for characterization and standardized testing. Scholars are working together to create reference points for assessing the characteristics of biomimetic nanocomposite materials, promoting inter-study comparability, and aiding in the development of industry-wide guidelines.

11.6.2.3 Durability Studies

Comprehensive durability studies are the main focus of ongoing research to comprehend the long-term performance of biomimetic nanocomposites. Studies on fatigue, environmental exposure, and accelerated aging are being used to shed light on the materials' long-term stability and dependability, which is important information for high-performance and structural applications.

11.6.2.4 Integration Strategies

Interdisciplinary research efforts are underway to address integration challenges by developing advanced bonding techniques and compatibility-enhancing additives. Collaborations between materials scientists, engineers, and experts in related fields are fostering a holistic approach to the seamless integration of biomimetic nanocomposites with existing materials and technologies.

11.6.2.5 Regulatory Compliance and Safety Assessments

To allay regulatory worries and guarantee the safety of biomimetic nanocomposites, scientists are hard at work performing extensive risk analyses and toxicity investigations. Comprehending the effects on the environment and possible health hazards linked to these substances is essential for managing regulatory processes and winning over the public.

11.6.2.6 Cost-Effective Solutions

Research on economical sourcing and production techniques is in progress to ensure the economic viability of biomimetic nanocomposites. Reducing production costs and improving market competitiveness require a focus on recycling technologies, optimizing manufacturing processes, and using sustainable biomimetic components.

11.6.3 Future Trends in the Field

Biomimetic nanocomposites have a bright future ahead of them, with expected developments and breakthroughs that could completely transform several industries. The creation of self-healing nanocomposites, which take their cue from biological systems that can self-heal damage, is one prominent trend. Innovative polymers and nanomaterials that can start repair processes are being investigated by researchers to create materials with longer lifespans and greater durability [7, 41].

The incorporation of nanoscale sensors into biomimetic nanocomposites for real-time structural health monitoring is an intriguing new direction. This development would allow for ongoing evaluation of material conditions, enabling preventative maintenance and guaranteeing peak performance in vital applications like infrastructure and aircraft.

A new trend in biomimetic nanocomposites is dynamic adaptability, where materials are engineered to change shape in response to external stimuli. These materials, which mimic the adaptability found in nature, may find use in wearable technology and robotics to create flexible and responsive structures [41–43].

Biomimetic nanocomposites are expected to be major players in the future thanks to artificial intelligence (AI). Innovation is anticipated to accelerate with the use of AI algorithms in materials design and optimization processes. Through the analysis of large datasets, prediction of material behaviors, and recommendation of ideal combinations, machine learning algorithms can accelerate the discovery of new biomimetic materials with previously unheard-of properties [44, 45].

The creation of biomimetic nanocomposites from renewable resources is becoming more popular in the field of sustainability. Researchers are working to develop biomimetic materials that support global efforts to move towards a more sustainable and circular economy by investigating bio-based feedstocks and environmentally friendly manufacturing processes. Another frontier is the meeting point of nanotechnology and biotechnology. Biomimetic nanocomposites have the potential to replicate the structural characteristics of natural materials as well as their functional attributes, like energy storage or photosynthesis. Technological advances in energy conversion, storage, and harvesting may result from this [46–52].

11.7 CONCLUSION

This book chapter concludes with a thorough and perceptive investigation of the revolutionary possibilities of biomimetic nanocomposites in the field of orthopedic applications. This chapter deftly examines the urgent problems with conventional orthopedic materials, like metals and polymers, emphasizing the need for creative solutions that go beyond their constraints. The need for materials that can blend in with the biological environment seamlessly emphasizes how crucial biomimicry is to the design of nanocomposite structures.

A detailed analysis of the principles of biomimetic nanocomposites is presented, with a focus on how orthopedics can benefit from them. These cutting-edge materials have improved mechanical strength, regenerative potential, and biocompatibility by imitating natural tissue structures and applying biomimetic design principles. A thorough review of the properties of nanocomposite materials that are essential to orthopedic success is given in this chapter. These properties include optimized integration with the musculoskeletal system, tailored nanoscale control, and stimulation of regenerative responses.

As the chapter explores particular examples motivated by the inventiveness of nature, like bone structure, cartilage, spider silk, sea shells, gecko feet, and coral skeletons, biomimetic design principles become apparent as a cutting-edge methodology. The creation of nanocomposites that closely resemble the complexity and functionality of living tissues is facilitated by the careful examination of these natural blueprints. The thorough characterization of biomimetic nanocomposites, including their structural, mechanical, biological, chemical, and dynamic features, is essential. Detailed characterization becomes essential to verify the safety, effectiveness, and functionality of these novel materials and to successfully integrate them into the intricate biological environments of orthopedic applications.

The final section of the chapter discusses the field's future trends, present difficulties, and ongoing research projects. It highlights the integration of nanoscale sensors for real-time monitoring, the potential advancements in self-healing nanocomposites, and the role of artificial intelligence in accelerating innovation. The chapter offers insights into ongoing research efforts aimed at overcoming obstacles such as complex manufacturing processes and standardization issues, while also acknowledging these challenges. All things considered, this chapter provides a thorough overview, shedding light on the rapidly changing field of biomimetic nanocomposites and their critical role in transforming orthopedic interventions for better patient outcomes and long-term musculoskeletal health.

REFERENCES

1. Deng Yongjun, Zhou Chao, Fu Lifeng, Huang Xiaogang, Liu Zunyong, Zhao Jiayi, Liang Wenqing, Shao Haiyan. (2023). A Mini-review on the Emerging Role of Nanotechnology in Revolutionizing Orthopedic Surgery: Challenges and the Road Ahead. *Frontiers in Bioengineering and Biotechnology.* https://doi.org/10.3389/fbioe.2023.1191509

2. Dakhelallah Faisal, Al-Shalawi, Hanim Azmah, Ariff Mohamed, Jung Yongwon, Khairol Mohd, Mohd Anuar, Dermot Ariffin, Maha Brabazon, Al-Osaimi Obaid. (2023). Biomaterials as Implants in the Orthopedic Field for Regenerative Medicine: Metal versus Synthetic Polymers. *Polymers.* https://doi.org/10.3390/polym15122601

3. R. Sung, Ji Choi, Kwon Won, Soo Kyung, Hak Suk, Kim Sun, Hwan Seong, Si Moon, Park Young, Lee Byoungho. (2023). The Clinical Use of Osteobiologic and Metallic Biomaterials in Orthopedic Surgery: The Present and the Future. *Materials.* https://doi.org/10.3390/ma16103633

4. R. Dua, J. Vadivel, I. Khurana, et al. (2023). Development of Smart Metallic Orthopedic and Dental Implants Based on Biomimetic Design. *Research Square.* https://doi.org/10.21203/rs.3.rs-2927067/v1.

5. Aleksandar Radunovic, Ognjen Radunović, Maja Vulovic, Milan Aksić. (2023). Biomimetics in Orthopedic Surgery and Traumatology. *Engineering Materials.* https://doi.org/10.1007/978-3-031-17269-4_8

6. K. G. Gareev., Denis S. Grouzdev, Veronika V. Koziaeva, Nikita O. Sitkov, Huile Gao, Tatiana M. Zimina, Maxim Shevtsov. (2022). Biomimetic Nanomaterials: Diversity, Technology, and Biomedical Applications. *Nanomaterials.* https://doi.org/10.3390/nano12142485

7. S. Chakraborty, D. Bera, L. Roy, C. K. Ghosh. (2023). Biomimetic and Bioinspired Nanostructures. In: M. Sen, M. Mukherjee (eds) *Bioinspired and Green Synthesis of Nanostructures.* https://doi.org/10.1002/9781394174928.ch15

8. Deng Yongjun, Zhou Chao, Fu Lifeng, Huang Xiaogang, Liu Zunyong, Zhao Jiayi, Liang Wenqing, Shao Haiyan. (2023). A Mini-review on the Emerging Role of Nanotechnology in Revolutionizing Orthopedic Surgery: Challenges and the Road Ahead. *Frontiers in Bioengineering and Biotechnology.* https://doi.org/10.3389/fbioe.2023.1191509

9. Chen Ming Qi. (2022). Recent Advances and Perspective of Nanotechnology-Based Implants for Orthopedic Applications. *Frontiers in Bioengineering and Biotechnology*. https://doi.org/10.3389/fbioe.2022.878257

10. F. V. Vincent Julian, A. Bogatyreva Olga, R. Bogatyrev Nikolaj, Bowyer Adrian, Pahl Anja-Karina. (2006). Biomimetics: Its Practice and Theory. *Journal of the Royal Society Interface*, 3471–3482. http://doi.org/10.1098/rsif.2006.0127

11. Li Pengju, Kim Sae-Seung, Tian Bozhi. (2022). Nanoenabled Trainable Systems: From Biointerfaces to Biomimetics. *ACS Nano*. https://doi.org/10.1021/acsnano.2c08042

12. Ashwani Kumar, Mangey Ram, Yogesh Kumar Singla. (2022). *Advanced Material for Biomechanical Applications*. Publisher Taylor & Francis and CRC Press, ISBN: 9781032054490. https://doi.org/10.1201/9781003286806.

13. Arbind Prasad, Ashwani Kumar, Kishor Kumar Gajrani. (2022). *Biodegradable Composites for Packaging Application*. Publisher Taylor & Francis and CRC Press, ISBN: 978103231511. https://doi.org/10.1201/9781003227908.

14. Ashwani Kumar, Yatika Gori, Avinash Kumar, Chandan Swaroop Meena, Nitesh Dutt. (2022). *Advanced Materials for Biomedical Applications*. Taylor & Francis and CRC Press, ISBN: 9781003344810. https://doi.org/10.1201/9781003344810.

15. Arbind Prasad, Ashwani Kumar, Manoj Gupta. (2023). *Advanced Materials and Manufacturing Techniques in Biomedical Applications*. Publisher Wiley Scrivener, ISBN: 9781394166190. https://doi.org/10.1002/9781394166985.

16. Sandeep Bhoi, Arbind Prasad, Ashwani Kumar, Rudra Bubai Sarkar, Bidyanand Mahto, Chandan Swaroop Meena, Chandan Pandey. (2022). Experimental Study to Evaluate the Wear Performance of UHMWPE and XLPE Material for Orthopedics Application. *Bioengineering*, 9, 676. https://doi.org/10.3390/bioengineering9110676.

17. Arun Kumar Singh Gangwar, P. Sudhakar Rao, Ashwani Kumar. (2021). Bio-Mechanical Design and Analysis of Femur Bone. *Materials Today: Proceedings*, 44, Part 1, 2179–2187, ISSN 2214-7853. https://doi.org/10.1016/j.matpr.2020.12.282.

18. Shuai Liu, Jiangming Yu, Yan-Chang Gan, Xiao-Zhong Qiu, Zhe-Chen Gao, Huanting Wang, Yuan Xiong, Guohui Liu, Si En Lin, Alec McCarthy, Johnson V. John, Daixu Wei, Honghao Hou. (2023). Biomimetic Natural Biomaterials for Tissue Engineering and Regenerative Medicine: New Biosynthesis Methods, Recent Advances, and Emerging Applications. *Military Medical Research*. https://doi.org/10.1186/s40779-023-00448-w

19. L. F. Cano Salazar, J. A. Claudio Rizo, T. E. Flores Guía, D. A. Cabrera Munguía. (2023). Nanocomposites Comprise of Collagen and Acrylate-Derived Polymers for Biomedical Applications. In: F. Avalos Belmontes, F. J. González, M. A. López-Manchado (eds) *Green-Based Nanocomposite Materials and Applications. Engineering Materials*. Springer, Cham. https://doi.org/10.1007/978-3-031-18428-4_9

20. S. Chaudhary, O. Vryonis, A. S. Vaughan, T. Andritsch, M. Feuchter. (2022). Dynamic Mechanical Response in Epoxy Nanocomposites Incorporating Various Nano-Silica Architectures. 2022 IEEE 4th International Conference on Dielectrics (ICD), Palermo, Italy, pp. 86–89. https://doi.org/10.1109/ICD53806.2022.9863531

21. Melika Shahhosseini, Anjelica Kucinic, Peter Beshay, Wolfgang Pfeifer, Carlos Castro. (2022). *Dynamic and Mechanical Applications of DNA Nanostructures in Biophysics, DNA Origami: Structures, Technology, and Applications*. Wiley. https://doi.org/10.1002/9781119682561.ch5

22. Li Cheng-Hui. (2023). Physicochemical Characterization of Nanobiocomposites. https://doi.org/10.5772/intechopen.108818

23. Khizra Bano, Anam Munawar. (2023). Analytical Techniques for Characterization of Nanomaterials. Advances in Digital Crime, Forensics, and Cyber Terrorism Book Series. https://doi.org/10.4018/978-1-6684-8325 -1.ch003

24. Arun Kumar Singh Gangwar, P. Sudhakar Rao, Ashwani Kumar, Pravin P. Patil. (2019). Design and Analysis of Femur Bone: BioMechanical Aspects. *Journal of Critical Reviews*, 6, 4, 133–139, ISSN-2394-5125.

25. Arbind Prasad, Sudipto Datta, Ashwani Kumar, Manoj Gupta. (2023). Introduction to Next-Generation Materials for Biomedical Applications. In: Arbind Prasad, Ashwani Kumar, Manoj Gupta (eds) *Advanced Materials and Manufacturing Techniques for Biomedical Applications*. John Wiley & Sons, Chapter 01, pp. 01–24. https://doi.org/10.1002/9781394166985.ch1.

26. Sriparna De, Dipankar Das, Arbind Prasad, Ashwani Kumar, Dipankar Chattopadhyay. (2023). Insights into Multifunctional Smart Hydrogels in Wound Healing Applications. In: Arbind Prasad, Ashwani Kumar, Manoj Gupta (eds) *Advanced Materials and Manufacturing Techniques for Biomedical Applications*. John Wiley & Sons, Chapter 03, pp. 37–60. https://doi.org/10.1002/9781394166985.ch3

27. Avinash Kumar, Mohit Byadwal, Abhishek Kumar, Ashwani Kumar, Francis Luther King M. (2023). Laser Micromachining in Biomedical Industry. In: Avinash Kumar, Ashwani Kumar, Abhishek Kumar (eds) *Laser-based Technologies for Sustainable Manufacturing*. CRC Press: Boca Raton, FL, Chapter 08, pp. 169–206. https://doi.org/10.1201/9781003402398-8.

28. Avinash Kumar, Anka Datta, Ashwani Kumar, Abhishek Kumar. (2022). Recent Advancements and Future trends in Next-Generation Materials for Biomedical Applications. In: *Advanced Materials for Biomedical Applications*. CRC Press and Taylor & Francis, ISBN: 9781003344810. https://doi.org/10.1201/9781003344810-1.

29. Anka Datta, Avinash Kumar, Ashwani Kumar, Abhishek Kumar, Varun Pratap Singh. (2022). Advanced Materials in Biological Implants and Surgical Tools. In: *Advanced Materials for Biomedical Applications*. CRC Press and Taylor & Francis, ISBN: 9781003344810. https://doi.org/10.1201 /9781003344810-2.

30. Ashwani Kumar, Arun Kumar Singh Gangwar, Avinash Kumar, Chandan Swaroop Meena, Varun Pratap Singh, Nitesh Dutt, Arbind Prasad, Yatika Gori. (2022). Biomedical Study of Femur Bone Fracture and Healing. In: *Advanced Materials for Biomedical Applications*. CRC Press and Taylor & Francis, ISBN: 9781003344810. https://doi.org/10.1201/9781003344810-14.

31. Nicholas A. Kotov. (2023). Composites with High Omnidirectional Fracture Toughness Due to Helical Interlocking Fasteners Are Found in Gingko Seed Shells. *National Science Review*. https://doi.org/10.1093/nsr/nwad065

32. Anna Cecília, do Nascimento, Pereira Silvia, Lenyra Meirelles, Campos Titotto. (2023). Bioinspired Composites: Nature's Guidance for Advanced Materials Future. *Functional Composites and Structures.* https://doi.org/10.1088/2631-6331/acbc64

33. Darelius Elin. (2023). A Feasibility Study of the Bioinspired Green Manufacturing of Nanocomposite Materials. https://doi.org/10.1002/9781394174928.ch10

34. Yi-Chen, Li Jeng, Shiung Jan, Piotr Luliński, Hung-Yin Lin. (2022). Editorial: Applications of Biomimetic (composite) Materials. *Frontiers in Bioengineering and Biotechnology.* https://doi.org/10.3389/fbioe.2022.1020909

35. S. Haidar Z (ed.) (2023). *Biomimetics - Bridging the Gap. Biomedical Engineering.* IntechOpen. http://dx.doi.org/10.5772/intechopen.100667.

36. Subhash Singh, Sanjay K. Behura, Ashwani Kumar, Kartikey Verma. (2022). *Nanomanufacturing and Nanomaterials Design: Principles and Applications.* Publisher Taylor & Francis and CRC Press, ISBN: 9781032081687, ISBN: 9781003220602. https://doi.org/10.1201/9781003220602.

37. Ashwani Kumar, Yatika Gori, Nitesh Dutt, Yogesh Kumar Singla, Ambrish Maurya. (2021). *Advanced Computational Methods in Mechanical and Materials Engineering.* Publisher Taylor & Francis and CRC Press, ISBN: 9781032052915. https://doi.org/10.1201/9781003202233.

38. Arbind Prasad, Gourhari Chakraborty, Ashwani Kumar. (2022). Bio-based Environmentally Benign Polymeric Resorbable Materials for Orthopedic Fixation Applications. In: *Advanced Materials for Biomedical Applications.* CRC Press and Taylor & Francis, ISBN: 9781003344810. https://doi.org/10.1201/9781003344810-15.

39. Arbind Prasad, Gourhari Chakraborty, Ashwani Kumar, Kishor Kumar Gajrani. (2022). Introduction to Biodegradable Polymers. In: *Biodegradable Composites for Packaging Applications.* CRC Press and Taylor & Francis, ISBN: 978103227908. https://doi.org/10.1201/9781003227908-1.

40. Gourhari Chakraborty, Arbind Prasad, Ashwani Kumar. (2022). Processing of Biodegradable Composites. In: *Biodegradable Composites for Packaging Applications.* CRC Press and Taylor & Francis, ISBN: 978103227908. https://doi.org/10.1201/9781003227908-3.

41. Kausar Ayesha, Ishaq Ahmad, Malik Maaza, Patrizia Bocchetta. (2023). Self-Healing Nanocomposites—Advancements and Aerospace Applications. *Journal of Composites Science,* 7(4), 148. https://doi.org/10.3390/jcs7040148

42. Vishakha Sherawata, Anamika Saini, Priyanka Dalal, Deepika Sharma. (2023). A Decade of Biomimetic and Bioinspired Nanostructures, Bioinspired and Green Synthesis of Nanostructures: A Sustainable Approach. https://doi.org/10.1002/9781394174928.ch9

43. Yuan Liu, Gungun Lin, Mariana Medina-Sánchez, Maria Guix, Denys Makarov, Dayong Jin. (2023). Responsive Magnetic Nanocomposites for Intelligent Shape-Morphing Microrobots. *ACS Nano.* https://doi.org/10.1021/acsnano.3c01609

44. Kun Rok Park, Chi-Oh Song, Jinkyoo Park, Seunghwa Ryu. (2023). Multi-objective Bayesian Optimization for the Design of Nacre-Inspired Composites: Optimizing and Understanding Biomimetics Through AI. *Materials Horizons.* https://doi.org/10.1039/d3mh00137g

45. Honghao Chen, Yingzhe Zheng, Jiali Li, Lanyu Li, Xiaonan Wang. (2023). *AI for Nanomaterials Development in Clean Energy and Carbon Capture, Utilization and Storage (CCUS)*. ACS Nano. https://doi.org/10.1021/acsnano.3c01062.

46. Ashwani Kumar, Yatika Gori, Sachin Rana, Neelesh Kumar Sharma, Brijesh Yadav. (2022). FEA of Humerus Bone Fracture and Healing. In: *Advanced Materials for Biomechanical Applications*. CRC Press and Taylor & Francis, ISBN: 9781032054490. https://doi.org/10.1201/9781003286806-14.

47. Ashwani Kumar, Deepak Prasad Mamgain, Himanshu Jaiswal, Pravin P. Patil. (2015). Modal Analysis of Hand Arm Vibration (Humerus Bone) for Biodynamic Response Using Varying Boundary Conditions Based on FEA. *Springer Book Series: Advances in Intelligent Systems and Computing*, 308, 169–176. https://doi.org/10.1007/978-81-322-2012-1_18. Series ISSN- 2194-5357.

48. Ramesh Kumar, Arbind Prasad, Ashwani Kumar. (2023). *Sustainable Smart Manufacturing Processes in Industry 4.0*. Publisher Taylor & Francis and CRC Press, ISBN: 9781003436072. https://doi.org/10.1201/9781003436072.

49. Ramesh Kumar, Ashwani Kumar, Laxmi Kant, Arbind Prasad, Sandeep Bhoi, Chandan Swaroop Meena, Varun Pratap Singh, Aritra Ghosh. (2023). Experimental and RSM-based Process-Parameters Optimisation for Turning Operation of EN36B Steel. *Materials*, 16, 339. https://doi.org/10.3390/ma16010339.

50. Sandeep Bhoi, Ashwani Kumar, Arbind Prasad, Chandan Swaroop Meena, Rudra Bubai Sarkar, Bidyanand Mahto, Aritra Ghosh. (2022). Performance Evaluation of Different Coating Materials in Delamination for Micro-Milling Applications on High-Speed Steel Substrate. *Micromachines*, 13, 1277. https://doi.org/10.3390/mi13081277.

51. Atanu Kumar Paul, Arbind Prasad, Ashwani Kumar. (2022). Review on Artificial Neural Network and its Application in the Field of Engineering. *Journal of Mechanical Engineering: PRAKASH*, 1(1), 53–61. https://doi.org/10.56697/JMEP.2022.1107.

52. Gourhari Chakraborty, Vivek Pandey, Arbind Prasad, Ashwani Kumar. (2023). Introduction to Sustainable Manufacturing for Industries 4.0. In: Ramesh Kumar, Arbind Prasad, Ashwani Kumar (eds) *Sustainable Smart Manufacturing Processes in Industry 4.0*. CRC Press: Boca Raton, FL, Chapter 01, pp. 01–17. https://doi.org/10.1201/9781003436072-1.

Functional Nano-manufactured Bio-composite in Healthcare Applications

Francis Luther King M, Thillikkani S,
Raja K, and Srinivasan V

INTRODUCTION

The field of nanotechnology encompasses the scientific and technical disciplines that focus on the creation, composition, and examination of materials and devices with a functional structure at the nanoscale, which is equivalent to one billionth of a meter. This requires the use of both materials and tools. At these dimensions, the ability to manipulate the essential characteristics of a substance or technology relies on considering the individual molecules and their interconnecting molecular groups. The manipulation of a molecular structure allows for the manipulation of macroscopic characteristics [1]. Nanotechnology has seldom been used and developed in the domain of construction and building materials. The commercial use of nanotechnology in concrete is still in its nascent stage, with only a limited number of items successfully brought to market [2]. Nanotechnology involves the creation, processing, characterization, and preparation of devices, systems, and production methods with dimensions ranging from 0.1 to 100 nm. These products exhibit unique and greatly improved physical, chemical, and biological properties, functions, phenomena, and processes. Nanotechnology is now most widely used in several fields such as nanocomposites, nano-biotechnology, nano-systems, nano-electronics, and nanostructured materials (Figure 1). Due to the exceptional thermal conductivity, nonlinear optical properties, and electrochemical reactivity of nanoparticles (NPs), they have garnered significant interest in research for their potential applications [3].

12.1 NANOCOMPOSITES

To improve the dynamic performance, nanocomposites include one or more distinct NPs into the matrix material. Metals, including iron, titanium, and magnesium, as well as ceramics like alumina, glass, and porcelain, are often used as the primary ingredients in nanocomposites. Examples of nanocomposites include epoxy, nylon, polyepoxide, and polyetherimide. The NPs may be classified as natural, accidental, or synthetic nanoparticles

DOI: 10.1201/9781003470311-12

based on their origin. Naturally occurring or naturally derived nanomaterials are found in the environment, such as volcanic dust, lunar dust, magneto-tactic microorganisms, and minerals. Incidental NPs are generated due to anthropogenic industrial operations such as coal combustion and welding emissions. To obtain nanomaterials of the desired shape and size, one may use crystal growth, chemical synthesis, or lithographic etching of a larger sample to create smaller subunits known as NPs [4–5]. Bio-nanocomposites, sometimes referred to as BNCs, are a specific category of materials that consist of naturally occurring polymers (biopolymers) combined with inorganic nano particles. The term "bio-nanocomposite," introduced in 2004, is sometimes referred to as nano-biocomposites (NCs), green composites, or bio-hybrids. Bio-nanocomposites are notable for their ability to disperse at the nanoscale, with dimensions less than 1,000 nm.

12.1.1 ZnO/TiO$_2$ Nanocomposites

ZnO/TiO2 bio-nanocomposites are composite materials that consist of zinc oxide (ZnO) and titanium dioxide (TiO$_2$) nanoparticles (NPs) embedded in a biopolymer matrix. Recently, there has been a significant amount of interest in them due to their unique characteristics and potential applications in the field of biomedicine. Zinc oxide/titanium dioxide bio-nanocomposites may be produced using many techniques, including in situ polymerization, melt blending, and solution mixing. The process of solution mixing entails dispersing ZnO and TiO$_2$ nanoparticles in a solvent and then combining them with a biopolymer solution. Melt blending is the process of combining ZnO and TiO$_2$ nanoparticles with a biopolymer while it is in a liquid condition. The process of in situ polymerization entails the creation of a biopolymer structure when ZnO and TiO$_2$ NPs are present. This includes the analysis and evaluation of ZnO/TiO$_2$ bio-nanocomposites, as well as their potential applications in the field of biomedicine [6]. Zinc oxide (ZnO) and titanium dioxide (TiO$_2$) are well recognised as photocatalytic substances that may use light energy to facilitate chemical processes. The incorporation of zinc oxide (ZnO) and titanium dioxide (TiO$_2$) nanoparticles in a nanocomposite may significantly augment the photocatalytic activity, hence rendering it highly efficient for various applications such as water purification, air pollution mitigation, and self-cleaning surfaces. The ZnO/TiO$_2$ nanocomposite has potential applications in electrical and optoelectronic devices [7]. Zinc oxide nanoparticles (ZnO NPs) increase the electrical conductivity of the composite, while titanium dioxide nanoparticles (TiO$_2$ NPs) contribute to favourable optical characteristics. Due to its unique properties, this combination is well-suited for use in solar cells, sensors, and photovoltaic systems. Zinc oxide nanoparticles (ZnO NPs) have been extensively researched due to their antibacterial and antimicrobial characteristics [8]. The addition of ZnO nanoparticles (NPs) to the TiO$_2$ matrix enhances the antibacterial properties of the resultant nanocomposite. This makes it suitable for many applications in healthcare, food packaging, and antimicrobial coatings. Energy storage applications may also be investigated for the ZnO/TiO$_2$ nanocomposite. The nanocomposite formed by combining ZnO and TiO$_2$ has favourable electrochemical characteristics, resulting in enhanced energy storage capacity and cycle stability. Consequently, this composite material is well-suited for use in batteries and supercapacitors [9].

12.1.2 Characterization of ZnO/TiO$_2$ Bio-nanocomposites

Characterization of ZnO/TiO$_2$ bio-nanocomposites is necessary to ascertain their physical, chemical, and biological attributes. Scanning electron microscopy (SEM), transmission electron microscopy (TEM), X-ray diffraction (XRD), Fourier transform infrared spectroscopy (FTIR), and thermal analysis are techniques used to analyse the properties of ZnO/TiO$_2$ bio-nanocomposites [10]. The purpose of SEM is to analyse and describe the dimensions and structure of nanocomposites. X-ray diffraction analysis (XRD) is used to identify the metallic properties of particles under investigation, determine atomic dimensions, and ascertain the arrangement of atoms and molecules inside materials. Furthermore, due to its ability to penetrate deeply, XRD may provide insights into the overall structure of the material. UV-visible spectroscopy is used to track the precise kinetics of the production of the ZnO/TiO$_2$ nanocomposite. Fourier transform infrared spectroscopy (FTIR) is used to analyse the relationship between the intensity of infrared light, the wavelength of light, and the vibrational characteristics of chemical functional groups [11]. The ZnO–TiO$_2$ nanocomposite was imaged using electron microscopy at the nanometer scale, achieving a magnification of 38,700× at room temperature. The NPs vary in size, ranging from 50 to 200 nm. The ZnO–TiO$_2$ nanoparticles have a size range of 60–200 nm, while the thickness of the nanosheets falls between 50 and 100 nm. The X-ray diffraction (XRD) patterns obtained using an X-ray, sophisticated scientific XRD system indicate the level of crystallisation of the sample in a powdered form. The source frequency used was 1.54 Å [12]. The XRD examination identifies the presence of ZnO–TiO$_2$ powder at room temperature and reveals that the sample also includes ZnTiO$_3$ with a little degradation of sulphate hydrate. The peak has a full width at half maximum (FWHM) of 0.192° and a d-spacing of 1.48. According to Scherrer's formula, the minimum particle size is 50 nm. The FTIR spectra of TiO$_2$ has a wide band ranging from 470 to 865 cm^{-1} due to the overlapping of many bands associated with the Ti–O–Ti and Ti–O vibration modes [13]. The sharp peak at 675 cm^{-1} is attributed to the Ti–O stretching. The dominant peaks found in ZnO between 460 and 540 cm^{-1} are attributed to the stretching mode of Zn–O [14]. The H–O–H and O–H stretching and bending vibrations exhibited signals within the ranges of 3,000–3,800 and 1,600–1,650 cm^{-1}, respectively, as shown by the peaks detected between 1,600 and 700 cm^{-1} [15]. The diffuse reflectance spectra (DRS) were measured in the wavelength range of 300–700 nm. The DRS analysis reveals that the photocatalysts TiO2, ZnO, B–ZnO, ZnO/TiO$_2$, and B–ZnO/TiO$_2$ exhibit optical absorption at a wavelength of 400 nm. The photocatalysts exhibit a high level of reflectance at visible wavelengths. An abrupt rise in reflectance has been seen for TiO2, ZnO, B–ZnO, ZnO/TiO$_2$, and B–ZnO/TiO$_2$ near the retention edge at wavelengths of 414, 440, 430, 455, and 411 nm, respectively [7].

12.1.3 Chitosan with Metal Nanomaterials for Bone Tissue Engineering

12.1.3.1 Chitosan–Silver Nanocomposites

Silver nanoparticles (AgNPs) have garnered significant interest in the field of bone-related implant research owing to their inherent antibacterial capabilities. Xie et al. (2019) created composites of silver nanoparticles (AgNPs) incorporated with polydopamine–hydroxyapatite–chitosan by introducing AgNPs into hybrid materials. This resulted in a notable decrease in microbial infection at the site of implantation [16]. Polydopamine and chitosan are crucial in facilitating the regulated release of AgNPs at the implanted location and also serve as biocompatible scaffolds. Wang et al. (2019) created a system that included hydroxyapatite and silver-based composites. They then applied this system onto titanium implants and chitosan using electrodeposition. The purpose was to control the release of silver ions and calcium ions [17]. The biocomposite, composed of chitosan, graphene oxide, and hydroxyapatite, was infused with silver and antimicrobial medicines. In addition, a single-step electrodeposition technique was used to coat biocomposites onto titanium. The incorporation of graphene oxide and chitosan has been shown to enhance both the mechanical strength and cell adhesion. Significantly, the biocomposites that were created have exceptional antibacterial efficacy [18]. A fibrillar collagen–chitosan matrix loaded with AgNP was used to facilitate biomineralization by the application of a simulated bodily fluid (SBF) solution. The composites that were created demonstrate enhanced mineralization and notable antibacterial properties [19]. An induction plasma-spray coating method was used to coat titanium with hydroxyapatite. Subsequently, the hydroxyapatite was polished using silver and silica. The evaluation of acemannan release from the coating material was also conducted in the SBF solution. Acemannan was discovered to be released in a sustained way. Additionally, an in vitro research examining cell interactions with osteoblasts shown that the generated substance promotes cell proliferation. Furthermore, experiments conducted on a rat distal femur model demonstrate a substantial increase in new bone formation. In addition, notable antibacterial characteristics against *Staphylococcus epidermidis* have been discovered [20]. The electrophoretic deposition approach was used to generate coating materials that consist of chitosan, bioactive glass, and AgNPs. The generated substance was applied onto stainless steel 316 substrates. Moreover, the fabricated material exhibits the production of apatite in simulated body fluid (SBF) and it promotes the proliferation of MG-63 osteoblast-like cells. Furthermore, it was shown that there has antibacterial action against *Staphylococcus aureus* [21].

12.1.3.2 Chitosan–Gold Nanocomposites

Gold nanoparticles (AuNPs) have been intensively researched for their uses in tissue engineering, medication delivery, diagnostics, and bioimaging. This is because they are biocompatible, can be adjusted in size, and have the capability to encapsulate various therapeutic agents. Gold nanoparticles regulate the process of osteoclastic differentiation [22–24]. The osteogenic characteristics of AuNPs were seen in vitro cell contact with mesenchymal stem cells via the p38 MAPK signalling pathway [25]. The use of gold nanoparticles (AuNPs) has shown encouraging outcomes in promoting the differentiation of bone marrow mesenchymal stem cells into osteogenic lineages. This effect is likely attributed to the size and inherent characteristics of the AuNPs. In their work, Mahmoud et al. (2020) investigated the effectiveness of several materials including AuNPs, hydroxyapatite nanoparticles, chitosan nanoparticles, gold hydroxyapatite-based nanocomposites, and chitosan–hydroxyapatite-based nanocomposites in promoting bone regeneration. The osteogenic differentiation capability of these nanoparticles was evaluated by studying the interaction between the nanoparticles and mesenchymal stem cells generated from bone marrow in a laboratory setting. The alizarin red S test also verifies the formation of mineralized nodules. In addition, qRT-PCR study demonstrates an upregulation of gene expression for runt-related transcription factor 2 and bone morphogenic protein 2. The in vitro biological experiments demonstrate that AuNPs have exceptional osteoinductive capabilities [26]. Choi et al. (2015) conducted a research study where they created chitosan-mobilized AuNPs to address bone deficiencies. Chitosan was used as a reducing agent to synthesize AuNPs. The AuNPs that were created enhance the process of osteogenic differentiation in human adipose-derived mesenchymal stem cells. The cell growth was proven by the alamarBlue assay. In addition, the qRT-PCR study revealed an increase in the expression of alkaline phosphatase, bone sialoprotein, and osteocalcin genes. The alizarin red S test was conducted by cultivating human adipose-derived mesenchymal stem cells with chitosan-conjugated AuNPs. This test demonstrated that the produced nanoparticles enhance the process of osteogenic differentiation in human adipose-derived mesenchymal stem cells, as confirmed by the observed calcium deposition. The Western blot analysis validated the protein expression of human adipose-derived mesenchymal stem cells that is associated with β-catenin signaling in the osteogenic process [27].

12.1.3.3 Chitosan–Copper Nanocomposites

Multiple study findings have substantiated the osteogenic characteristics of copper nanoparticles (CuNPs). Hydrogels that may be injected into the body that include copper together with bioactive nanoparticles, chitosan, glycerophosphate, and silk fibroin were created with the purpose of promoting bone repair. Additionally, in vitro biological experiments conducted using MC3T3-E1 cells provide evidence of the osteogenic characteristics of the created hydrogel. Furthermore, a series of tests were performed on rat calvarial bone abnormalities for a duration of eight weeks. The confirmation of new bone formation in the damaged area is supported by microscale computational micrographs and staining test results [28]. Ning et al. (2019) synthesised copper ions combined with mesoporous silica nanoparticles (MSN) and chitosan, which were modified with glycyl-L-histidyl-L-lysine. In addition, the composite was examined for the release of copper ions by immersing it in a buffer solution. Furthermore, MC3T3-E1 cells were subjected to biological tests. Research has shown that the created substance is compatible with living organisms and promotes the activation of genes related to bone formation. In addition, notable antibacterial activities against *Escherichia coli* and *Staphylococcus aureus* were achieved [29]. Lu et al. (2018) conducted a research where they created a scaffolding system using copper ions combined with carboxymethyl chitosan and alginate. This system was designed specifically for repairing bone tissue. The scaffolds had a porosity size ranging from 45 to 107 μm, with an average size of 73.06 ± 21.13 μm. MC3T3-E1 cells were subjected to in vitro biological tests. The biological experiments demonstrate that the constructed scaffold enhances both cell adhesion and proliferation. Furthermore, improvements in alkaline phosphatase activity, stimulation of mineralization, and increased expression of osteogenic genes were detected. Experiments were conducted on Sprague Dawley rats in a living organism. Microscale computational analysis and histology investigation indicate the presence of newly produced bone. Furthermore, the constructed scaffold exhibited exceptional antibacterial efficacy against *Staphylococcus aureus* [30]. The freeze-drying approach was used to construct scaffolds made of nanocopper–zinc combined with nanohydroxyapatite, gelatin, and chitosan, with the aim of enhancing their osteogenic capabilities. The scaffolds were fabricated with a diameter of 8 mm and a thickness of 2.5 mm. The porosity varies between 97.8% and 99.5%, with a pore size ranging from 113 to 143 μm. The scaffolds were tested for their osteogenic capacities by conducting in vitro cell contact experiments with mouse embryonic fibroblasts [31]. Tripathi et al. (2012) conducted a research to examine the bone-forming characteristics of a scaffold made up of nanocopper-zinc, chitosan, and nanohydroxyapatite. The osteogenic capabilities of the scaffold that was created were verified using biological experiments using rat osteoprogenitor cells. Furthermore, the scaffold exhibits remarkable antibacterial efficacy against *Staphylococcus aureus* and *Escherichia coli* [32].

12.1.3.4 Chitosan–Titanium Oxide Nanocomposites

Titanium and titanium-based alloys are commonly used in the biomedical field, particularly in bone tissue engineering, due to their exceptional bio-compatibility, superior corrosion resistance, substantial structural rigidity, and ability to withstand body fluids [33,34]. A recent research has shown that modifications applied to the surface of titanium oxide (TiO2) nanotubes may alter their properties, significantly affecting cell adhesion and antibacterial efficacy. Consequently, the combination of antibiotic medicines with a surface-modified TiO2-based drug delivery system in synthetic bone implants may promote bone repair and simultaneously hinder bacterial infection. In addition, the use of coating materials containing TiO2 may enhance drug stabilisation, resulting in a sustained drug release profile over an extended period of time [35]. Lai et al. (2018) used the electrochemical anodization procedure to fabricate TiO2 nanotubes. Naringin was introduced into TiO2 nanotubes by direct deposition, followed by subsequent encapsulation with chitosan layers. The system exhibited a sustained release of naringin over an extended period of time. The in vitro biological studies conducted on osteoblasts demonstrated their viability and an increase in alkaline phosphatase activity. Furthermore, the use of Alizarin red S staining tests successfully identified the formation of mineralized nodules [36]. Gentamicin drug combination was coated onto TiO2 nanotubes on a Ti substrate. In addition, a self-assembly approach was used to coat the TiO2-gentamicin composite with a mixture of alginate and chitosan. Biological studies were conducted on osteoblasts derived from the calvaria bones of newborn rats. The cells exhibited viability and proliferation in the presence of the synthesised composite material. Furthermore, there was a rise in alkaline phosphatase activity. In addition, a remarkable antibacterial activity was demonstrated against Staphylococcus aureus and Escherichia coli [37]. Lai et al. (2017) synthesised TiO2 nanotubes that were loaded with melatonin. Afterwards, a spin-based layer-by-layer method was used to apply chitosan and gelatin-based films. Moreover, a laboratory investigation examining the interaction between cells in a controlled environment found that the created biocomposite material had remarkable ability to promote the formation of bone tissue [38]. Chen et al. (2013) created TiO2 nanotubes that contained selenium and were coated with chitosan in a separate research investigation. The generated biocomposite has been shown to possess antibacterial, anticancer, and osteogenic characteristics, as revealed by further analysis [39].

12.1.3.5 Chitosan–Zinc Oxide Nanocomposites

Zinc has been included as a trace element in composites for bone tissue engineering applications because to its ability to enhance bone density and reduce bone loss. The objective of this work was to replicate the natural bone matrix by modifying montmorillonite clay with chitosan/hydroxyapatite–zinc oxide nanocomposites. The nanocomposites achieve a mechanical strength of 30.13 ± 0.16 MPa. This composite exhibits antibacterial effectiveness against both gram-negative and gram-positive bacterial species, such as *Escherichia coli*, *Lysinibacillus fusiformis*, and *Bacillus cereus*. The cytotoxicity of the substance was assessed using an in vitro proliferation assay using MG-63 cells. The results suggest that the nonhazardous chemicals are suitable for use in applications involving the engineering of bone tissue [40]. A novel composite consisting of palladium, zinc oxide, and hydroxyapatite was synthesised and then coated with varying amounts of chitosan (0.125 and 0.25 g) in order to enhance its compressive strength and toughness. The composites were assessed for their antibacterial efficacy against gram-negative bacteria (*Pseudomonas aeruginosa*), and the findings demonstrate remarkable activity and suppression of bacterial proliferation at a concentration of 25 µg/mL. The bioactivity of the composites was assessed by simulated tests of bodily fluids. The findings indicate that the composites have the ability to generate hydroxyapatite bone mineral crystals with a calcium to phosphorus ratio of 1.67 [41]. Huang et al. (2017) developed a nanocomposite consisting of chitosan and gelatin with integrated zinc to mitigate the occurrence of surgical site infections. The nanocomposites were applied as a coating on titanium substrates and shown effective antibacterial properties against *Escherichia coli* and *Staphylococcus aureus* bacterial species. The reaction of the nanocomposites was assessed in vitro using rat bone marrow stromal cells. The findings indicate that the composites exhibited an increased proliferation rate with the introduction of the zinc trace element. Moreover, the findings suggest a decrease in cytotoxicity and a notable level of activity in the enzymatic alkaline phosphatase test [42]. The alkaline phosphatase experiment was conducted on mouse embryonic fibroblasts, and the observed rise in activity on the 21st day indicates a conducive environment for cell growth and specialisation. Two male rabbits were subjected to an in vivo research by creating two 25 mm longitudinal incisions on their right and left dorsum. The bioimplants were inserted and evaluated 4 weeks post surgery. On the 14th day, histological analysis indicated cellular infiltration inside the cavities.

12.1.3.6 Chitosan and Biosilica

Due to their exceptional biocompatibility and capacity for cell proliferation, silica-based biomaterials are extensively used in bone tissue engineering. Furthermore, the combination of biodegradability and enhanced mechanical strength renders them very adaptable for use as a synthetic bone implant. Furthermore, materials that are specifically designed with silica, such as mesoporous bioactive glass, have remarkable capabilities for promoting bone formation [43, 44]. Tamburaci and colleagues created scaffolding systems that include diatomite and chitosan. The composite material exhibits remarkable cell proliferation, mineralization, and alkaline phosphatase activity on MG-63 cells, Saos-2 cells, and human osteoblasts, indicating its importance in the field of bone tissue engineering [45].

The nanocomposites containing chitosan and biosilica, such as chitosan/octa(tetramethylammonium)polyhedral silsesquioxane, chitosan–nanoSiO$_2$–chondroitin sulphate, chitosan–nanoSiO$_2$–gelatin, and chitosan–bioglass/hydroxyapatite/halloysite nanotubes, exhibit exceptional osteogenic properties [46–49]. The production of chitosan and silica-based microspheres included the use of sol–gel techniques, followed by emulsification and cross-linking processes. Subsequently, the vancomycin hydrochloride was enclosed inside the microspheres. The in vitro biomineralisation assays demonstrate the production of apatite on the microspheres' surface. Furthermore, a sustainable drug release profile was identified. This discovery demonstrates that the microspheres that were created have great potential for use in bone tissue engineering [50].

12.2 APPLICATIONS

12.2.1 Biosafety of Nanocomposites

Nanocomposites are composite materials composed of nanoparticles (NPs) and a matrix material. They have garnered considerable interest across other disciplines owing to their distinct characteristics and prospective uses. Nevertheless, in the context of biosafety, it is important to evaluate the possible hazards linked to the use of nanocomposites in order to guarantee their secure implementation [51]. Biosafety of nanocomposites may be achieved by meticulously choosing appropriate components and implementing surface changes. Nanocomposites consist of intrinsically biocompatible materials, indicating a little likelihood of inflicting damage to living beings. Biocompatible materials, such as certain polymers or ceramics, have undergone thorough examination and experimentation to determine their compatibility with biological systems [52]. Surface modification of nanocomposites may be used to improve their biosafety, as seen in Figure 5. Surface modifications may include the application of a protective layer of biocompatible substances, such as polymers or bioactive compounds, onto the NPs or nanofillers. This is done to avoid direct interaction between the NPs and the surrounding biological environment. Surface modification may mitigate possible toxicity and enhance the overall biosafety of the nanocomposite. Nanocomposites may be engineered to enclose or transport bioactive molecules, such as medications or growth hormones, in a regulated way [53]. The capacity to regulate the release of therapeutic substances enables precise delivery to specific targets, while reducing their overall exposure and possible harm to the body. Nanocomposites may be deliberately designed to possess precise dimensions and surface characteristics that improve their ability to provide biological safety. By manipulating the dimensions and electrostatic properties of nanoparticles (NPs), it is feasible to limit their contact with cells or tissues and mitigate the potential for harmful biological consequences. Certain nanocomposites may be engineered to possess biodegradability, indicating their ability to decompose gradually into harmless byproducts that can be readily removed from the body. Biodegradable nanocomposites are very advantageous in medical contexts due to their ability to progressively decompose and be substituted by natural tissue as part of the healing process [54].

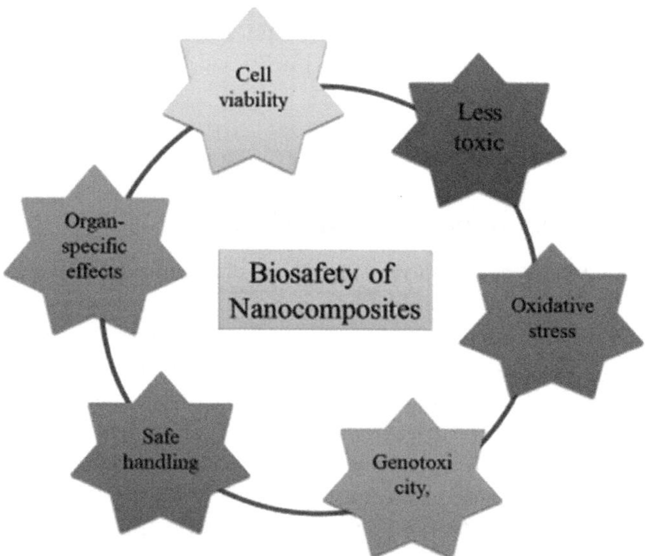

Figure 12.1 Applications of ZnO NPs.

12.2.2 Applications of ZnO NPs

Zinc oxide nanoparticles (ZnO NPs) have been used in several sectors such as rubber, biosensors, food additives, pigments, and electrical materials. Multiple research studies have shown the impact of ZnO nanoparticles on bacteria. The experiment included using an ammonium carbonate solution and a zinc acetate solution to generate the precursors necessary for the production of ZnO NPs. Zinc oxide nanoparticles were generated by the process of calcination. Enhancing the compatibility between ZnO nanoparticles and an organic matrix may be achieved by surface treatment with oleic acid. Covalent bonds were produced due to chemical interactions between surface hydroxylic groups and organic molecules of ZnO NPs. On the other hand, silica provides protection for ZnO nanoparticles. The catalytic activity of ZnO NPs was dramatically reduced due to an interfacial chemical interaction with SiO_2 [55]. Zinc oxide has exceptional chemical and physical characteristics, such as a high electrochemical coupling coefficient, a wide range of radiation absorption, and remarkable chemical stability. Various techniques have been used to produce ZnO nanoparticles. The chemical and physical characteristics of ZnO nanoparticles, including their dimensions, uniformity in size, morphology, surface condition, crystal lattice, arrangement on a substrate, and capacity to disperse, play a vital role in several applications. Consequently, many production techniques have been developed [56] and implemented, including a controlled precipitation plan. Zinc acetate and ammonium carbonate were used for the precipitation of zinc oxide $(Zn(CH_3COO)2 \cdot H_2O)$. Lanje et al. [57] used a straightforward precipitation technique to synthesise zinc oxide. The production of ZnO nanoparticles should be a single-step process conducted on a massive scale, ensuring the absence of any undesired contaminants. Zinc (Zn) is a vital component for the human body, nevertheless, it is crucial to acknowledge that excessive quantities of zinc may truly be poisonous. Zinc is essential for a range of biological activities, including enzyme functionality, immune system reinforcement, and wound recovery. However, similar to several other nutrients, it adheres to a U-shaped dose–response relationship, indicating that both insufficiency and surplus might have negative consequences. Zinc oxide nanoparticles (NPs) find use in several dental treatments such as restorative dentistry, endodontics, regenerative endodontics, periodontics, prosthodontics, orthodontics, oral medicine, cancer diagnostics, dental implantology, preventative dentistry, and biomedical waste management [58]. Zinc oxide nanoparticles (ZnO NPs) have shown potential as an alternative to titanium oxide nanoparticles (TiO_2 NPs) in several energy conservation and transportation applications, such as batteries, solar cells, semiconductors, photocatalysis, decontamination, and biosensing [59]. Recently, there has been much research on metal oxide nanoparticles (NPs) as nano-antibiotics for enhanced sanitation, particularly against drug-resistant bacteria and parasites [60]. When exposed to intense ultra-violet (UV) radiation, these particles interfere with the oxidative stress in microorganisms [61]. While ZnO is a chemical based on Zn that is generally believed to be regulated by the US Food and Drug Administration [62], it is necessary to confirm the safety of ZnO NPs. It is essential to conduct an inquiry and mitigate any hazards to both the environment and human well-being [63].

12.2.3 Application of TiO$_2$ NPs

Titanium is highly favoured because to its solid chemical structure, bio-compatibility, and versatile physical, optical, and electrical capabilities. The photocatalytic properties of this substance have been used in many environmental applications for the purpose of eliminating pollutants from both water and air [64]. Titanium dioxide exists in three distinct crystalline forms: anatase, rutile, and brookite [65]. Antase TiO2 functions mainly as a photocatalyst when exposed to UV light and has a crystalline structure resembling a tetragonal sphere with dipyramidal forms. Additionally, we see crystals of TiO$_2$ having a tetragonal structure of the rutile type, exhibiting a prismatic shape. This particular titanium is mostly used as a pigment for white paint. Brookite-type TiO$_2$ has a crystalline orthorhombic structure. TiO$_2$ is a versatile component that is used in many products such as sunscreen lotions and paint pigments [66]. Additionally, it is employed in solar cells, capacitors, electrochemical electrodes, and even as a culinary flavouring ingredient and in toothpaste [67]. The anatase type of TiO2 nanoparticles is often chosen for its robust photocatalytic activity, larger specific surface area, lack of toxicity, photochemical stability, and customer preference. Furthermore, the potential energy of photo-generated electrons is higher because to the stronger negative conduction band edge potential [68]. Titanium dioxide (TiO$_2$) and zinc oxide (ZnO) nanoparticles (NPs) are often used in bio-nanocomposites due to their distinct physical and chemical properties. ZnO and TiO$_2$ nanoparticles have been shown to possess antibacterial properties, making them very suitable for use as coatings on medical equipment to facilitate wound healing. Furthermore, ZnO/TiO$_2$ bio-nanocomposites have shown potential in the fields of drug delivery, tissue engineering, and biosensor applications [66]. ZnO/TiO$_2$ bio-nanocomposites have the potential to be used for medication delivery, enabling the precise and regulated release of pharmaceuticals to particular locations inside the body. The use of ZnO/TiO$_2$ bio-nanocomposites has shown an enhancement in the absorption and discharge of medications, resulting in enhanced therapeutic effectiveness [69]. ZnO/TiO$_2$ bio-nanocomposites have potential use as scaffolds in tissue engineering for the purpose of tissue regeneration. Adding ZnO and TiO$_2$ nanoparticles to the biopolymer matrix might enhance the mechanical robustness and biocompatibility of the scaffolds [70]. Bio-nanocomposites consisting of ZnO and TiO_2 may serve as biosensors to detect biomolecules, offering exceptional sensitivity and selectivity. Integrating ZnO and TiO2 nanoparticles into the biopolymer matrix might enhance the functionality of the biosensors by improving their detection limits and response times [71]. The use of ZnO/TiO_2 bio-nanocomposites has great promise in the field of biomedicine. Antimicrobial uses utilise them as antibacterial agents for wound healing and as coatings for medical equipment to avoid infections. ZnO/TiO_2 bio-nanocomposites have the ability to transport medications to precise locations inside the body, enabling precise and regulated release. Within the field of tissue engineering, scaffolds may serve as structures that support the growth of new tissue, enhancing both the mechanical resilience and compatibility with living organisms. Biosensors may be used to detect biomolecules with exceptional sensitivity and selectivity [72]. In summary, ZnO/TiO_2 bio-nanocomposites have exceptional potential in the field of biomedicine owing to their distinctive characteristics and prospective uses. Additional investigation is required to enhance their efficiency for certain purposes and to guarantee their safety and compatibility with living organisms for medical use [73].

12.2.4 Antimicrobial Activity of ZnO/TiO_2 Nanocomposites

ZnO/TiO_2 bio-nanocomposites have shown potent antibacterial properties against a wide range of pathogens, including bacteria, fungus, and viruses. The antibacterial activities of ZnO/TiO_2 bio-nanocomposites originate from the distinctive physical and chemical characteristics of the nanoparticles (NPs), which have the ability to harm the microbial cell membrane and interfere with cellular processes [74]. Zinc oxide (ZnO) and titanium dioxide (TiO_2) nanoparticles (NPs) have antibacterial properties via distinct processes, as seen in Figure 6. Upon exposure to moisture, ZnO nanoparticles (NPs) liberate zinc ions (Zn2+), leading to the initiation of oxidative stress, interference with cellular processes, and impairment of the microbial cell membrane. Titanium dioxide nanoparticles (TiO2 NPs) produce reactive oxygen species (ROS), namely hydroxyl radicals, when exposed to ultraviolet (UV) radiation. These ROS have the potential to harm microbial DNA and proteins [75]. The use of ZnO and TiO_2 in a nanocomposite configuration may provide synergistic outcomes, leading to heightened antibacterial efficacy. The coexistence of both substances may produce a wider range of reactive oxygen species (ROS), resulting in heightened harm to microbial cells. Moreover, the use of ZnO may boost the photocatalytic activity of TiO_2, hence increasing its effectiveness in creating reactive oxygen species (ROS) [76]. Multiple research have shown the antibacterial properties of ZnO/TiO_2 bio-nanocomposites in diverse applications. For instance, ZnO/TiO$_2$ bio-nanocomposites have shown significant efficacy in inhibiting bacterial growth and facilitating the process of wound healing. ZnO/TiO$_2$ bio-nanocomposites have shown the ability to hinder the proliferation of oral bacteria and impede the development of biofilms in dental settings. ZnO/TiO$_2$ bio-nanocomposites have shown efficacy in preventing bacterial adhesion and development on the surface of medical device coatings, hence lowering the likelihood of infection [77]. The assessment of the antibacterial efficacy of ZnO/TiO$_2$ bio-nanocomposites may be conducted by many techniques, including disc diffusion tests, minimum inhibitory concentration (MIC) assays, and time-kill studies. These experiments may provide useful data on the efficacy of the bio-nanocomposites against certain pathogens and the ideal dose necessary for their application. It is crucial to acknowledge that while ZnO/TiO$_2$ bio-nanocomposites have effective antibacterial properties, their potential for causing harm to human health, such as cytotoxicity and long-term consequences, must be thoroughly assessed. Furthermore, it is crucial to verify the biocompatibility of the bio-nanocomposites and confirm that they do not have any detrimental effects on the host tissue [78]. The effectiveness of silicate/(ZnO–TiO2) NCMs in killing microorganisms was evaluated utilising the disc diffusion test method. The silicate/(ZnO-TiO$_2$) NCM dispersions were quickly immersed in small sterile filter paper discs and let to dry fully. The surface of a nutrient agar plate was uniformly coated with a 100 L bacterial solution that had been cultivated overnight. Discs were placed on the side of the plate opposite to where the bacteria were located, and this side contained silicate/(ZnO–TiO2) NCM. In order to affix the sheets to the agar, a volume of 3 liters of sterilised water was placed on top of them. Following a 24-hour incubation period at temperatures of 37°C and 28°C for the bacterial and fungal plates, respectively, the area around the disc where growth was inhibited was observed [79]. Nanoparticles generated from Hibiscus rosa-sinensis extract and ZnO/TiO$_2$ nanocomposites were reported to have antibacterial properties against both Gram-positive bacteria, such as Staphylococcus species, and gram-negative bacteria, such as *E. coli*. Zinc oxide nanoparticles (NPs) were synthesised utilising an extract of *Hibiscus rosa-sinensis*. These NPs exhibited small zones of inhibition against *E. coli* and *Staphylococcus aureus*, indicating limited antibacterial activity. The effectiveness of the ZnO/TiO2 nanocomposite against *S. aureus* and *E. coli* has been increased by enhancing its inhibitory zone [80].

12.2.5 Antidiabetic Activity of ZnO/TiO$_2$ Nanocomposites

An investigation has been conducted on the characteristics of ZnO/TiO2 nanocomposites, namely their ability to combat diabetes and act as antioxidants. The synthesis of ZnO/TiO2 nanocomposites was conducted, and subsequently, their antioxidant and anti-diabetic activities were evaluated. The nanocomposites exhibited significant antioxidant activity in vitro, as shown by both the ferric-reducing antioxidant power test and the DPPH radical scavenging experiment. Furthermore, the nanocomposites exhibited antidiabetic action by inhibiting the enzymes amylase and glucosidase, which play a role in glucose digestion. According to experts, ZnO/TiO2 nanocomposites might potentially be used as a natural alternative to pharmaceutical anti-inflammatory and antioxidant drugs [81]. The researchers assessed the ability of ZnO/TiO2 nanocomposites to function as antidiabetic agents in streptozotocin-induced diabetic rats (Figure 7). The nanocomposites were orally supplied for a duration of 21 days [82], and their impact on blood glucose levels and antioxidant status were assessed. The findings demonstrated that the nanocomposites had a substantial impact on lowering blood glucose levels and enhancing the antioxidant status in rats with diabetes. According to the scientists, the nanocomposites' capacity to eliminate harmful free radicals and control the process of glucose metabolism is responsible for their antidiabetic and antioxidant properties [83]. The effectiveness of ZnO/TiO2 nanocomposites in safeguarding pancreatic beta cells from oxidative stress was assessed. The nanocomposites demonstrated a reduction in oxidative stress and an enhancement in cell viability in beta cells when exposed to hydrogen peroxide. The authors proposed that the nanocomposites may hold promise for therapeutic use in diabetes therapy by safeguarding pancreatic beta cells from oxidative harm [71].

12.2.6 Anticancer Activity of ZnO/TiO$_2$ Nanocomposites

The potential anticancer efficacy of ZnO/TiO2 nanocomposites has been investigated. A research conducted in 2017 included the creation and evaluation of ZnO/TiO2 nanocomposites for their ability to inhibit the growth of human breast cancer cells (MCF-7) in the field of materials science and engineering. The nanocomposites significantly impeded the proliferation and migration of MCF-7 cells, leading to a notable increase in cell mortality (Figure 8). The scientists postulated that the ability of the nanocomposites to generate reactive oxygen species (ROS) and induce apoptosis in cancer cells may be responsible for their anticancer effects [71]. The anti-cancer effects of four non-additive cell cultures, specifically the MD-231 human breast adenocarcinoma cell line, CHO Chinese hamster ovary cells, HeLa human cervical cancer cell line, and B16-F10 *Mus musculus* cutaneous melanoma cell line, were assessed using the 3-(4,5-dimethylthiazol-2-yl)-2,5-diphenyltetrazolium bromide (MTT) assay. Each well was allocated varying amounts of the control solution (PBS) and the nanocomposites (1, 3, 10, 30, and 100 g mL^{-1}). The duration of incubation was 24 hours at a temperature of 37°C with a carbon dioxide concentration of 5%. Following incubation, the wells were washed twice with PBS prior to the addition of 100 L of MTT and a further 4-hour incubation period. The formazan crystals resulting from mitochondrial activity were eliminated by using acidified isopropanol (0.1% Tris-HCl in isopropanol). The samples underwent analysis at a wavelength of 562 nm using a plate reader. The experiments were replicated and each replication was conducted five times to control for pipetting mistakes. Only samples with a ZNP/TNP ratio of 1:1 were used in this experiment [84]. A separate research, published in the *International Bio-deterioration & Biodegradation* journal in 2020, examined the possible anticancer effects of ZnO/TiO2 nanocomposites on A549 human lung cancer cells. The nanocomposites exhibited pronounced cytotoxicity in A549 cells, leading to substantial cell death, as well as suppressing their proliferation and colony formation. The scientists proposed that the nanocomposites' capacity to produce reactive oxygen species (ROS) and cause DNA damage in cancer cells may account for their anticancer properties [85]. The potential anticancer efficacy of ZnO/TiO2 nanocomposites against human cervical cancer cells (HeLa) was assessed in a 2019 research published in the *Journal of Inorganic Biochemistry*. The nanocomposites exhibited pronounced cytotoxicity against HeLa cells, effectively impeding their proliferation and migration. According to the scientists, the nanocomposites' capacity to produce reactive oxygen species (ROS) and trigger programmed cell death (apoptosis) in cancer cells is believed to be responsible for their anticancer effects [86].

12.2.7 Anti-larval Activity

Michael and colleagues (87) first introduced the brine prawn test, which was subsequently improved by Ghufran and colleagues (88). This test is an effective tool for identifying many hazardous substances. For a considerable time, it has been used to examine the harmful effects on cells of dental materials, pesticides, heavy metals, plant extracts, and fungal toxins [89]. Extracting the physiologically active compounds from the plant extract is a valuable approach [90]. Presently, several experts are intrigued by the cytotoxicity of nanomaterials towards *Artemia salina* larvae. Due to the test's need for just a little amount of NPs, this approach is straightforward, cost-effective, and appealing. Various animal models are now used for in vivo testing to investigate the cytotoxic effects of exposure to nanoparticles. The techniques used to introduce individuals to NPs include injection, cutaneous application, inhalation, and oral administration [91]. Researchers used in vitro techniques to evaluate the harmful effects of NPs, since in vivo studies are costly and time-consuming. Pharmaceutical research currently often assesses the toxicity of various drugs using a species of brine prawns known as *Artemia salina* [92]. Since there is no need for sterile preparations in this scenario, A. salina tests may be utilised instead of the less reliable

MTT assay or animal serum can be used [93]. Since its creation by Michael and his colleagues in 1959, the brine shrimp test has been widely used by many labs as a method for promptly evaluating toxicity [86, 94]. Artemia is a valuable test organism for toxicity testing because to its affordability, simplicity, and efficient screening procedure. The brine shrimp eggs are gathered specifically for the purpose of conducting a cytotoxic test on them. Subsequently, the eggs are maintained at a temperature of 28°C for a period of time. Egg hatching is expedited by using synthetic saline solution and a heat source maintained at a temperature of 37°C. This approach was successful while using 96-well plates. By using a Pasteur pipette, recently hatched nauplii are carefully chosen and introduced into individual wells. The test sample is inserted into each well and the volume is calibrated. After a 24-hour incubation period, the brine shrimp are extracted from the 96-well plates and then enumerated using a microscope. The percentage of deceased prawns in each well is computed after a 24-hour incubation period [95].

Scientists have conducted experiments to assess the harmful effects of chemical nanoparticles on brine prawns. Regarding these NPs and their interactions with brine shrimp, there are several frameworks available for promotion. Madhav et al. [96] created spherical ZnO nanoparticles with an average diameter of 114.36 nm via chemical synthesis. This work demonstrates that the interaction between established NPs and *Artemia salina* is detrimental, as it leads to the generation of oxidative stress and considerable disruption of proteolytic enzymes. The escalating fatality rate served as evidence of the harmful effects of zinc oxide nanoparticles. This study also revealed that nanoparticles (NPs) had an uneven shape and had an average diameter of 63.13 nm [97]. Furthermore, an examination has been conducted to assess the potential ability of ZnO/TiO$_2$ nanocomposites to inhibit the growth of mosquito larvae. In a study published in Environmental Chemical Engineering in 2018, researchers developed and evaluated the larvicidal efficacy of ZnO/TiO$_2$ nanocomposites against the Aedes aegypti mosquito, which is responsible for transmitting dengue disease. When the nanocomposites were present at a concentration of 50 ppm, they exhibited a substantial larvicidal effect, leading to the complete mortality of all larvae. According to the scientists, the capacity of the nanocomposites to harm the cellular membrane of mosquito larvae and result in their death may be the reason for their larvicidal function [98]. A separate investigation, published in the Journal of Cluster Science in 2020, assessed the ability of ZnO/TiO$_2$ nanocomposites to combat the larvae of the Anopheles stephensi mosquito, which is known to transmit malaria. When the nanocomposites were present at a concentration of 100 ppm, they demonstrated potent anti-larval activity, leading to the complete mortality of the larvae. According to the authors, the nanocomposites have the ability to hinder the growth and development of mosquito larvae, which is why they exhibit anti-larval action [99]. In a study published in the *Journal of Hazardous Materials* in 2021, the larvicidal efficacy of ZnO/TiO_2 nanocomposites against the filariasis vector mosquito Culex quinquefasciatus was investigated. At a concentration of 20 parts per million (ppm), the nanocomposites demonstrated significant larvicidal activity, resulting in the death of all larvae. The authors suggest that the larvicidal impact of the nanocomposites may be attributed to their ability to impair the nervous system of mosquito larvae and inhibit the production of certain proteins [100].

12.3 CONCLUSION

In general, the synthesis of ZnO/TiO_2 nanocomposites can be achieved through physical, chemical, and biological means. However, biological methods are considered to be safer, more environmentally friendly, and more cost-effective compared to physical and chemical approaches. Plant-based ZnO/TiO_2 nanocomposites are synthesised and subsequently subjected to character analysis in a biological process. Following characterization, nanocomposites can be utilised in a multitude of biological applications. The quantity of biomedical applications in various processes, including medication administration, biosensors, tissue engineering, and gene delivery, is increasing on a daily basis. The toxicity properties of ZnO/TiO_2 make it a powerful alternative to antibiotics and an effective tool against numerous drug-resistant microorganisms. The results of this analysis will aid future research in exploring new methodological and clinical relationships in this field.

REFERENCES

1. Bittnar Z, Bartos PJ, Nemecek J, Smilauer V, Zeman J. *Nanotechnology in Construction. Proceedings of the NICOM3.* Springer Science & Business Media; 2009. doi:10.1007/978-3-642-00980-8
2. Scrivener KL, Kirkpatrick RJ. Innovation in use and research on cementitious material. Cem *Concr Res.* 2008;38(2):128–36. doi:10.1016/j.cemconres.2007.09.025
3. Silva GA. Introduction to nanotechnology and its applications to medicine. *Surg Neurol.* 2004;61(3):216–20. doi:10.1016/j.surneu.2003.09.036
4. Thostenson ET, Li C, Chou T-W. Nanocomposites in context. *Compos Sci Technol.* 2005;65(3–4):491–516. doi:10.1016/j.compscitech.2004.11.003
5. Pande V, Sanklecha V. Bionanocomposite: A review. *Austin J Nanomed Nanotechnol.* 2017;5(1):1045.
6. Navarro-Gázquez P, Muñoz-Portero M, Blasco-Tamarit E, Sánchez-Tovar R, García-Antón J. Synthesis and applications of TiO2/ZnO hybrid nanostructures by ZnO deposition on TiO2 nanotubes using electrochemical processes. *Rev Chem Eng.* 2022. doi:10.1515/revce-2021-0105.

7. Upadhyay GK, Rajput JK, Pathak TK, Kumar V, Purohit LP. Synthesis of ZnO: TiO2 nanocomposites for photocatalyst application in visible light. *Vacuum.* 2019;160:154–63. doi:10.1016/j.vacuum.2018.11.026

8. Abdullah SM, Kolo K, Sajadi SM. Greener pathway toward the synthesis of lichen-based ZnO@ TiO2@ SiO2 and Fe3O4@ SiO2 nanocomposites and investigation of their biological activities. *Food Sci Nutr.* 2020;8(8):4044–54. doi:10.1002/fsn3.1661

9. Rheima AM, Hussain DH, Abed HJ. Fabrication of a new photo-sensitized solar cell using TiO2\ZnO Nanocomposite synthesized via a modified sol-gel Technique. *IOP Conf Ser Mater Sci Eng.* 2020, November;928(5):052036. doi:10.1088/1757-899X/928/5/052036

10. Hu H, Onyebueke L, Abatan A. Characterizing and modeling mechanical properties of nanocomposites-review and evaluation. *J Miner Mater Charact Eng.* 2010;9(04):275. doi:10.4236/jmmce.2010.94022

11. Rasmussen MK, Pedersen JN, Marie R. Size and surface charge characterization of nanoparticles with a salt gradient. *Nat Commun.* 2020;11(1):2337. doi:10.1038/s41467-020-15889-3

12. Molla MAI, Furukawa M, Tateishi I, Katsumata H, Suzuki T, Kaneco S. Photocatalytic decolorization of dye with self-dye-sensitization under fluorescent light irradiation. *Chem Eng.* 2017;1:8. doi:10.3390/chemengineering1020008

13. Shaikh SF, Mane RS, Min BK, Hwang YJ, Joo OS. D-sorbitol-induced phase control of TiO2 nanoparticles and its application for dye-sensitized solar cells. *Sci Rep.* 2016;6:20103. doi:10.1038/srep20103

14. Ahmed AZ, Islam MM, Islam MMu, Masum SM, Islam R, Molla MAI. Fabrication and characterization of B/Sn-doped ZnO nanoparticles via mechanochemical method for photocatalytic degradation of rhodamine B. *Inorg Nano-Met Chem.* 2020;51(10):1369–78. doi:10.1080/24701556.2020.1835976

15. Mousa HM, Alenezi JF, Mohamed IMA, Yasin AS, Hashem AFM, Abdal-hay A. Synthesis of TiO2@ZnOheterojunction Dye photodegradation wastewater. *Treat J Alloy Compd.* 2021;886:161169. doi:10.1016/j.jallcom.2021.161169

16. Xie K, Zhou Z, Guo Y, Wang L, Li G, Zhao S, Liu X, Li J, Jiang W, Wu S, Hao Y. Long-term prevention of bacterial infection and enhanced osteoinductivity of a hybrid coating with selective silver toxicity. *Adv. Healthcare Mater.* 2019;8(5):1801465. doi:10.1002/adhm.201801465

17. Wang X, Yan L, Ye T, Cheng R, Tian J, Ma C, Wang Y, Cui W. Osteogenic and antiseptic nanocoating by in situ chitosan regulated electrochemical deposition for promoting osseointegration. *Mater. Sci. Eng. C* 2019;102:415–26. doi:10.1016/j.msec.2019.04.060

18. Stevanović M, Djošić M, Janković A, Rhee KY, Mišković-Stanković V. Electrophoretically deposited hydroxyapatite-based composite coatings loaded with silver and gentamicin as antibacterial agents-Review. Journal of the Serbian Chemical Society. *J. Serb Chem Soc.* 2019;84:1287–304. doi:10.2298/jsc190821092s

19. Socrates R, Prymak O, Loza K, Sakthivel N, Rajaram A, Epple M, Narayana Kalkura S. Biomimetic fabrication of mineralized composite films of nanosilver loaded native fibrillar collagen and chitosan. *Mater Sci Eng C* 2019;99:357–66. doi:10.1016/j.msec.2019.01.101

20. Banerjee D, Bose S. Effects of aloe vera gel extract in doped hydroxyapatite-coated titanium implants on in vivo and in vitro biological properties. *ACS Appl. Bio Mater.* 2019;2:3194–202. doi:10.1021/acsabm.9b00077

21. Pishbin F, Mouriño V, Gilchrist JB, McComb DW, Kreppel S, Salih V, Ryan MP, Boccaccini AR. Single-step electrochemical deposition of antimicrobial orthopaedic coatings based on a bioactive glass/chitosan/nano-silver composite system. *Acta Biomater.* 2013;9:7469–79. doi:10.1016/j.actbio.2013.03.006

22. Sul OJ, Kim JC, Kyung TW, Kim HJ, Kim YY, Kim SH, Kim JS, Choi HS. Gold nanoparticles inhibited the receptor activator of nuclear factor-κb ligand (RANKL)-induced osteoclast formation by acting as an antioxidant. *Biosci Biotechnol Biochem.* 2010;74:2209–13. doi:10.1271/bbb.100375

23. Gera S, Sampathi S, Dodoala S. Role of nanoparticles in drug delivery and regenerative therapy for bone diseases. Curr. *Drug Delivery* 2017;14:904–16. doi:10.2174/1567201813666161230142123

24. Rao SH, Harini B, Shadamarshan RPK, Balagangadharan K, Selvamurugan N. Natural and synthetic polymers/bioceramics/bioactive compounds-mediated cell signalling in bone tissue engineering. *Int J Biol Macromol.* 2018;110:88–96. doi:10.1016/j.ijbiomac.2017.09.029

25. Yi C, Liu D, Fong CC, Zhang J, Yang M. Gold nanoparticles promote osteogenic differentiation of mesenchymal stem cells through p38 MAPK pathway. *ACS Nano* 2010;4:6439–48. doi:10.1021/nn101373r

26. Mahmoud NS, Ahmed HH, Mohamed MR, Amr KS, Aglan HA, Ali MAM, Tantawy MA. Role of nanoparticles in osteogenic differentiation of bone marrow mesenchymal stem cells. *Cytotechnology* 2020;72:1–22. doi:10.1007/s10616-019-00353-y

27. Choi SY, Song MS, Ryu PD, Lam ATN, Joo SW, Lee SY. Gold nanoparticles promote osteogenic differentiation in human adipose-derived mesenchymal stem cells through the Wnt/β-catenin signaling pathway. *Int J Nanomed.* 2015;10:4383–92. doi:10.2147/ijn.s78775

28. Wu J, Zheng K, Huang X, Liu J, Liu H, Boccaccini AR, Wan Y, Guo X, Shao Z. Thermally triggered injectable chitosan/silk fibroin/bioactive glass nanoparticle hydrogels for in-situ bone formation in rat calvarial bone defects. *Acta Biomater.* 2019;91:60–71. doi:10.1016/j.actbio.2019.04.023

29. Ning C, Jiajia J, Meng L, Hongfei Q, Xianglong W, Tingli L. Electrophoretic deposition of GHK-Cu loaded MSN-chitosan coatings with pH-responsive release of copper and its bioactivity. *Mater Sci Eng C* 2019;104:109746.

30. Lu Y, Li L, Zhu Y, Wang X, Li M, Lin Z, Hu X, Zhang Y, Yin Q, Xia H, Mao C. Multifunctional copper-containing carboxymethyl chitosan/alginate scaffolds for eradicating clinical bacterial infection and promoting bone formation. *ACS Appl Mater Interfaces* 2018;10:127–38. doi:10.1021/acsami.7b13750

31. Forero JC, Roa E, Reyes JG, Acevedo C, Osses N. Development of useful biomaterial for bone tissue engineering by incorporating nano-copper-zinc alloy (nCuZn) in chitosan/gelatin/nano-hydroxyapatite (Ch/G/nHAp) scaffold. *Materials* 2017;10:1177. doi:10.3390/ma1010117

32. Tripathi A, Saravanan S, Pattnaik S, Moorthi A, Partridge NC, Selvamurugan N. Bio-composite scaffolds containing chitosan/nano-hydroxyapatite/nano-copper–zinc for bone tissue engineering. *Int J Biol Macromol.* 2012;50:294–9. doi:10.1016/j.ijbiomac.2011.11.013

33. Kulkarni M, Mazare A, Gongadze E, Perutkova Š, Kralj-Iglič V, Milošev I, Schmuki P, Iglič A, Mozetič M. Titanium nanostructures for biomedical applications. *Nanotechnology* 2015;26:062002. doi:10.1088/0957-4484/26/6/062002

34. Khorasani AM, Goldberg M, Doeven EH, Littlefair GJ. Titanium in biomedical applications—properties and fabrication: a review. *Biomater Tissue Eng.* 2015;5:593–619. doi:10.1166/jbt.2015.1361

35. Kunrath MF, Leal BF, Hubler R, de Oliveira SD, Teixeira ER. Antibacterial potential associated with drug-delivery built TiO2 nanotubes in biomedical implants. *AMB Express* 2019;9:51. doi:10.1186/s13568-019-0777-6

36. Lai M, Jin Z, Yan M, Zhu J, Yan X, Xu KJ. The controlled naringin release from TiO2 nanotubes to regulate osteoblast differentiation. *Biomater Appl.* 2018;33:673–80. doi:10.1177/0885328218809239

37. Liu P, Hao Y, Zhao Y, Yuan Z, Ding Y, Cai K. Surface modification of titanium substrates for enhanced osteogenetic and antibacterial properties. *Colloids Surf B* 2017;160:110–116. doi:10.1016/j.colsurfb.2017.08.044

38. Lai M, Jin Z, Tang Q, Lu M. Sustained release of melatonin from TiO2 nanotubes for modulating osteogenic differentiation of mesenchymal stem cells in vitro. *J. Biomater Sci Polym Ed.* 2017;28:1651–64. doi:10.1080/09205063.2017.1342334

39. Chen X, Cai K, Fang J, Lai M, Hou Y, Li J, Luo Z, Hu Y, Tang L. Fabrication of selenium-deposited and chitosan-coated titania nanotubes with anticancer and antibacterial properties. *Colloids Surf B* 2013;103:149–57. doi:10.1016/j.colsurfb.2012.10.022

40. Bhowmick A, Banerjee SL, Pramanik N, Jana P, Mitra T, Gnanamani A, Das M, Kundu PP. Organically modified clay supported chitosan/hydroxyapatite-zinc oxide nanocomposites with enhanced mechanical and biological properties for the application in bone tissue engineering. *Int J Biol Macromol.* 2018;106:11–19. doi:10.1016/j.ijbiomac.2017.07.168

41. Heidari F, Tabatabaei FS, Razavi M, Lari RB, Tavangar M, Romanos GE, Vashaee D, Tayebi L. 3D construct of hydroxyapatite/zinc oxide/palladium nanocomposite scaffold for bone tissue engineering. *J Mater Sci Mater Med.* 2020;31:85. doi:10.1007/s10856-020-06409-2

42. Huang P, Ma K, Cai X, Huang D, Yang X, Ran J, Wang F, Jiang T. Enhanced antibacterial activity and biocompatibility of zinc-incorporated organic-inorganic nanocomposite coatings via electrophoretic deposition. *Colloids Surf B* 2017;160:628–38. doi:10.1016/j.colsurfb.2017.10.012

43. Eivazzadeh-Keihan R, Chenab KK, Taheri-Ledari R, Mosafer J, Hashemi SM, Mokhtarzadeh A, Maleki A, Hamblin MR. Recent advances in the application of mesoporous silica-based nanomaterials for bone tissue engineering. *Mater Sci Eng C* 2020;107:110267. doi:10.1016/j.msec.2019.110267

44. Shadjou N, Hasanzadeh M. Bone tissue engineering using silica-based mesoporous nanobiomaterials: Recent progress. *Mater Sci Eng C* 2015;55:401–9. doi:10.1016/j.msec.2015.05.027

45. Tamburaci S, Tihminlioglu F. Biosilica incorporated 3D porous scaffolds for bone tissue engineering applications. *Mater Sci Eng C* 2018;91:274–91. doi:10.1016/j.msec.2018.05.040

46. Kavya KC, Dixit R, Jayakumar R, Nair SV, Chennazhi KP. Synthesis and characterization of chitosan/chondroitin sulfate/nano-SiO2 composite scaffold for bone tissue engineering. *J Biomed Nanotechnol.* 2012;8:149–60. doi:10.1166/jbn.2012.1363

47. Kavya KC, Jayakumar R, Nair S, Chennazhi KP. Fabrication and characterization of chitosan/gelatin/nSiO2 composite scaffold for bone tissue engineering. *Int J Biol Macromol.* 2013;59:255–63. doi:10.1016/j.ijbiomac.2013.04.023

48. Tamburaci S, Tihminlioglu F. Chitosan-hybrid poss nanocomposites for bone regeneration: The effect of poss nanocage on surface,morphology, structure and in vitro bioactivity. *Int J Biol Macromol.* 2020;142:643–57. doi:10.1016/j.ijbiomac.2019.10.006

49. Molaei A, Yousefpour M. Preparation of Chitosan-based nanocomposites and biomedical investigations in bone tissue engineering. *Int J Polym Mater Polym Biomater.* 2019;68:701–13. doi:10.1080/00914037.2018.1493683

50. Niu N, Teng SH, Zhou HJ, Qian HS. Synthesis, Characterization, and In Vitro Drug Delivery of Chitosan-Silica Hybrid Microspheres for Bone Tissue Engineering. *J Nanomater.* 2019:7425787. doi:10.1155/2019/7425787

51. Pattnaik S, Swain K, Lin Z. Graphene and graphene-based nanocomposites: biomedical applications and biosafety. *J Mater Chem B.* 2016;4(48):7813–31. doi:10.1039/C6TB02086K

52. Castillo RR, Vallet-Regí M. Functional mesoporous silica nanocomposites: biomedical applications and biosafety. *Int J Mol Sci.* 2019;20(4):929. doi:10.3390/ijms20040929

53. Gudkov SV, Burmistrov DE, Lednev VN, Simakin AV, Uvarov OV, Kucherov RN, et al. Biosafety construction composite based on iron oxide nanoparticles and PLGA. *Inventions.* 2022;7(3):61. doi:10.3390/inventions7030061

54. Verma R, Kumar Gupta S, Lamba NP, Singh BK, Singh S, Bahadur V, et al. Graphene and graphene based nanocomposites for bio-medical and bio-safety applications. *ChemistrySelect.* 2023;8(6):e202204337. doi:10.1002/slct.202204337

55. Srivastava V, Gusain D, Sharma YC. Synthesis, characterization and application of zinc oxide nanoparticles (n-ZnO). *Ceram Int.* 2013;39(8):9803–8.

56. Hong R, Pan T, Qian J, Li H. Synthesis and surface modification of ZnO nanoparticles. *Chem Eng J.* 2006;119(2–3):71–81

57. Lanje AS, Sharma SJ, Ningthoujam RS, Ahn J-S, Pode RB. Low temperature dielectric studies of zinc oxide (ZnO) nanoparticles prepared by precipitation method. *Adv Powder Technol.* 2013;24(1):331–5.

58. Pushpalatha C, Suresh J, Gayathri VS, Sowmya SV, Augustine D, Alamoudi A, et al. Zinc oxide nanoparticles: A review on its applications in dentistry. *Front Bioeng Biotechnol.* 2002;10:818.

59. Yu X, Marks TJ, Facchetti A. Metal oxides for optoelectronic applications. *Nat Mater.* 2016;15(4):383–96.

60. Abd-El-Aziz AS, Agatemor C, Etkin N. Antimicrobial resistance challenged with metal-based antimicrobial macromolecules. *Biomaterials.* 2017;118:27–50.

61. Jin SE, Hwang W, Lee HJ, Jin HE. Dual UV irradiation-based metal oxide nanoparticles for enhanced antimicrobial activity in Escherichia coli and M13 bacteriophage. *Int J Nanomed.* 2017;12:8057–70.

62. Liu J, Rojas-Andrade MD, Chata G, Peng Y, Roseman G, Lu JE, et al. Photo-enhanced antibacterial activity of ZnO/graphene quantum dot nanocomposites. *Nanoscale.* 2018;10(1):158–66.

63. Jin SE, Jin JE, Hwang W, Hong SW. Photocatalytic antibacterial application of zinc oxide nanoparticles and self-assembled networks under dual UV irradiation for enhanced disinfection. *Int J Nanomed.* 2019;14:1737.

64. Pavasupree S, Jitputti J, Ngamsinlapasathian S, Yoshikawa S. Hydrothermal synthesis, characterization, photocatalytic activity and dye-sensitized solar cell performance of mesoporous anatase TiO2 nanopowders. *Mat Res Bull.* 2008;43:149–57.

65. Puma GL, Bono A, Krishnaiah D, Collin JG. Preparation of titanium dioxide photocatalyst loaded onto activated carbon support using chemical vapor deposition: A review paper. *J Haz Mat.* 2008;157:209–19.

66. Meacock G, Taylor KA, Knowles MJ, Himonides A. The improved whitening of minced cod flesh using dispersed titanium dioxide. *J Sci Food Agr.* 1997;73(2):221–5.

67. Macwan D, Dave PN, Chaturvedi S. A review on nano-TiO2 sol–gel type syntheses and its applications. *J Mater Sci.* 2011;46:3669–86.

68. Suresh J, Pradheesh G, Alexramani V, Sundrarajan M, Hong SI. Green synthesis and characterization of zinc oxide nanoparticle using insulin plant (Costus pictus D. Don) and investigation of its antimicrobial as well as anticancer activities. *Adv Nat Sci Nanosci Nanotechnol.* 2018;9(1):015008.

69. Kaleji B, Mousaei M, Halakouie H, Ahmadi A. Sol-gel synthesis of ZnO nanoparticles and ZnO-TiO2-SiO2 nanocomposites and their photo-catalyst investigation in methylene blue degradation. *J Nanostruct.* 2015;5(3):219–25.

70. Jinga S-I, Zamfirescu A-I, Voicu G, Enculescu M, Evanghelidis A, Busuioc C. PCL-ZnO/TiO2/HAp electrospun composite fibers with applications in tissue engineering. *Polymers.* 2019;11(11):1793.

71. Liang Z, Zhang X. Zn–ZnO@ TiO2 nanocomposite: A direct electrode for nonenzymatic biosensors. *J Mater Sci.* 2018;53(10):7138–49.

72. Mazabuel-Collazos A, Gómez CD, Rodríguez-Páez J. ZnO-TiO2 nanocomposites synthesized by wet-chemical route: Study of their structural and optical properties. *Mater Chem Phys.* 2019;222:230–45.

73. Elderdery AY, Alhamidi AH, Elkhalifa AM, Althobiti MM, Tebien EM, Omer NE, et al. Synthesis and characterization of ZnO–TiO2–chitosan–escin metallic nanocomposites: Evaluation of their antimicrobial and anticancer activities. *Green Process Synth.* 2022;11(1):1026–39.

74. Lee M, Han S-I, Kim C, Velumani S, Han A, Kassiba AH, et al. ZrO2/ZnO/TiO2 nanocomposite coatings on stainless steel for improved corrosion resistance, biocompatibility, and antimicrobial activity. *ACS Appl Mater Interfaces.* 2022;14(11):13801–11.

75. Daou I, Moukrad N, Zegaoui O, Rhazi Filali F. Antimicrobial activity of ZnO-TiO2 nanomaterials synthesized from three different precursors of ZnO: influence of ZnO/TiO2 weight ratio. *Water Sci Technol.* 2018;77(5):1238–49.

76. Sirotkin N, Khlyustova A, Costerin D, Naumova I, Titov V, Agafonov A. Applications of plasma synthesized ZnO, TiO2, and Zn/TiOx nanoparticles for making antimicrobial wound-healing viscose patches. *Plasma Process Polym.* 2022;19(1):2100093.

77. Omidi S, Sedaghat S, Tahvildari K, Derakhshi P, Motiee F. Biosynthesis of silver nanocomposite with Tarragon leaf extract and assessment of antibacterial activity. *J Nanostruct Chem.* 2018;8:171–8.

78. Ali MM, Haque MJ, Kabir MH, Kaiyum MA, Rahman M. Nano synthesis of ZnO–TiO2 composites by sol-gel method and evaluation of their antibacterial, optical and photocatalytic activities. *Res Mater.* 2021;11:100199.

79. Dhanalakshmi R, Pandikumar A, Sujatha K, Gunasekaran P. Photocatalytic and antimicrobial activities of functionalized silicate sol–gel embedded ZnO–TiO2 nanocomposite materials. *Mater Exp.* 2013;3(4):291–300.

80. Abd El-Kader M, Elabbasy M, Adeboye AA, Zeariya MG, Menazea A. Morphological, structural and antibacterial behavior of eco-friendly of ZnO/TiO2 nanocomposite synthesized via Hibiscus rosa-sinensis extract. *J Mater Res Technol.* 2021;15:2213–20.

81. Suganthi N, Thangavel S, Kannan K. Hibiscus subdariffa leaf extract mediated 2-D fern-like ZnO/TiO2 hierarchical nanoleaf for photocatalytic degradation. *Flat Chem.* 2020;24:100197.

82. Chauhan P, Mahajan S, Prasad GBKS. Preparation and characterization of CS-ZnO-NC nanoparticles for imparting anti-diabetic activities in experimental diabetes. *J Drug Deliv Sci Technol.* 2019;52:738–47.

83. Gharpure S, Akash A, Ankamwar B. A review on antimicrobial properties of metal nanoparticles. *J Nanosci Nanotechnol.* 2020;20(6):3303–39.

84. Chakra CS, Rajendar V, Rao KV, Kumar M. Enhanced antimicrobial and anticancer properties of ZnO and TiO2 nanocomposites. *3 Biotech.* 2017;7:1–8.

85. Dyshlyuk L, Babich O, Ivanova S, Vasilchenco N, Atuchin V, Korolkov I, et al. Antimicrobial potential of ZnO, TiO2 and SiO2 nanoparticles in protecting building materials from biodegradation. *Int Biodeter Biodegrad.* 2020;146:104821.

86. Pragathiswaran C, Smitha C, Barabadi H, Al-Ansari MM, Al-Humaid LA, Saravanan M. TiO2@ ZnO nanocomposites decorated with gold nanoparticles: Synthesis, characterization and their antifungal, antibacterial, anti-inflammatory and anticancer activities. *Inorg Chem Commun.* 2020;121:108210.

87. Michael A, Thompson C, Abramovitz M. Artemia salina as a test organism for bioassay. *Science.* 1956;123(3194):464–4.

88. Ghufran M, Rehman AU, Ayaz M, Ul-Haq Z, Uddin R, Azam SS, et al. New lead compounds identification against KRas mediated cancers through pharmacophore-based virtual screening and in vitro assays. *J Biomol Struct Dyn.* 2022;1–15.

89. Sasidharan ATK, Elyas KK. Research article anti-fungal potential and brine shrimp lethality assay of in vitro raised clones of celastrus paniculatus. *As J Biol Sci.* 2019;12(4):877–83.

90. Teng H, Deng H, Zhang C, Cao H, Huang Q, Chen L. The role of flavonoids in mitigating food originated heterocyclic aromatic amines that concerns human wellness. *Food Sci Hum Wellness.* 2023;12(4):975–85. doi:10.1016/j.fshw.2022.

91. Suh WH, Suslick KS, Stucky GD, Suh Y-H. Nanotechnology, nanotoxicology, and neuroscience. *Prog Neurobiol.* 2009;87(3):133–70.

92. Costa-Lotufo LV, Khan MTH, Ather A, Wilke DV, Jimenez PC, Pessoa C, et al. Studies of the anticancer potential of plants used in Bangladeshi folk medicine. *J Ethnopharmacol.* 2005;99(1):21–30.

93. Mclaughlin JL, Rogers LL, Anderson JE. The use of biological assays to evaluate botanicals. *Drug Inf J.* 1998;32(2):513–24.

94. Vanhaecke P, Persoone G, Claus C, Sorgeloos P. Proposal for a short-term toxicity test with Artemia nauplii. Ecotox Environ Saf. 176 Muhammad et al. *Int J Biosci* 1981;5(3):382–7.

95. Khalil AT, Ovais M, Ullah I, Ali M, Shinwari ZK, Maaza M. Physical properties, biological applications and biocompatibility studies on biosynthesized single phase cobalt oxide (Co3O4) nanoparticles via Sageretia thea (Osbeck.). *Arab J Chem.* 2020;13(1):606–19.

96. Madhav M, David SEM, Kumar RS, Swathy J, Bhuvaneshwari M, Mukherjee A, et al. Toxicity and accumulation of Copper oxide (CuO) nanoparticles in different life stages of Artemia salina. *Environ Toxicol Pharmacol.* 2017;52:227–38.

97. Zhu S, Luo F, Chen W, Zhu B, Wang G. Toxicity evaluation of graphene oxide on cysts and three larval stages of Artemia salina. *Sci Total Environ.* 2017a;595:101–9.

98. Aadil KR, Pandey N, Mussatto SI, Jha H. Green synthesis of silver nanoparticles using acacia lignin, their cytotoxicity, catalytic, metal ion sensing capability and antibacterial activity. *J Environ Chem Eng.* 2019;7(5):103296.

99. Harun NH, Mydin RBS, Sreekantan S, Saharudin KA, Basiron N, Aris F, et al. Bactericidal capacity of a heterogeneous TiO2/ZnO nanocomposite against multidrug-resistant and non-multidrug-resistant bacterial strains associated with nosocomial infections. *ACS Omega.* 2020;5(21):12027–34.

100. Khalid AD, Iqbal SS, Buzdar SA, Ahmad M. Structural, optical and cytotoxic behavior of titanium dioxide nanoparticles and its nanocomposites with zinc oxide. *J Nanoscope.* 2021;2(2):185–97.

Chapter 13

Degradation Studies of Resorbable Materials for Biomedical Applications

*Vishnuvarthanan Mayakrishnan
and Preethi Arul Murugan*

13.1 INTRODUCTION

In the domain of biomedical engineering and healthcare, the thoughtful choice of materials plays a pivotal role, determining the functionality, safety, and effectiveness of numerous medical devices, implants, and therapeutic interventions [1]. The intricate array of materials utilized in biomedical applications reflects a dedication to continuous innovation, combining scientific creativity with clinical necessities to confront diverse healthcare challenges.

Metals, known for their intrinsic strength, lasting durability, and compatibility with biological systems, have established a significant presence in the fields of orthopedics and dentistry [2]. Titanium, esteemed for its outstanding biocompatibility and resistance to corrosion, plays a pivotal role in orthopedic implants by seamlessly integrating with bone tissue and withstanding mechanical stresses. Likewise, stainless steel, possessing strong mechanical properties and sterilization capabilities, is employed in cardiovascular stents, surgical instruments, and orthopedic fixtures, showcasing the harmonious relationship between material characteristics and clinical requirements [3].

Ceramics, known for their exceptional bioactivity and similarity to natural biological substances, have become crucial components in orthopedic and dental applications [4]. Hydroxyapatite, which replicates the mineral composition of bone, promotes osseointegration and bone regeneration. This makes it indispensable in coatings for orthopedic implants and substitutes for bone grafts. Alumina, distinguished by its outstanding hardness, biocompatibility, and resistance to wear, is prominent in dental prosthetics and joint replacements. This highlights the crucial role of material characteristics in determining clinical performance.

On the contrary, the introduction of polymers has marked a new era characterized by versatility and adaptability in biomedical applications [5]. These polymers including biodegradable ones like polylactic acid (PLA) and poly(lactic-co-glycolic acid) (PLGA) as well as elastomeric types such as silicone. Polymers offer a diverse range of options customized for specific

DOI: 10.1201/9781003470311-13

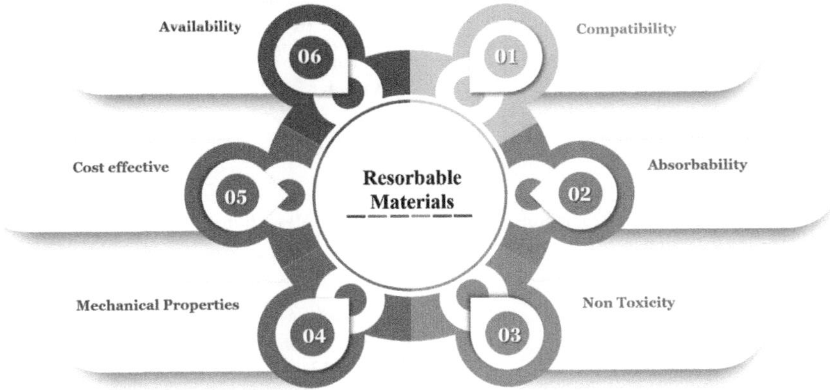

Figure 13.1 Properties of resorbable materials.

clinical contexts. Biodegradable polymers, being inherently temporary, act as foundations for drug delivery systems and scaffolds for tissue engineering. They gradually dissolve as therapeutic goals are achieved, eliminating the need for surgeries to retrieve implants. Meanwhile, silicone, known for its flexibility, biocompatibility, and durability, is widely used in medical devices like catheters, seals, and prosthetic components, encapsulating the essence of adaptability in material design [6]. The collaboration of materials extends to the domain of composites, combining the distinctive characteristics of various materials to generate improved functionalities and performance metrics. Composite materials, exemplified by carbon-fiber reinforced polymers and bioceramic composites, are carefully crafted to leverage synergistic effects. This optimization aims to enhance mechanical strength, biological integration, and functional versatility, particularly in specialized biomedical applications like orthopedic implants and cardiovascular devices.

13.2 RESORBABLE MATERIALS

Resorbable materials have emerged as a groundbreaking category within the biomedical field, offering revolutionary solutions that eliminate the necessity for subsequent removal surgeries and promote superior tissue regeneration [7].

Unlike traditional materials that persist indefinitely in the body, resorbable materials undergo gradual degradation and assimilation, imitating natural healing processes and enabling temporary support or therapeutic interventions. Encompassing various materials such as biodegradable polymers, ceramics, and composites, resorbable materials are precisely designed to display customized degradation profiles, ensuring optimal performance

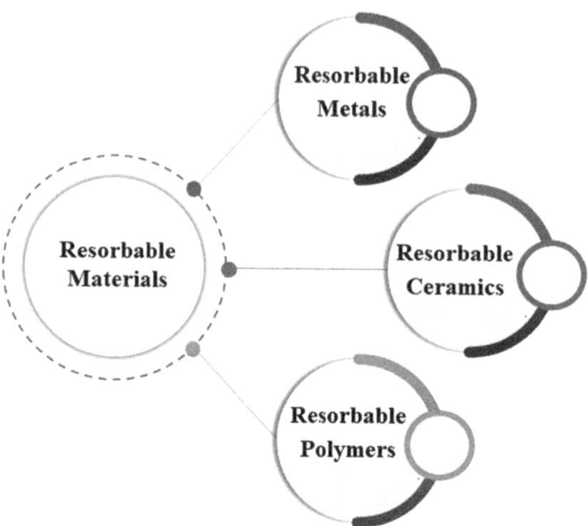

Figure 13.2 Classification of resorbable materials.

and biocompatibility across diverse clinical scenarios. Their transient nature, marked by gradual dissolution and metabolic clearance, facilitates seamless integration with native tissues, reducing inflammatory responses and promoting optimal healing outcomes. Additionally, the inherent adaptability and tunability of resorbable materials empower clinicians and researchers to tailor material properties, degradation kinetics, and functional attributes to align with specific therapeutic goals and patient requirements [8]. As a harbinger of innovation in biomedical engineering, bioabsorbable materials epitomize the convergence of advanced materials science, clinical creativity, and patient-centered care, signaling a paradigm shift towards transient yet impactful biomedical solutions.

13.2.1 Resorbable Metals

Resorbable metals signify a revolutionary breakthrough in the field of biomaterials, surpassing conventional paradigms of implant design and therapeutic approaches [9]. These metals, known for their inherent ability to degrade and assimilate within the body, mark the onset of a transformative era in applications related to orthopedics, cardiovascular interventions, and dentistry. This in-depth examination clarifies the complexities, progressions, and consequences associated with bioabsorbable metals, emphasizing their crucial influence in shaping the trajectory of biomedical engineering in the future.

The distinctive feature of resorbable metals lies in their capability to experience controlled degradation, eliminating the requirement for subsequent removal surgeries and minimizing enduring complications linked

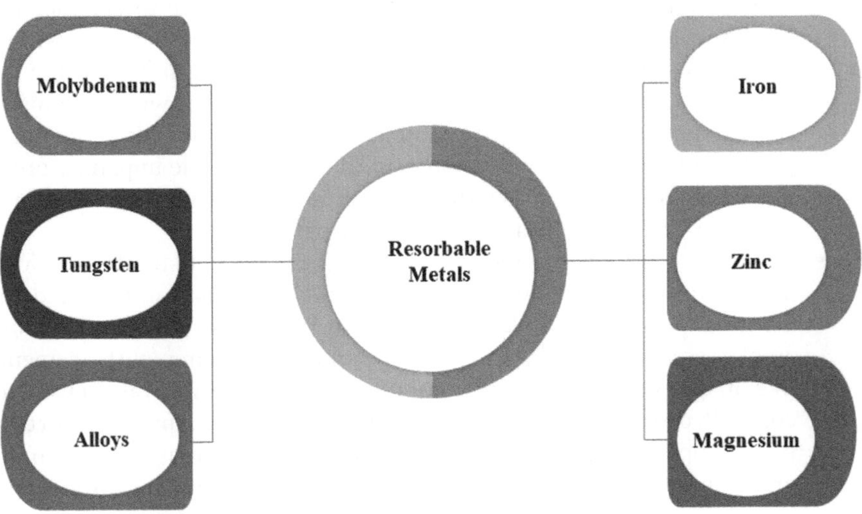

Figure 13.3 Resorbable metals.

to permanent implants. Mainly composed of alloys based on magnesium, these resorbable metals showcase mechanical properties similar to those of natural bone. This similarity enables optimal load-bearing capacities and the distribution of physiological stress. The controlled degradation kinetics, influenced by alloy composition, microstructural features, and environmental factors, guarantee gradual assimilation and metabolic clearance, aligning with the inherent healing and remodeling processes of the human body [10].

- **Iron:** Iron-based resorbable metals are a class of materials that have gained significant attention in the field of biomedical engineering, particularly in the development of implantable devices [11]. These metals are designed to degrade over time within the human body, eliminating the need for a second surgery to remove the implant. One of the key advantages of iron-based resorbable metals is their biocompatibility. Iron is an essential element in the human body and is involved in various physiological processes. As a result, implants made from iron-based resorbable metals tend to have minimal adverse effects on the surrounding tissues. The degradation process of these metals is carefully controlled to match the healing time of the specific tissue or bone in which the implant is placed. This controlled degradation is typically achieved through alloying iron with other elements, such as manganese or zinc, which helps in modulating the corrosion rate. Iron-based resorbable metals find applications in orthopedic implants, such as screws, plates, and scaffolds for bone repair. As the metal gradually degrades, it is replaced by the natural bone tissue, promoting the regeneration of the damaged area. Various studies have been taken place to enhance the mechanical properties and degradation kinetics of these materials. The goal is to strike a balance between the initial strength needed for the implant to fulfill its function and the gradual breakdown of the material as the body heals. The iron-based resorbable metals represent a promising avenue in the development of biodegradable implants, offering a solution that reduces the need for additional surgeries and provides a more natural healing process for patients.

- **Zinc:** Zinc resorbable metals are designed for implantable devices, gradually breaking down within the body, eliminating the need for secondary surgeries [12]. Their inherent biocompatibility stems from zinc's essential role in human physiology. Alloying with elements like magnesium or calcium modulates the corrosion rate, ensuring controlled degradation aligns with tissue healing. Applied in orthopedic implants, such as screws and plates, these materials promote gradual integration with natural tissues, aiding the regeneration process. Ongoing research focuses on refining mechanical properties and degradation kinetics, emphasizing the delicate balance between initial strength for functionality and controlled breakdown to support natural healing.

- **Molybdenum:** Resorbable molybdenum materials, integral in biomaterials research, are tailored for implantable devices, gradually decomposing within the body to obviate additional surgeries [13]. Biocompatibility is inherent to molybdenum's properties, ensuring minimal adverse reactions. Alloying with elements like zinc or magnesium regulates the corrosion rate, aligning with tissue healing. Predominantly used in orthopedic implants like screws and plates, these materials facilitate natural tissue integration, promoting effective regeneration. Ongoing research concentrates on refining mechanical properties and degradation kinetics, striking a balance between initial strength and controlled breakdown. This discreet process ensures seamless integration, underscoring molybdenum's potential as a resorbable biomaterial.

- **Tungsten:** Tungsten resorbable materials, a significant focus in biomaterials, are engineered for implantable devices, gradually degrading within the body, eliminating the need for subsequent surgeries [14]. Their biocompatibility is derived from tungsten's unique properties, and careful alloying with elements like titanium ensures a controlled corrosion rate, aligning with tissue healing timelines. Commonly used in orthopedic applications, such as screws and pins, these materials facilitate natural tissue integration, supporting effective regeneration. Ongoing research aims to enhance mechanical properties and degradation kinetics, emphasizing a delicate balance between initial strength and controlled breakdown. This discreet process remains undetectable, ensuring seamless integration within the human body.

- **Magnesium:** Magnesium and its alloys are notable examples of resorbable metals widely used in biomedical applications [15]. These materials possess the unique capability to undergo controlled degradation within the physiological environment, eliminating the need for subsequent removal surgeries. Specifically, magnesium-based alloys, including but not limited to Mg-Zn, Mg-Ca, and Mg-Sr, are actively explored for their resorbable properties. Pure magnesium (Mg): Renowned for its ability to undergo controlled degradation, pure magnesium is utilized in a variety of medical implants. Magnesium–zinc (Mg-Zn) alloys: Combinations of magnesium and zinc in alloy form are under scrutiny for their capacity to degrade in a controlled manner within the human body. Magnesium–calcium (Mg-Ca) alloys: Alloys that meld magnesium and calcium are being examined for their resorbable characteristics, with a particular focus on applications in orthopedics. Magnesium–strontium (Mg-Sr) alloys: Alloys incorporating both magnesium and strontium are the subject of investigation due to their resorbable properties and potential advantages, particularly in the field of orthopedics.

13.2.1.1 Degradation Mechanisms

The degradation mechanism of resorbable metals involves a controlled process where the material gradually breaks down within the physiological environment [16]. Specifically, for magnesium-based alloys, which are commonly used as resorbable metals, the degradation mechanism unfolds through a series of steps:

13.2.1.1.1 Initial Corrosion

Upon implantation, the resorbable metal, such as a magnesium alloy, initiates contact with bodily fluids. The metal surface undergoes corrosion, leading to the formation of metal ions.

13.2.1.1.2 Ion Release

Corrosion results in the release of magnesium ions and other alloying elements into the surrounding tissue. The controlled release of ions is a critical aspect of the resorption process.

13.2.1.1.3 Phagocytosis and Cellular Response

Cells in the vicinity, particularly macrophages, phagocytize the degraded material and react to the released ions. This interaction triggers cellular responses involved in the natural healing and tissue remodeling processes.

13.2.1.1.4 Gradual Absorption

The resorbable metal continues to degrade gradually, allowing for the absorption of degradation by-products by surrounding cells and tissues.

13.2.1.1.5 Metabolic Clearance

Ultimately, the by-products are metabolically cleared from the body, completing the degradation process. This clearance aligns with the body's natural ability to process and eliminate substances.

The alloy composition, microstructure, and environmental factors play crucial roles in modulating the kinetics of the degradation process, ensuring that it aligns with the desired therapeutic outcomes and avoids undesirable side effects. This controlled degradation mechanism is a key feature of resorbable metals, as it provides temporary support or intervention while minimizing long-term complications associated with permanent implants.

13.2.1.2 Clinical Applications

Resorbable metals find extensive application across various clinical settings, including orthopedic fixation, cardiovascular interventions, and craniofacial implants. Particularly in orthopedics, the use of resorbable magnesium-based implants like screws, plates, and intramedullary nails has gained considerable recognition [17]. These implants play a crucial role in stabilizing fractures, promoting bone healing, and subsequently degrading within the body, eliminating the need for additional retrieval surgeries. The temporary nature of these implants reduces the risks associated with permanent metallic residues, lessening the chances of inflammatory responses, infections, and biomechanical mismatches [18]. Consequently, this contributes to optimal healing outcomes and the restoration of functional capabilities.

13.2.1.3 Advancements and Challenges

While resorbable metals hold significant transformative promise, their practical application in clinical settings requires careful attention to material characteristics, degradation kinetics, and reactions within host tissues [19]. The inherent biocompatibility, mechanical strength, and degradation patterns of these metals are intricately influenced by factors such as alloy composition, changes in microstructure, and environmental conditions. As a result, continuous research efforts focus on enhancing alloy formulations, improving processing methods, and understanding the complex interaction between material properties and biological responses.

Overcoming challenges related to corrosion control, mechanical stability, and inflammatory reactions requires creative approaches, such as surface alterations, adjustments to alloy compositions, and the incorporation of bioactive coatings or polymers [20]. Additionally, the effective implementation of resorbable metals in clinical applications requires thorough preclinical assessments, extended follow-up studies, and continuous refinements. These measures are essential to guarantee safety, efficacy, and optimal performance in various clinical situations during the translational process.

13.2.1.4 Future Perspectives

The growing field of resorbable metals anticipates a future abundant with possibilities for innovation, cooperation, and groundbreaking progress in biomedical engineering. Current research initiatives, which include activities in alloy design, degradation kinetics, and interactions with host tissues, aim to clarify fundamental mechanisms, enhance material performance, and facilitate clinical application [21]. The intersection of materials science, bioengineering, and clinical medicine promotes collaborative efforts across disciplines, nurturing a dynamic environment for innovation, the sharing of knowledge, and the emergence of transformative developments.

The resorbable metals represent the intersection of scientific innovation, clinical needs, and patient-centered care within the field of biomedical engineering [22]. Their transformative potential, diverse applications, and continual advancements emphasize the crucial role of resorbable metals in influencing the future of orthopedic treatments, cardiovascular therapies, and craniofacial reconstructions. As the range of possibilities widens, the steadfast commitment to excellence, innovation, and transformative solutions propels the field of resorbable metals to unprecedented levels. This contributes to the development of enhanced therapeutic approaches, improved patient outcomes, and lasting contributions to global advancements in healthcare.

13.2.2 Resorbable Ceramics

Resorbable ceramics, an emerging category of biomaterials, have transformed the field of regenerative medicine, orthopedic procedures, and dental reconstructions [23]. These ceramics, known for their compatibility with the body, bioactivity, and ability to support bone growth, represent the intersection of advanced materials science and biomedical engineering. This detailed discussion explores the complexities, progressions, and significance of resorbable ceramics, emphasizing their critical contribution to shaping the future of biomedical applications.

Resorbable ceramics, primarily consisting of calcium phosphates, showcase seamless integration with the body's natural environment, promoting optimal tissue regeneration, bone formation, and remodeling [24].

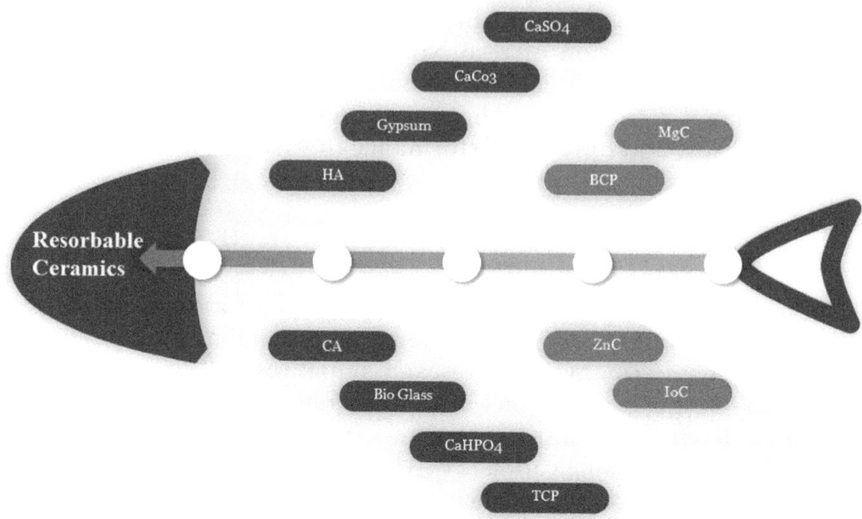

Figure 13.4 Resorbable ceramics.

Hydroxyapatite (HA), a key mineral in bones, stands out as a quintessential resorbable ceramic due to its structural similarity to native bone and inherent bioactivity. Furthermore, tricalcium phosphate (TCP) and biphasic calcium phosphates (BCP), combining hydroxyapatite and β-tricalcium phosphate phases, demonstrate improved solubility, osteoconductivity and controlled degradation profiles. This versatility caters to a variety of clinical needs and therapeutic goals.

- **Hydroxyapatite (HA):** A principal mineral in bone, HA is a resorbable ceramic known for its structural resemblance to native bone and inherent bioactivity.
- **Gypsum:** Gypsum, a notable biomaterial, is employed in medical applications for its gradual dissolution within the body, eliminating the need for implant removal surgeries. Its biocompatibility and controlled breakdown make it a promising candidate for temporary medical devices.
- **Calcium Carbonate:** Calcium carbonate ($CacO_3$) serves as a promising biomaterial, gradually dissolving in the body and offering potential applications in temporary medical devices.
- **Calcium Sulfate:** Calcium sulfate (CaSO4) possessing osteoinductive and osteoconductive characteristics, can be adjusted to achieve a controllable degradation speed using sintering methods. This feature enhances its potential as a viable choice for addressing bone defects in the context of repair.

- **Carbonate apatite:** Carbonate apatite (CA) specifically carbonated hydroxyapatite (CHAp), demonstrates heightened resorption compared to pure hydroxyapatite (HAp) because of its increased solubility, a critical factor contributing to its resorbable nature.
- **Bioactive Glass:** An innovative and exceptionally bioactive glass composition with resorbable properties has been created, exhibiting promise for use in tissue engineering. The structure and solubility of this bio glass are impacted by elements like surface topography and matrix structure. Additionally, there is a proposal for the development of a resorbable UV-transparent phosphate glass optical fiber, as evidenced by in-vitro tests revealing dissolution kinetics spanning approximately a month. Notably, high-strength bioresorbable glass fibers have demonstrated continuous resorption and the formation of a calcium phosphate layer in in-vitro degradation assessments.
- **Dicalcium Phosphate Dihydrate:** Dicalcium Phosphate Dihydrate (CaHPO4) is a flexible substance with possible uses in biomineralization and biomedicine. Its potential extends to the creation of controlled-release matrix-type tablets for highly water-soluble drugs, presenting itself as a more straightforward and cost-effective option.
- **Tricalcium Phosphate (TCP):** TCP is a resorbable ceramic that exhibits enhanced solubility, osteoconductivity, and is often used in conjunction with HA for various clinical applications.
- **Biphasic Calcium Phosphates (BCP):** BCP is a composite resorbable ceramic that combines both hydroxyapatite and β-tricalcium phosphate phases. It offers improved versatility with enhanced solubility and osteoconductivity.
- **Magnesium-based Ceramics:** Resorbable ceramics based on magnesium exhibit potential for applications in orthopedic and dental implants. This is attributed to their enhanced mechanical characteristics and decreased sintering temperature.
- **Iron Oxide Ceramics:** Iron oxide-based resorbable ceramics is good for their biocompatibility and controlled degradation, present potential advancements in the development of biodegradable implants for medical applications.
- **Zinc-based Ceramics:** Zinc-based resorbable ceramics, such as zinc-tin-oxide and zinc orthostannate, have been thoroughly examined for their characteristics and potential uses, necessitating additional investigation to understand their viability in the biomedical field, particularly for the creation of resorbable bone implants.

13.2.2.1 Degradation Mechanisms

The inherent degradation processes of resorbable ceramics are regulated by the release of ions, surface dissolution, and subsequent interactions with cells [25]. In this process, the ceramic matrix undergoes gradual resorption, leading to new bone formation and physiological remodeling. Following implantation, resorbable ceramics set off a series of biomineralization events. During these events, calcium and phosphate ions are released, promoting the development of a biologically active hydroxyapatite layer. This bioactive interface supports cellular adhesion, proliferation, and differentiation, facilitating a smooth integration with the host tissue and promoting optimal osseointegration.

The degradation mechanism of resorbable ceramics involves several key steps that contribute to their gradual breakdown within the physiological environment:

13.2.2.1.1 Ion Release

Resorbable ceramics release ions, particularly calcium and phosphate, as part of their degradation process.

13.2.2.1.2 SURFACE DISSOLUTION

The ceramic matrix experiences surface dissolution, where the material gradually breaks down at the surface level.

13.2.2.1.3 CELLULAR INTERACTIONS

Following surface dissolution, cellular interactions come into play. The released ions contribute to the formation of a biologically active hydroxyapatite layer.

13.2.2.1.4 BIOMINERALIZATION

A cascade of biomineralization events occurs, facilitated by the released ions. This leads to the creation of a layer of biologically active hydroxyapatite on the ceramic surface.

13.2.2.1.5 NEW BONE FORMATION

The presence of the biologically active hydroxyapatite layer fosters cellular adhesion, proliferation, and differentiation. This, in turn, contributes to new bone formation.

13.2.2.1.6 PHYSIOLOGICAL REMODELING

The gradual resorption of the ceramic matrix, accompanied by new bone formation, is part of the physiological remodeling process. This degradation mechanism ensures that resorbable ceramics integrate seamlessly with the host tissue, fostering optimal osseointegration and supporting the overall goal of facilitating tissue regeneration.

13.2.2.2 Clinical Applications

The applications of resorbable ceramics in clinical settings are diverse, covering orthopedic implants, bone graft substitutes, dental reconstructions, and systems for controlled drug release. In orthopedic contexts, resorbable ceramic-based scaffolds and bone graft substitutes, enriched with bioactive signals and growth factors, stimulate improved osteogenesis, angiogenesis, and tissue regeneration [26]. This, in turn, supports processes like fracture healing, bone augmentation, and functional restoration. In dental practices, resorbable ceramics, including hydroxyapatite coatings and biphasic calcium phosphate composites, contribute to periodontal regeneration, preservation of alveolar bone, and enhanced stability of implants. The overall result is enhanced clinical outcomes and increased satisfaction among patients.

13.2.2.3 Advancements and Challenges

While resorbable ceramics hold significant transformative potential, their practical application in clinical settings requires careful optimization, thorough validation, and continuous refinements to guarantee safety, effectiveness, and performance across a variety of applications [27]. Addressing challenges related to mechanical strength, degradation rates, and interactions with host tissues necessitates the development of innovative strategies. These may include modifications to the ceramics, formulation of composite materials, and integration with bioactive agents or nanoparticles. The intersection of materials science, ceramic engineering, and biomedical research stimulates collaborative efforts across disciplines, creating a dynamic environment that fosters innovation, the exchange of knowledge, and the emergence of groundbreaking developments.

13.2.2.4 Future Perspectives

The evolving field of resorbable ceramics anticipates a future rich with prospects for innovation, collaboration, and transformative advancements in biomedical engineering. Continuing research efforts, including the design of ceramics, understanding degradation kinetics, and interactions with host tissues, aim to clarify fundamental mechanisms, enhance material performance, and facilitate practical application in clinical settings [28]. The intersection of materials science, bioengineering, and clinical medicine propels the domain of resorbable ceramics to unprecedented levels, fostering improved therapeutic methods, enhanced patient outcomes, and lasting contributions to advancements in global healthcare.

Resorbable ceramics symbolize the convergence of scientific innovation, clinical necessities, and patient-focused care within the field of biomedical engineering [29]. The transformative possibilities, diverse applications, and continuous advancements emphasize the crucial role of resorbable ceramics in influencing the future of regenerative medicine, orthopedic procedures, and dental reconstructions. As the range of possibilities broadens, the unwavering commitment to excellence, innovation, and transformative solutions propels the field of resorbable ceramics to unprecedented levels, facilitating improved therapeutic approaches, enhanced patient outcomes, and lasting contributions to advancements in global healthcare.

13.2.3 Resorbable Polymers

Resorbable polymers have become a fundamental element in biomaterials, embodying the concept of temporary yet influential solutions across a range of biomedical applications [30]. These polymers, known for their inherent biocompatibility, customizable degradation patterns, and adaptable functionalities, have driven significant progress in areas such as drug delivery systems, scaffolds for tissue engineering, and implantable devices. This thorough examination delves into the complexities, progressions, and consequences associated with resorbable polymers, highlighting their crucial role in transforming the field of biomedical engineering.

Resorbable polymers, spanning a diverse range of both synthetic and natural compositions, are intricately crafted to display customized degradation kinetics [31]. This ensures optimal therapeutic release, seamless tissue integration, and eventual assimilation within the body's natural environment. In the contemporary context, synthetic polymers like polylactic acid (PLA) [32], poly(lactic-co-glycolic acid) (PLGA) [33], and poly(caprolactone) (PCL) [34] predominate due to their consistent properties, modifiable degradation profiles, and adaptability in processing and fabrication. In contrast, natural polymers such as collagen, gelatin, and chitosan draw on inherent biological motifs and extracellular matrix components, promoting improved cell interactions, tissue regeneration, and physiological remodeling.

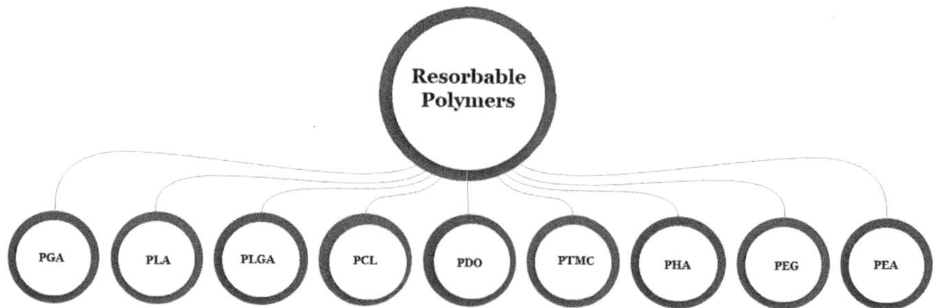

Figure 13.5 Resorbable polymers.

- **Polyglycolic Acid (PGA):** PGA is a biodegradable polymer that has attracted interest for its potential applications in diverse fields, such as drug delivery and tissue engineering. Its environmentally friendly nature and further adds to its appeal as a sustainable option.
- **Polylactic Acid (PLA):** PLA is a synthetic polymer derived from renewable sources like cornstarch. It is widely employed in drug delivery systems, sutures, and tissue engineering due to its biocompatibility.
- **Poly(lactic-co-glycolic Acid) (PLGA):** PLGA, a copolymer of lactic acid and glycolic acid, is known for its tunable degradation rates. It finds applications in drug delivery, tissue engineering, and surgical sutures.
- **Poly(caprolactone) (PCL):** PCL, a synthetic polyester, degrades more slowly than PLA or PLGA. It is used in controlled drug release, wound healing, and tissue engineering applications.
- **Polydioxanone (PDO):** PDO, a synthetic and biocompatible polymer, is commonly utilized in surgical sutures. It degrades through hydrolysis and is valued for its high tensile strength.
- **Poly (trimethylene carbonate) (PTMC):** PTMC is a flexible and degradable polymer with possible uses in soft tissue regeneration and drug delivery. Variants of PTMC, derived from 2,2-bis(methylol)propionic acid, can undergo additional functionalization through organocatalytic transesterification.
- **Polyhydroxyalkanoates (PHA):** Polyhydroxyalkanoates (PHAs) constitute a category of biodegradable polymers with varied uses in fields such as medicine, agriculture, and packaging. PHAs, exemplified by polymers like 3-hydroxybutyrate-co-3-hydroxyvalerate, are sourced from renewable materials and hold promise as resorbable polymers.
- **Polyethylene Glycol (PEG):** Polyethylene glycol stands out as a resorbable polymer known for its strong biocompatibility, offering promising prospects in the realms of gene and drug delivery applications.
- **Polyesteramides (PEA):** Resorbable polymers known as polyesteramides have been created with a substantial quantity of end groups and multifunctionality, rendering them well-suited for a variety of applications. Specifically, those derived from diacid monomers exhibit diverse properties, including biodegradability, expanding their potential applicability.
- **Polysaccharides:** Natural polysaccharides like chitosan, alginate, and hyaluronic acid are employed as resorbable polymers known for their biocompatibility. They play roles in drug delivery and tissue engineering.
- **Protein-based Polymers:** Proteins such as collagen and gelatin are utilized as resorbable polymers due to their biocompatibility and similarity to natural extracellular matrix components. Applications include tissue engineering and drug delivery.

13.2.3.1 Degradation Mechanisms

The inherent degradation mechanisms of resorbable polymers are dictated by processes involving hydrolysis and enzymes where polymer chains experience scission, resulting in a gradual breakdown and eventual removal from the host tissue [35]. Polymers that degrade hydrolytically, like PLA and PLGA, undergo cleavage of ester bonds, enabling stepwise degradation and metabolic integration into harmless byproducts such as water and carbon dioxide. On the other hand, polymers responsive to enzymes, like gelatin and chitosan are susceptible to proteolytic cleavage induced by host enzymes. This prompts location-specific degradation, influencing tissue responses in a controlled manner. The degradation mechanism of resorbable polymers involves a gradual breakdown process within the physiological environment. The steps typically include:

13.2.3.1.1 Water Uptake

Resorbable polymers are designed to be hydrophilic, allowing them to absorb water from the surrounding environment.

13.2.3.1.2 Hydrolysis

The absorbed water initiates hydrolysis, a chemical reaction where the polymer chains are cleaved into smaller fragments through the breaking of chemical bonds.

13.2.3.1.3 Oxidation

The oxidative degradation of resorbable polymers involves a gradual breakdown induced by reactive oxygen species, impacting their structural integrity over time.

13.2.3.1.4 Enzymatic Degradation

Enzymatic degradation of resorbable polymers occurs through specific enzymatic activities, where enzymes break down the polymer chains into biocompatible byproducts, a crucial mechanism in tailoring the biodegradability of the polymers.

13.2.3.1.5 Polymer Chain Cleavage

Hydrolysis leads to the cleavage of polymer chains, forming smaller fragments and soluble by-products.

13.2.3.1.6 Water-Soluble By-Products

The by-products generated during hydrolysis are water-soluble, allowing for their gradual clearance from the body through natural metabolic processes.

13.2.3.1.7 Assimilation and Elimination

The smaller polymer fragments are assimilated and metabolized by the body or eliminated through excretion pathways. This controlled degradation mechanism ensures that the resorbable polymers gradually disintegrate, aligning with the body's natural processes and avoiding long-term accumulation of foreign materials. The specifics of the degradation process can vary depending on the type of resorbable polymer and its intended applications.

13.2.3.2 Clinical Applications

The applications of resorbable polymers in clinical settings are diverse, covering a range of uses such as drug-eluting stents, biodegradable sutures, scaffolds for tissue engineering, and systems for controlled drug release. In cardiovascular procedures, stents made from resorbable polymers, coated with substances that inhibit cell growth, contribute to optimal blood vessel openness, prevent excessive tissue thickening, and subsequently break down [36]. This eliminates the long-term risks associated with permanent metallic residues. In orthopedic and craniofacial reconstructions, resorbable polymer scaffolds, containing bioactive signals and growth factors, support the formation of bone and cartilage, promoting tissue regeneration. Consequently, this aids in functional restoration and leads to improved patient outcomes.

13.2.3.3 Advancements and Challenges

While resorbable polymers hold significant transformative promise, their transition to clinical use demands careful optimization, thorough validation, and continuous refinements to guarantee safety, effectiveness, and performance across varied applications [37]. Challenges related to mechanical strength, degradation rates, and interactions with host tissues require innovative solutions, including modifications to the polymer, development of composite formulations, and integration with bioactive agents or nanoparticles. The intersection of materials science, polymer chemistry, and biomedical engineering stimulates collaborations across disciplines, creating a dynamic environment for innovation, the sharing of knowledge, and the emergence of groundbreaking developments.

13.2.3.4 Future Perspectives

The evolving field of resorbable polymers anticipates a future rich with prospects for innovation, collaboration, and transformative progress in biomedical engineering [38]. Continuing research initiatives, including the design of polymers, understanding degradation kinetics, and interactions with host tissues, aim to clarify fundamental mechanisms, enhance material performance, and facilitate practical application in clinical settings. The intersection of materials science, bioengineering, and clinical medicine propels the domain of resorbable polymers to unprecedented levels, facilitating improved therapeutic methods, enhanced patient outcomes, and lasting contributions to advancements in global healthcare.

The resorbable polymers symbolize the fusion of scientific innovation, clinical necessities, and patient-centered care within the domain of biomedical engineering. The transformative possibilities, diverse applications, and continuous advancements emphasize the crucial role of resorbable polymers in influencing the future of drug delivery systems, strategies for tissue engineering, and the development of implantable devices [39]. As the range of possibilities broadens, the unwavering commitment to excellence, innovation, and transformative solutions drives the field of resorbable polymers to unprecedented levels, facilitating improved therapeutic approaches, enhanced patient outcomes, and lasting contributions to advancements in global healthcare.

13.3 CONCLUSION

In conclusion, the advancements in resorbable materials represent a substantial leap forward in the realm of biomedical applications, leading to significant enhancements in patient care and treatment approaches. This chapter looked into the complicated world of studying how these materials break down, giving us a better understanding of how they work in biomedical engineering. Resorbable materials are crucial in today's medicine because they can break down on their own inside the body. Since they don't last forever, there's no need for extra surgeries to take them out. This makes them useful for things like temporary support, delivering medicine, and helping tissues grow back. In the end, these materials are a versatile solution that improves how we care for patients and treat diseases. So, it's important to really understand how these materials break down in the body. This means looking at things like what they're made of how fast they break down, how well they get along with our bodies, and how our tissues react to them. To do this, scientists use advanced techniques to closely study the materials, checking out their physical and chemical properties, molecular structures, and how they change shape during the breakdown process. These observations are important because they help to figure out how different things, like what the material is made of or how strong it is affect how it breaks down.

REFERENCES

1. Altayyar, Saleh S. "The essential principles of safety and effectiveness for medical devices and the role of standards." *Medical Devices: Evidence and Research* 13 (2020): 49–55.
2. Al-Shalawi, Faisal Dakhelallah, Azmah Hanim Mohamed Ariff, Dong-Won Jung, Mohd Khairol Anuar Mohd Ariffin, Collin Looi Seng Kim, Dermot Brabazon, and Maha Obaid Al-Osaimi. "Biomaterials as Implants in the Orthopedic Field for Regenerative Medicine: Metal versus Synthetic Polymers." *Polymers* 15, 12 (2023): 2601.
3. Bandopadhyay, Shantanu, Nabamita Bandyopadhyay, Sarfaraz Ahmed, Vivek Yadav, and Rakesh K. Tekade. "Current research perspectives of orthopedic implant materials." *Biomaterials and Bionanotechnology* (2019): 337–374.
4. Vaiani, Lorenzo, Antonio Boccaccio, Antonio Emmanuele Uva, Gianfranco Palumbo, Antonio Piccininni, Pasquale Guglielmi, Stefania Cantore, Luigi Santacroce, Ioannis Alexandros Charitos, and Andrea Ballini. "Ceramic Materials for Biomedical Applications: An Overview on Properties and Fabrication Processes." *Journal of Functional Biomaterials* 14, 3 (2023): 146.
5. Grada, Ayman, and Kate Weinbrecht. "Next-generation sequencing: Methodology and application." *Journal of Investigative Dermatology* 133, 8 (2013): 1–4.
6. Zare, Mina, Erfan Rezvani Ghomi, Prabhuraj D. Venkatraman, and Seeram Ramakrishna. "Silicone-based biomaterials for biomedical applications: Antimicrobial strategies and 3D printing technologies." *Journal of applied polymer science* 138, 38 (2021): 50969.
7. Vach Agocsova, Sara, Martina Culenova, Ivana Birova, Leona Omanikova, Barbora Moncmanova, Lubos Danisovic, Stanislav Ziaran, Dusan Bakos, and Pavol Alexy. "Resorbable biomaterials used for 3D scaffolds in tissue engineering: A review." *Materials* 16, 12 (2023): 4267.
8. Ramezani, Maziar, and Zaidi Mohd Ripin. "4D printing in biomedical engineering: Advancements, challenges, and future directions." *Journal of functional biomaterials* 14, 7 (2023): 347.
9. Toong, Daniel Wee Yee, Jaryl Chen Koon Ng, Yingying Huang, Philip En Hou Wong, Hwa Liang Leo, Subbu S. Venkatraman, and Hui Ying Ang. "Bioresorbable metals in cardiovascular stents: Material insights and progress." *Materialia* 12 (2020): 100727.
10. Stephen, Meera, Ali Nawaz, Sang Yeon Lee, Prashant Sonar, and Wei Lin Leong. "Biodegradable materials for transient organic transistors." *Advanced Functional Materials* 33, 6 (2023): 2208521.
11. Zivic, Fatima, Nenad Grujovic, Eva Pellicer, Jordi Sort, Slobodan Mitrovic, Dragan Adamovic, and Maja Vulovic. "Biodegradable metals as biomaterials for clinical Practice: Iron-based materials." *Biomaterials in Clinical Practice: Advances in Clinical Research and Medical Devices* 1 (2018): 225–280.
12. Yang, Nan, Jeffrey Venezuela, Sharifah Almathami, and Matthew Dargusch. "Zinc-nutrient element based alloys for absorbable wound closure devices fabrication: Current status, challenges, and future prospects." *Biomaterials* 280 (2022): 121301.

13. Morsada, Zinnat, Md Milon Hossain, M. Tauhidul Islam, Md Ahsanul Mobin, and Shumit Saha. "Recent progress in biodegradable and bioresorbable materials: From passive implants to active electronics." *Applied Materials Today* 25 (2021): 101257.

14. Fernandes, Catarina, and Irene Taurino. "Biodegradable molybdenum (mo) and tungsten (w) devices: One step closer towards fully-transient biomedical implants." *Sensors* 22, 8 (2022): 3062.

15. Pogorielov, Maksym, Eugenia Husak, Alexandr Solodivnik, and Sergii Zhdanov. "Magnesium-based biodegradable alloys: Degradation, application, and alloying elements." *Interventional Medicine and Applied Science* 9, 1 (2017): 27–38.

16. Liu, Yang, Yufeng Zheng, Xie-Hui Chen, Jian-An Yang, Haobo Pan, Dafu Chen, Luning Wang et al. "Fundamental theory of biodegradable metals—definition, criteria, and design." *Advanced Functional Materials* 29, 18 (2019): 1805402.

17. Wang, Jia-Li, Jian-Kun Xu, Chelsea Hopkins, Dick Ho-Kiu Chow, and Ling Qin. "Biodegradable magnesium-based implants in orthopedics—a general review and perspectives." *Advanced science* 7, 8 (2020): 1902443.

18. Bandyopadhyay, Amit, Indranath Mitra, Stuart B. Goodman, Mukesh Kumar, and Susmita Bose. "Improving biocompatibility for next generation of metallic implants." *Progress in Materials Science* 133 (2023): 101053.

19. Khan, Ahsan Riaz, Navdeep Singh Grewal, Chao Zhou, Yuan Kunshan, Hai-Jun Zhang, and Zhang Jun. "Recent advances in biodegradable metals for implant applications: Exploring in vivo and in vitro responses." *Results in Engineering* 20 (2023): 101526.

20. Prasad, Karthika, Olha Bazaka, Ming Chua, Madison Rochford, Liam Fedrick, Jordan Spoor, Richard Symes et al. "Metallic biomaterials: Current challenges and opportunities." *Materials* 10, 8 (2017): 884.

21. Oliver, Alexander A., Malgorzata Sikora-Jasinska, Ali Gökhan Demir, and Roger J. Guillory II. "Recent advances and directions in the development of bioresorbable metallic cardiovascular stents: Insights from recent human and in vivo studies." *Acta Biomaterialia* 127 (2021): 1–23.

22. Hermawan, Hendra. "Updates on the research and development of absorbable metals for biomedical applications." *Progress in Biomaterials* 7 (2018): 93–110.

23. Vaiani, Lorenzo, Antonio Boccaccio, Antonio Emmanuele Uva, Gianfranco Palumbo, Antonio Piccininni, Pasquale Guglielmi, Stefania Cantore, Luigi Santacroce, Ioannis Alexandros Charitos, and Andrea Ballini. "Ceramic Materials for Biomedical Applications: An Overview on Properties and Fabrication Processes." *Journal of Functional Biomaterials* 14, 3 (2023): 146.

24. Barrère, Florence, Clemens A. van Blitterswijk, and Klaas de Groot. "Bone regeneration: Molecular and cellular interactions with calcium phosphate ceramics." *International journal of nanomedicine* 1, 3 (2006): 317.

25. Langstaff, S., M. Sayer, T. J. N. Smith, and S. M. Pugh. "Resorbable bioceramics based on stabilized calcium phosphates. Part II: Evaluation of biological response." *Biomaterials* 22, 2 (2001): 135–150.

26. Campana, Vincenzo, G. I. U. S. E. P. P. E. Milano, E. Pagano, Marta Barba, Claudia Cicione, Giampiero Salonna, Wanda Lattanzi, and Giandomenico Logroscino. "Bone substitutes in orthopaedic surgery: From basic science to clinical practice." *Journal of Materials Science: Materials in Medicine* 25 (2014): 2445–2461.

27. Vaiani, Lorenzo, Antonio Boccaccio, Antonio Emmanuele Uva, Gianfranco Palumbo, Antonio Piccininni, Pasquale Guglielmi, Stefania Cantore, Luigi Santacroce, Ioannis Alexandros Charitos, and Andrea Ballini. "Ceramic materials for biomedical applications: An overview on properties and fabrication processes." *Journal of Functional Biomaterials* 14, 3 (2023): 146.

28. Amini, Ami R., Cato T. Laurencin, and Syam P. Nukavarapu. "Bone tissue engineering: Recent advances and challenges." *Critical Reviews™ in Biomedical Engineering* 40, 5 (2012).

29. Tartsch, Jens, and Markus B. Blatz. "Ceramic dental implants: An overview of materials, characteristics, and application concepts." *Compendium of Continuing Education in Dentistry (Jamesburg, NJ: 1995)* 43, 8 (2022): 482–488.

30. Vacaras, Sergiu, Mihaela Baciut, Ondine Lucaciu, Cristian Dinu, Grigore Baciut, Liana Crisan, Mihaela Hedesiu et al. "Understanding the basis of medical use of poly-lactide-based resorbable polymers and composites—a review of the clinical and metabolic impact." *Drug Metabolism Reviews* 51, 4 (2019): 570–588.

31. Pappalardo, Daniela, Torbjörn Mathisen, and Anna Finne-Wistrand. "Biocompatibility of resorbable polymers: A historical perspective and framework for the future." *Biomacromolecules* 20, 4 (2019): 1465–1477.

32. Stemberg, Frank, and Axel Wilke. "Evaluation of bioresorbable polymers of lactic acid in a culture of human bone marrow cells." *Journal of Biomaterials Science, Polymer Edition* 12, 2 (2001): 171–184.

33. Yao, Chang, Matt Hedrick, Gyan Pareek, Joseph Renzulli, George Haleblian, and Thomas J. Webster. "Nanostructured polyurethane-poly-lactic-co-glycolic acid scaffolds increase bladder tissue regeneration: An in vivo study." *International Journal of Nanomedicine* 8, 1 (2013): 3285–3296.

34. Al-Namnam, N. M., K. H. Kim, W. L. Chai, K. O. Ha, C. H. Siar, and W. C. Ngeow. "A biocompatibility study of injectable poly (caprolactone-trifumarate) for use as a bone substitute material." *Frontiers in Life Science* 8, 3 (2015): 215–222.

35. Pothupitiya, Jinal U., Christy Zheng, and W. Mark Saltzman. "Synthetic biodegradable polyesters for implantable controlled-release devices." *Expert Opinion on Drug Delivery* 19, 10 (2022): 1351–1364.

36. Rodriguez-Arias, Juan J., Luis Ortega-Paz, and Salvatore Brugaletta. "Durable polymer everolimus-eluting stents: History, current status and future prospects." *Expert Review of Medical Devices* 17, 7 (2020): 671–682.

37. Joseph, Jasmin, Ramesh Parameswaran, and Unnikrishnan Gopalakrishna Panicker. "Recent advancements in blended and reinforced polymeric systems as bioscaffolds." *International Journal of Polymeric Materials and Polymeric Biomaterials* 72, 11 (2023): 834–855.

38. Hoffmann, J., K. Friedrich, M. Evstatiev, and U. Finkc. "A totally bioresorbable fibrillar reinforced composite system: Structure and properties." *International Journal of Polymeric Materials* 50, 3–4 (2001): 469–482.

39. Ravi Kumar, Majeti N. V., and Neeraj Kumar. "Polymeric controlled drug-delivery systems: Perspective issues and opportunities." *Drug Development and Industrial Pharmacy* 27, 1 (2001): 1–30.

Chapter 14

Nanobiocomposites in Wound Healing

Divya Thakur, Deepika Kaushal, Rajender Kumar, Vinay Chauhan, and Manish Kumar

14.1 INTRODUCTION

Three layers make up skin: the stratum corneum (epidermis), which is mostly formed of keratinocytes; the dermis (connective tissue); and the hypodermis (subcutaneous layer), which is made of fat tissue and provides the body with mechanical and thermal protection (Suarato et al., 2018). Wounds are fractures or flaws in the skin that can result from thermal or physicochemical injury. Adults typically get scars from the wound healing process, which is a non-healing mass of fibrotic tissue (Gurtner et al., 2008). The risk of managing and caring of wounds are increased by anthropogenic and lifestyle variables. Chronic wounds and sepsis risk, which have a high death rate, continue to be key healthcare problems despite medical breakthrough. Biocomposites and biomaterials prepared from silk fibers, alginate, chitin, cellulose, collagen, hyaluronate and gelatin are rising popularly due to their biocompatibility, bioactive behavior, antibacterial, immunomodulatory, and angiogenic capabilities (Osmani et al., 2021).

In order to repair complete functional tissues by utilizing innovative bio composites or artificial scaffolds, an alternative and successful strategy known as skin tissue engineering has been developed (Macneil, 2008). In addition to acting as a temporary barrier against external infection, the scaffolds can also act as an inductive pattern that directs skin cell remodelling and resulting penetration and incorporation of host tissues (Zhong et al., 2010). A perfect tissue artificial scaffold must have sufficient physical and mechanical strength, but also have the proper surface microstructures and biochemistry to promote cell adhesion, proliferation and differentiation (Yildirimer et al., 2012). For facilitating skin wound healing several biocomposite scaffolds made of organic and inorganic components are used (Ninan et al., 2015). A variety of engineered nanocomposites (size ranging <500 nm) based on ceramic, polymeric and metallic nanomaterials are

DOI: 10.1201/9781003470311-14

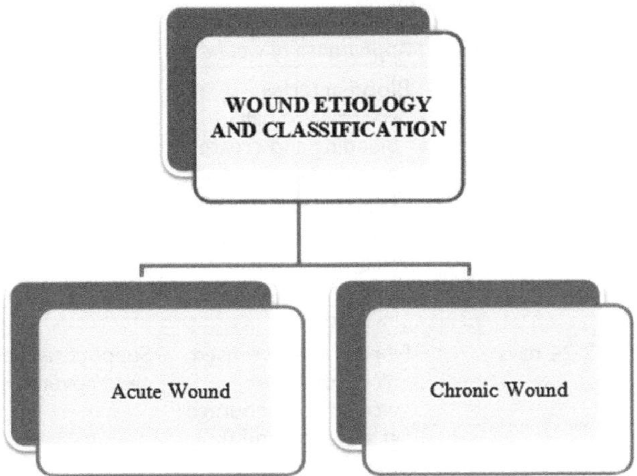

Figure 14.1 Wound etiology and classification.

utilized for infection prevention and both acute and chronic wound healing (Parani et al., 2016).

14.2 WOUND ETIOLOGY AND CLASSIFICATION

14.2.1 Acute Wound

A wound that emerges suddenly and heals through the phases as antici-pated. Acute wounds include things like small cuts, bites, lacerations, abra-sions, and surgical wounds.

14.2.2 Chronic Wound

A wound that takes longer than 4 to 6 weeks to heal or heals slowly. Chronic wounds include things like ischemic ulcers, venous ulcers, pressure ulcers, and non-healing or infected surgical or traumatic wounds.

14.3 PHASES OF WOUND HEALING

Different phases of wound healing including Haemostasis, Inflammation, Proliferation and Remodeling are described in Table 14.1.

Table 14.1 Physiology of wound healing

Stages	Time interval	Appearance of wound	Goal of wound management
Haemostasis	Within first few seconds	Blood arteries contract to halt bleeding and create blood clots	Stop bleeding
Inflammation	0-4 days	Together, neutrophils and macrophages clear away waste and protect against infection.	Remove toxins and avoid illness
Proliferation	2-24 days	Fibrous tissue is used to rebuild the wound to encourage granulation and fix the wound	Support tissue development and cover the wound
Remodeling	24 days-1 year	Epithelial tissue develops in wet healing environment.	Prevent growing epithelial tissue

14.4 MATERIALS AND METHODS FOR VARIOUS NANO-BASED BIOCOMPOSITES IN WOUND HEALING

14.4.1 Collagen–Nanosilver (Co-AgNP) Biocomposites

Due to unique physicochemical and biological characteristics, metal based silver nanoparticles (AgNP) have shown significant recognition from researchers in the field of wound healing. Since years, silver has been employed frequently for its medicinal properties (Konop et al., 2016). Silver nanoparticle-based topical creams were applied to the skin or mucous membranes allows it to enter the body have demonstrated efficacy as antibacterial to treat chronic infections throughout the healing process (Firdhouse & Lalitha, 2015). The use of silver nanoparticles with biopolymer-based biomaterials (AgNP-BM) for the treatment of wounds is safe and non-cytotoxic. AgNP biomaterials have good wound healing potential while limiting the development of microbes at the wound site. AgNP and biomaterials based on biopolymers can be used as dressing material for wound because of their high levels of biocompatibility and biodegradability in physiological environments (Subagio et al., 2020). The most contemporary technique for healing many skin infections caused by thermal or physical trauma has been treated by wound bandage, ensuring that the healing process goes without any difficulties (Ghasemzadeh et al., 2014).

14.4.1.1 Materials

Electrospinning setup and test materials were the primary resources used in this investigation. Materials for the electrospinning setup comprise a 30kV electric voltage source, a device collector, a 60 mL syringe pump, conductor, a spray system and a collector. Test material for electrospinning includes PVA, collagen, silver nitrate and distilled water. A spinneret is typically used in the electrospinning system together with syringe pumps, grounded collectors, as alternating current sources (Subagio et al., 2020).

14.4.1.2 Methods

PVA is regarded as a base substance that may be coupled with the primary substance. 2 g of PVA powder were used to make a 15 mL PVA solution, which was then homogenized for 3 hours with the aid of a magnetic stirrer at a temperature of 80°C. 1 g of collagen crystals was mixed for two hours with the help of a magnetic stirrer using 10 mL of deionized water to make collagen solution containing 0.5 M acetic acid. Then agitate PVA and collagen solutions for 3 hours. Similarly, polyvinyl alcohol solution is combined with nanosilver (dropwise addition) to create the solution of PVA-AgNP. The identical mixture of 2 g of PVA, 1 g of collagen and dropwise addition of nanosilver was added to create a PVA-collagen-AgNP solution over the course of 8 hours (Subagio et al., 2020).

Collagen is the easiest available protein, which accounts for one-third of the body's total protein by weight, which is essential for the extracellular matrix (Shoulders & Raines, 2009). Collagen dressings have a wide range of advantages in wound care, including boosting fibroblast synthesis, leukocytes, macrophages, epithelial cells, fibronectin bioavailability, and eventually preserve chemicals and a temperature controlled environment to speed up wound healing (Rangaraj et al., 2011). AgNP pads made of collagen are excellent options for enhancing wound repair processes because of their strong antibacterial activity. In addition to its antibacterial properties, AgNP plays a key role in the regulation of collagen deposition and enhanced fibril alignment throughout the wound healing process (Kwan et al., 2011).

The following requirements must be met by wound dressings: they must provide a moist environment around the wound, provide mechanical defence, promote the exchange of gases, allow removal without pain or damage, be harmless and beneficial in preventing bacterial growth, and hasten the wound healing process (Ge et al., 2014). Bacterial infection can still happen even when the wound is covered by a bandage because of the wet environment inside it, which provides microorganisms space to live and nutrients to grow (Devanesan et al., 2018). As a result, numerous antiseptics have been developed for use in wound dressing, including chitosan, curcumin, and silver nanoparticles (AgNP) (Rigo et al., 2013).

Because of its demonstrated high efficiency, utilising AgNP is the most convenient method among them. Small positively charged silver ions generated by AgNP are easily attracted by negatively charged surfaces of bacterial cell membranes, in contrast to other antibacterial agents. Once they enter, they capture the bacteria, stop the respiratory cycle, and kill the bacterium (Sulaiman et al., 2015). Therefore, AgNP possesses antibacterial effects against many infections.

14.4.2 Chitosan Nanofiber Biocomposites

Chitin, a naturally occurring polymer, is hydrolyzed to produce chitosan, a cationic natural polymer with a linear arrangement (Moeini et al., 2020). It is frequently used in scaffolds for the healing of wound and therapeutic medical purposes because of its biodegradability, biocompatibility, cell transplantation ability, as well as antibacterial and antifungal potentials (Nikbakht et al., 2019). Chitosan wound management products, such as ChitoSorb (ChitoTech), ChitoGauze Pro (HemCon), KytoCel (Aspen Medical), and Opticell (Medline), are employed to cure serious conditions of burnt skin, open wounds, and severe wounds due to its natural source and wound healing capacity (Bombaldi de Souza et al., 2020). Additionally, nanofibrous chitosan scaffolds are important in the healing of wounds because they have a good impact on the reproduction of the fragmentary layer (R. Ahmed et al., 2018). However, there are several drawbacks to its use as a wound dressing, such as limited mechanical strength and inadequate antimicrobial activities, which are insufficient for efficient wound dressing (Al-Musawi et al., 2020).

14.4.2.1 Materials

Materials for the synthesis of chitosan nanofiber includes chitosan (90% deacetylated), Acetic acid, deionized water, silver oxide(Ag_2O) and zinc oxide (ZnO) nanoparticles and PEO (900,000 g/mol).

14.4.2.2 Methods

14.4.2.2.1 Preparation of Chitosan/PEO Solution with Silver Nanoparticles

Chitosan and PEO solutions should be made separately in acetic acid to create the chitosan/PEO solution. In order to synthesize a chitosan solution (3 wt%), mix 0.3 g of chitosan with 80% acetic acid. The solution was mixed with a magnetic stirrer at 700 rpm for 16 hours at room temperature. Similarly, PEO solution (3wt%) was prepared. To create a homogeneous solution, 0.3 g of PEO was mixed with 0.5 M acetic acid and agitated (400 rpm) for 8 hours at room temperature; after separate preparation, PEO and chitosan solution were combined in a 9:1 weight ratio and agitated for 12 hours at room temperature at 400 rpm. The chitosan solution was then supplemented with the appropriate amounts of silver nanoparticles for each bacterium based on MIC. After that, the produced solution was poured into a syringe and placed in an electrospinning machine with the parameters of 20 kV electric voltage, a distance of needle from collector 14 cm, and collector rotation 700 rpm. The electrospinning process was carried out using the acquired parameters for 6 hours to produce nanofibrous mats embellished with silver nanoparticles and of the suitable thickness (Bagheri et al., 2022).

14.4.2.2.2 Preparation of Chitosan/PEO Solution with Zinc Oxide Nanoparticles

Using the same parameters as the electrospinning of the silver scaffold, zinc oxide polymeric solution was electrospun. The minimum inhibition concentration (MIC) of each bacterium was used to determine the concentration of zinc nanoparticles, which was then subsequently incorporated to the chitosan solution in order to create the nanofibers containing these particles.

14.4.2.2.3 Preparation of Chitosan/PEO Solution with Silver and Zinc Oxide Nanoparticles

Chitosan solution was mixed with different concentrations of silver and zinc nanoparticles based on the results of minimum inhibition concentration (MIC) for each bacteria to produce the nanofibrous mats. The stiffness of the nanofibrous mats is increased by cross-linking them with a 1% sodium tripolyphosphate (TPP) solution (Bagheri et al., 2022).

Growing interest has recently been seen in studies on nanofibrous scaffolds for tissue regeneration obtained from electrospinning polymers that are synthetic or natural alone or in combination with extracts from living plants and metallic nanomaterials (Abdul et al., 2016). Electrospinning is quite challenging due to the positively charged solution, intermolecular interactions and stiff chemical structure of chitosan (Desai et al., 2008). The most simple and effective method to enhance the ability of chitosan to electrospin is by combining chitosan with a polymer that has a high electrospinning potential for example; polyethylene oxide (Laschke et al., 2016).

14.4.3 Poly(vinyl alcohol)/Chitosan/Modified Graphene Oxide Biocomposite

Chitosan is typically employed in combination with other substances rather than in its pure form due to its limited mobility and low solubility in standard solvents as well as poor stability in biological environment (Berger et al., 2004). A synthetic water-soluble polymer called Poly(vinyl alcohol, or PVA) is ideally suited for application as a biomaterial due to its remarkable biocompatibility, nontoxicity, and lack of carcinogenicity (Kamoun et al., 2017). Polymer mixtures can improve the ductility and flexibility of other materials. An antibacterial sheet made of CS/oxidized pectin/PVA copolymer was created by Chetouani et al., and it showed potential as a wound dressing material due to its great swelling ratio and high mechanical characteristics (Chetouani et al., 2017). Gardenia is the source of genipin, a type of biological cross-linking agent. According to reports, genipin is a more effective cross linking agent for PVA/CS wound treatment than glutaraldehyde since the crosslinked PVA/CS hybrid hydrogels have superior mechanical properties and were 5,000–10,000 times less cytotoxic (Garnica-Palafox & Sánchez-Arévalo, 2016).

14.4.3.1 Materials

Materials used for the synthesis of PVA/CS/mGO are: graphene oxide (GO), Polyhexamethylene guanidine (PHMG), polyvinyl alcohol (PVA), Chitosan, which is 90% + deacetylated, Liquid paraffin (LP) and acetic acid (S. Chen et al., 2020).

14.4.3.2 Methods

An aqueous solution of PVA was created by dissolving it in dionized water and then treating it with an antifoaming agent LP with stirring at 90°C. To create a homogenous 1 wt% solution, CS was separately added to a 10 mg mL^{-1} acetic acid solution. One hour stirring was required for mixing the two polymer solutions at 80°C (50:50, v/v ratio). The mGO aqueous dispersions with mGO concentrations ranging from 0-4 mg mL^{-1} were made by sonicating it in distilled water. After that, the above-mentioned combined solution was vigorously agitated for 0.5 hours and then gradual addition of mGO was done. 5 mL of genipin solution was then dissolve in the above mixture, which was then heated to 60°C for 20 minutes before being reacted to produce a gel-like sample. To make the PVA/CS/mGO film, the mold was subsequently dried at 45°C in a vacuum oven. The film expands into a hydrogel when it takes up the saline or wound exudate. The PVA/CS/0.5 wt% PHMG was made by substituting a 0.5 wt% Polyhexamethylene guanidine (PHMG) solution for the mGO dispersion in the PVA/CS combination, which was then processed as usual (S. Chen et al., 2020).

A brand-new class of broad-spectrum antibacterial substances is emerging like Graphene materials. It's antibacterial modes of action involves physical annihilation, oxidative stress theory, mechanical wrapping, and nano knife effect, as well as lipid extraction (Karahan et al., 2018).

Graphene sheets are frequently utilised as supporting components in polymer matrices due to their excellent mechanical stiffness and vast surface area, in addition to their antibacterial characteristics (Qian et al., 2018). According to many previous studies, GO-based nanocomposites as dressing material may considerably speed up the healing of wounds by removing germs from the area (Applications, 2019). It is required to synthesise functionalized GO to strengthen their antibacterial effect since the changes in GO's chemical and physical features (such as shape, size, etc.), influence their antibacterial activity. There are currently several findings on increasing the antibacterial activity of GO by combining certain substances including bactericides, ZnO, and silver nanoparticles (AgNPs) (Liu et al., 2018). According to the combination of GO and CuO, PVA/CS/GO/CuO patches, for instance, enhanced wound-healing and antimicrobial activities (Venkataprasanna et al., 2020). Antibacterial activity significantly increased by nanofibrous membranes made of PVA/CS/GO composites that have been loaded with ciprofloxacin and ciprofloxacin hydrochloride (S. Chen et al., 2020).

Polyhexamethylene guanidine (PHMG) is a powerful antibacterial agent because guanidine inhibits the growth of bacteria by interacting electrostatically with their cationic and anionic groups on the surface. Dual-polymer made of polyethylene glycol (PEG) and PHMG and fluorinated graphene with guanidine modification exhibited strong antibacterial activity and a low grafting ratio (Park et al., 2020). The following factors may be used to explain the rationale behind the design of PVA/CS/mGO composite films:

1) PVA is a man-made, hydrophilic polymer that has excellent biocompatibility and increases the ductility and flexibility of CS.
2) CS is a naturally occurring biomaterial that promotes wound healing because it has antibacterial, antifungal, analgesic (painkiller), hemostatic, and mucoadhesive properties; and
3) GO possesses potent antibacterial activities that can be enhanced by PHMG grafting. Additionally, it could enhance the composite dressing's mechanical qualities.

14.4.4 Chitosan Nanobiocomposite Films Containing Gentamicin (GNT)

Chitosan has the beneficial potential to improve the tensile strength of wounded tissues and reduce swelling (Zeb et al., 2019). The fundamental features of colloidal particles that control the penetration of tissues and their medical advantages include EE%, particle size and zeta potential (Sharifi et al., 2019). It is suggested that increasing drug loading and decreasing particle size will boost the therapeutic benefits (Yokota & Kyotani, 2018).

14.4.4.1 Materials

Gentamicin can be prepared by using low molecular weight chitosan (CHI) with a deacetylation percentage of 75%, gentamicin (GNT), polysorbate, sodium tripolyphosphate (STPP), sodium hydroxide, and potassium dihydrogen phosphate (Asgarirad et al., 2021).

14.4.4.2 Methods

14.4.4.2.1 Ionic Gelation Method

Ionic gelation approach that relies on the electrochemical interaction among molecules with opposing charges was used to create CHI nanoparticles. Acetic acid solution of (1% v/v) was used to disseminate a low molecular weight CHI. The polymeric solution was stirred for 30 minutes at room temperature at 500 rpm. The polymer solution was then combined with 50 mg of GNT before dropwise addition of STPP aqueous solution. The electrostatic interaction between STPP and CHI causes colloidal particles to form as a result of the polymer thread bending. Centrifugation was used to clean the GNT-loaded nanoparticles (GNPs) to make sure the free medication was not adhered to their surface (Asgarirad et al., 2021).

THE ENCAPSULATION EFFICIENCY OF GNT LOADED NANOPARTICLES (GNPS)

The encapsulation efficiency percent (EE%) was calculated by using equation 1:

$$EE\% = (\text{Encapsulated GNT weight} / \text{Total GNT weight}) \times 100 \quad (1)$$

14.4.4.2 Casting Method

Using the casting technique as a basis, biocomposites were produced. A CHI solution was made by mixing a 1.2% w/w concentration of the polymer with a 1% v/v CH_3COOH solution for 60 minutes at constant stirring. The pH was adjusted to 5.5, then (0.5% w/w) glycerin was added as a plasticizer. To 2.5 mL polymer solution , 50 mg of GNT was supplemented along with 50 mg of GNPs which were dried in the freezer. The formulated ingredients were combined and then poured to a 35-mm-diameter petri plate. All formulations were dried on petri dishes during a 24-hour period at 40°C, after which they were kept in a controlled environment room at 25 °C and 50% RH (Asgarirad et al., 2021).

In hospitals and healthcare facilities, antimicrobial resistance is a major concern that is now affecting the entire world (Abebe et al., 2019). The solution to this problem is to increase the antibacterial potency of the active component using colloidal drug delivery techniques. By Ionic gelation method, the produced chitosan nanoparticles have demonstrated much more antibacterial activity than chitosan solutions (Qi et al., 2004). An aminoglycoside, i.e., gentamicin (GNT), has high effectiveness against inflammation brought on by gram-negative bacteria. Small ribosomal subunits are attacked by aminoglycosides, which bind to the 16s RNA and prevents the translation process in the production of proteins (Qi et al., 2004). Loading the GNT into the chitosan biocomposite can boost the drug's ability to enter the bacterial cytoplasm (Asgarirad et al., 2021).

14.4.5 Nano-ZnO Doped Calcium Phosphate– Chitosan–Alginate Biocomposites

Wound healing go through a number of interconnected and overlapping biochemical and cellular processes which involves the formation of the emerging collagen and fibroblastic cells, which causes the injured region to contract (Choi et al., 2017). Wounds change the concentration of several ions in cells, including calcium, zinc, and magnesium. A well-known function of CaP-NPs is as a controller of keratinocyte growth and differentiation in the homeostasis of mammalian skin (Kawai et al., 2011). When administered to the injured part, it reduces to Ca^{2+} ions. The precursor for the current keratinocyte and fibroblastic cells that are destroyed after damage is Ca^{2+} ion (Lansdown, 2002). Ca^{2+} ions released from the dressing material replace Na^+ ions from the wound fluid, which is crucial for the hemostasis phase of wound healing (Oliver & Blaine, n.d.). Materials made of calcium alginate are mostly used to treat wounds (O'Donoghue et al., 1997). In order to constrict injured regions and promote cell growth in a freshly constructed cellular structure with the same biophysical conditions, wound dressing biomaterials are utilized (Akturk et al., 2011). The best dressing biomaterials for wounds absorb exudates, function as a barrier for microorganisms and keep the necessary humidity in the injured area (Siritienthong et al., 2012). The interesting biological features of fibre polymers like chitosan (CS), are exploited in biomedical applications (Enescu & Olteanu, 2008). Wound healing materials synthesized by chitosan is very tempting because of its biological activities, non-toxicity, and antibacterial properties as well as its capacity to encourage hemostasis, absorb fluids, and accelerate tissue regeneration (Xiao et al., 2008). As an illustration, combining chitosan with sodium alginate (ALG) can improve the matrix's elasticity (Huang et al., n.d.). When divalent cations are present, such as Ca^{2+}, ALG may undergo cross-linking, resulting in biodegradable stable gels that are used as a substance for encapsulating cells and immobilisation. This fibrous polymer has the advantage of increasing flexibility and making it easier for nanoparticles to be released from the matrix. ZnO-NPs are utilised in biocomposites to offer antimicrobial action and limit the development of germs at the site of wounds because they are very stable and non-toxic (Guo et al., 2016). ZnO-NPs and CaP-NPs are embedded in a chitosan–alginate matrix when applied to a wound would have a low water permeability and an outstanding synergistic impact.

14.4.5.1 Materials

CS-ALG/CaP can be synthesized by using the materials: Shells of prawns which were processed in the lab to create the chitosan flake (CS). Sodium di-hydrogen phosphate (NaH_2PO_4), calcium L-lactate hydrate, acetic acid (CH_3COOH), NaOH, sodium tri-polyphosphate (TPP) ($Na_5P_3O_{10}$), ammonium hydroxide (NH_4OH), and zinc acetate dihydrate ($Zn(CH_3COO)_2.2H_2O$). All of the trials utilized double-distilled water (Rahman et al., 2020).

14.4.5.2 Methods

Take 500 mg of CS and mixed in 50 mL of CH_3COOH solution under constant stirring. In 50 mL of double-distilled water, 250 mg of ALG was mixed. ALG and CS were combined in a 1:2 weight ratio. To the CS ALG polymer mix solution, 100 mg ZnO nanoparticles and 500 mg CaP nanopartcles were mixed under constant stirring for 10 min at 200–300 rpm. To the above solution, 25 mL of an aqueous solution containing 4 mg mL^{-1} of TPP was mixed. The composite mix was precipitated out by adding a 1M 50 mL NaOH solution. The CS-ALG/CaP biocomposite mixture was repeatedly rinsed with deionized water to eliminate any leftover NaOH. At last freeze dryer was used to lyophilize the CS-ALG/CaP biocomposite at a temperature of –50°C and a vacuum of 20 Pa (Rahman et al., 2020).

To evaluate the ability to promote wound healing, CS-ALG/CaP biocomposite was put on the backs of male mice with deep wounds. As shown in Figure 14.2(a) there was no noticeable difference in the wound appearance in either case on the day 0 (the day surgery started). CS-ALG/CaP biocomposite heals wound more quickly than those treated with standard surgical gauge bandages, demonstrating the efficacy of the improved dressing. The wound healing ratios in the groups treated with biocomposites reached around 60% on day 5, compared to 5% in the control group (Figure 14.2 (b)). In contrast to the minimal tissue growth in the wound treated with gauge bandage, a substantial amount of granulation was visible at this time in the wound treated with the biocomposite. After 7 days of recovery, 90% of wound closure has been demonstrated by the treatment of CS-ALG/CaP biocomposite, compared to 20% closure in the control group, and a full closure (99% closure) after 10 days. Additionally, the biocomposite-treated skin that was developing seemed smoother and developed fewer scabs than

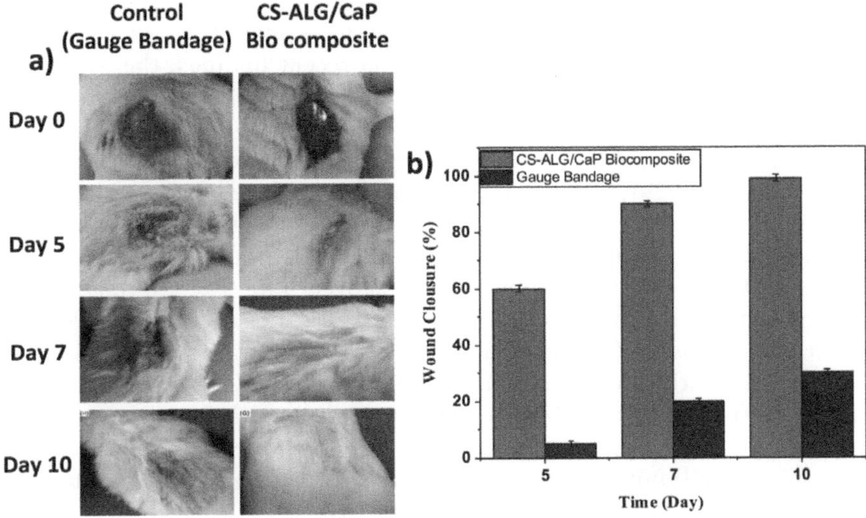

Figure 14.2 In vivo wound healing of cuts on the back of male mice. a) Illustrations of wounds treated with standard gauge bandage at 0, 5, 7 and 10 days andCS-ALG/CaP biocomposite respectively, b) the CS-ALG/CaP biocomposite's ability to heal wounds and control over time. (Reproduced with permission from (Rahman et al., 2020) Copyright 2020, Elsevier Publishers.)

the control skin. During this time, the control group only demonstrated 30% closure (Rahman et al., 2020).

According to a number of studies, alginate–ZnO (Shalumon et al., 2011), chitosan–ZnO (Guo et al., 2016), and calcium alginate (Lansdown & Path, n.d.) are possible biomaterials for quick wound healing. The incorporation of CaP-NPs will enable the release of Ca^{2+} ions through the chitosan–alginate fibrous matrix. As Ca^{2+} ions speed up cell division, chitosan and nano-ZnO will work together to protect the wound from bacterial assault.

14.5 RESULTS AND DISCUSSION

Under the ideal circumstances, the Co-AgNP nanofibers composite can be effectively generated by treating the solution in electrospinning machine. The electrospinning of PVA solutions with 15 and 20 wt% in water serves as the foundation for the development of the Co-AgNP film at a spraying distance of 20 cm and 25 kV of electric voltage (Subagio et al., 2020). The antimicrobial activity of silver (Ag_2O) and zinc oxide (ZnO) nanoparticles on wound infection gram-negative and gram-positive bacteria that should be embedded into nanofibers to produce nanofibrous mats were examined in order to achieve an appropriate and efficient concentration of nanoparticles. Antibiotics used as a control are tested against *E. coli*, *S. aureus*, and *Pseudomonas aeruginosa* at various doses of zinc oxide and silver nanoparticles. According to the recent findings, the Minimum inhibitory concentration for *E. coli* and *S. aureus* were 25 and 50 gmL^{-1}, respectively (Bagheri et al., 2022). The PVA/CS/mGO films displayed high biocompatibility and significantly increased antibacterial efficacy against *E. coli* and *S. aureus*, which may be due to the combined bactericidal effects of CS, GO, and PHMG, according to in vitro biological tests (S. Chen et al., 2020). In comparison to the other groups, the GNP biocomposite tested group had a considerably greater recovery rate ($P < 0.05$). Diffusion played a major role in regulating the release of drugs (GNT and GNPs) from biocomposites (Asgarirad et al., 2021). The antibacterial efficacy of the CS-ALG/CaP biocomposite against *S. enterica* and *E. coli* was analyzed based on the existence or absence of an inhibition diameter zone. *E. coli* had a larger zone of inhibition (25 mm), but *S. enterica* had a smaller zone of inhibition (10 mm). Compared to *E. coli*, *S. enterica* has a significantly thicker cell wall membrane (Rahman et al., 2020).

14.6 CONCLUSION

Wound healing is a challenging and complicated procedure of recreating damaged and devitalized cell structures and tissue layers. Hemostasis, inflammation, proliferation, and tissue remodeling are the four phases in the healing process of the skin. In this book chapter, recent progress on nano-based biocomposites and the alterations to make them more efficient for the wound healing have been discussed in details. Patients can safely use biopolymer-based (AgNP-BM) to heal wounds since they are non-cyto-toxic and harmless. They promote healthy wound healing while inhibiting the development of microorganisms at the wound site. Growing interest has recently been seen in studies on nanofibrous scaffolds for tissue regeneration made by electrospinning natural (chitosan) and artificial polymers alone or combining with metallic nanoparticles and bioactive plant extracts. According to many previous studies, GO-based nanocomposites can be utilized as bandages to considerably speed up the healing of wounds by removing germs from the area. A powerful broad-spectrum antibacterial agent with strong antibacterial action is polyhexamethylene guanidine (PHMG). An aminoglycoside gentamicin (GNT) exhibit excellent efficacy against infections caused by gram-negative bacteria. Alginate-ZnO, chitosan-ZnO, and calcium alginate are possible biomaterials for quick wound healing because they are very stable, non-toxic, and antimicrobial. DNG/Ch/CO dressings significantly reduced the risk of scarring. These cutting-edge nanobiocomposites dressings demonstrated flexibility, great association of strength and antimicrobial properties. They are non-allergic and non-toxic, and their manufacturing is easy, affordable and accessible.

They can be used as potential components for efficient wound treatment. Thus, this research area will continue to emerge in the upcoming years, and nano based biocomposites are needed to be explored more deeply.

REFERENCES

Abdul, S., Saood, S., & Sulaiman, G. M. (2016). Synthesis of biocompatible polymer blend for drug delivery in biomedical applications. *Engineering And Technology Journal, 34*(6, 842–851.

Abebe, M., Tadesse, S., Meseret, G., & Derbie, A. (2019). Type of bacterial isolates and antimicrobial resistance profile from different clinical samples at a Referral Hospital, Northwest Ethiopia: Five years data analysis. *BMC Research Notes, 12*(1). https://doi.org/10.1186/s13104-019-4604-6

Ahmed, R., Tariq, M., Ali, I., Asghar, R., Noorunnisa Khanam, P., Augustine, R., & Hasan, A. (2018). Novel electrospun chitosan/polyvinyl alcohol/zinc oxide nanofibrous mats with antibacterial and antioxidant properties for diabetic wound healing. *International Journal of Biological Macromolecules, 120,* 385–393. https://doi.org/10.1016/j.ijbiomac.2018.08.057

Akturk, O., Tezcaner, A., Bilgili, H., Deveci, M. S., Gecit, M. R., & Keskin, D. (2011). Evaluation of sericin/collagen membranes as prospective wound dressing biomaterial. *Journal of Bioscience and Bioengineering, 112*(3), 279–288. https://doi.org/10.1016/j.jbiosc.2011.05.014

Al-Musawi, S., Albukhaty, S., Al-Karagoly, H., Sulaiman, G. M., Alwahibi, M. S., Dewir, Y. H., Soliman, D. A., & Rizwana, H. (2020). Antibacterial activity of honey/chitosan nanofibers loaded with capsaicin and gold nanoparticles for wound dressing. *Molecules, 25*(20). https://doi.org/10.3390/molecules25204770

Applications, S. (2019). Two-dimensional graphene family material: Assembly, biocompatibility and sensors applications. *Sensors, 19*(13), 2966.

Asgarirad, H., Ebrahimnejad, P., Mahjoub, M. A., Jalalian, M., Morad, H., Ataee, R., Hosseini, S. S., & Farmoudeh, A. (2021). A promising technology for wound healing; in-vitro and in-vivo evaluation of chitosan nano-biocomposite films containing gentamicin. *Journal of Microencapsulation, 38*(2), 100–107. https://doi.org/10.1080/02652048.2020.1851789

Berger, J., Reist, M., Mayer, J. M., Felt, O., Peppas, N. A., & Gurny, R. (2004). Structure and interactions in covalently and ionically crosslinked chitosan hydrogels for biomedical applications. In *European Journal of Pharmaceutics and Biopharmaceutics* (Vol. 57, Issue 1, pp. 19–34). Elsevier. https://doi.org/10.1016/S0939-6411(03)00161-9

Bombaldi de Souza, R. F., Bombaldi de Souza, F. C., Bierhalz, A. C. K., Pires, A. L. R., & Moraes, Â. M. (2020). Biopolymer-based films and membranes as wound dressings. In *Biopolymer Membranes and Films* (pp. 165–194). Elsevier. https://doi.org/10.1016/B978-0-12-818134-8.00007-9

Chen, S., Wang, H., Jian, Z., Fei, G., Qian, W., Luo, G., Wang, Z., & Xia, H. (2020). Novel Poly(vinyl alcohol)/Chitosan/modified Graphene oxide Biocomposite for wound dressing application. *Macromolecular Bioscience, 20*(3). https://doi.org/10.1002/mabi.201900385

Chetouani, A., Elkolli, M., Bounekhel, M., & Benachour, D. (2017). Chitosan/oxidized pectin/PVA blend film: mechanical and biological properties. *Polymer Bulletin*, 74(10), 4297–4310. https://doi.org/10.1007/s00289-017-1953-y

Choi, H. J., Thambi, T., Yang, Y. H., Bang, S. I., Kim, B. S., Pyun, D. G., & Lee, D. S. (2017). AgNP and rhEGF-incorporating synergistic polyurethane foam as a dressing material for scar-free healing of diabetic wounds. *RSC Advances*, 7(23), 13714–13725. https://doi.org/10.1039/c6ra27322j

Desai, K., Kit, K., Li, J., & Zivanovic, S. (2008). Morphological and surface properties of electrospun chitosan nanofibers. *Biomacromolecules*, 9(3), 1000–1006. https://doi.org/10.1021/bm701017z

Devanesan, S., AlSalhi, M. S., Balaji, R. V., Ranjitsingh, A. J. A., Ahamed, A., Alfuraydi, A. A., AlQahtani, F. Y., Aleanizy, F. S., & Othman, A. H. (2018). Antimicrobial and cytotoxicity effects of synthesized silver nanoparticles from Punica Granatum peel extract. *Nanoscale Research Letters*, 13. https://doi.org/10.1186/s11671-018-2731-y

Enescu, D., & Olteanu, C. E. (2008). Functionalized Chitosan and its use in pharmaceutical, biomedical, and biotechnological research. *Chemical Engineering Communications*, 195(10), 1269–1291. https://doi.org/10.1080/00986440801958808

Firdhouse, M. J., & Lalitha, P. (2015). Biosynthesis of silver nanoparticles and its applications. In *Journal of Nanotechnology* (Vol. 2015). Hindawi Publishing Corporation. https://doi.org/10.1155/2015/829526

Garnica-Palafox, I. M., & Sánchez-Arévalo, F. M. (2016). Influence of natural and synthetic crosslinking reagents on the structural and mechanical properties of chitosan-based hybrid hydrogels. *Carbohydrate Polymers*, 151, 1073–1081. https://doi.org/10.1016/j.carbpol.2016.06.036

Ge, L., Li, Q., Wang, M., Ouyang, J., Li, X., & Xing, M. M. Q. (2014). Nanosilver particles in medical applications: Synthesis, performance, and toxicity. In *International Journal of Nanomedicine* (Vol. 9, Issue 1, pp. 2399–2407). Dove Medical Press Ltd. https://doi.org/10.2147/IJN.S55015

Ghasemzadeh, G., Momenpour, M., Omidi, F., Hosseini, M. R., Ahani, M., & Barzegari, A. (2014). Applications of nanomaterials in water treatment and environmental remediation. In *Frontiers of Environmental Science and Engineering* (Vol. 8, Issue 4, pp. 471–482). Higher Education Press. https://doi.org/10.1007/s11783-014-0654-0

Guo, Y. Y., Liu, B., Hu, B. B., Xiao, G. Y., Wu, Y. P., Sun, P. F., Zhang, X. L., Jia, Y. H., & Lu, Y. P. (2016). Antibacterial activity and increased osteoblast cell functions of zinc calcium phosphate chemical conversion on titanium. *Surface and Coatings Technology*, 294, 131–138. https://doi.org/10.1016/j.surfcoat.2016.03.085

Gurtner, G. C., Werner, S., Barrandon, Y., & Longaker, M. T. (2008). Wound repair and regeneration. In *Nature* (Vol. 453, Issue 7193, pp. 314–321). Nature Publishing Group. https://doi.org/10.1038/nature07039

Huang, Y., Yao, M., Zheng, X., Liang, X., Su, X., Zhang, Y., Lu, A., & Zhang, L. (n.d.). Subscriber access provided by NEW YORK MED COLL Effects of chitin whiskers on physical properties and osteoblast culture of alginate based nanocomposite hydrogels effects of chitin whiskers on physical properties and osteoblast culture of alginate 2 based nanocomposite hydrogels. http://pubs.acs.org

Kamoun, E. A., Kenawy, E. R. S., & Chen, X. (2017). A review on polymeric hydrogel membranes for wound dressing applications: PVA-based hydrogel dressings. In *Journal of Advanced Research* (Vol. 8, Issue 3, pp. 217–233). Elsevier B.V. https://doi.org/10.1016/j.jare.2017.01.005

Karahan, H. E., Wiraja, C., Xu, C., Wei, J., Wang, Y., Wang, L., Liu, F., & Chen, Y. (2018). Graphene materials in antimicrobial nanomedicine: Current status and future perspectives. *Advanced Healthcare Materials*, 7(13), 1701406. https://doi.org/10.1002/adhm.201701406

Kawai, K., Larson, B. J., Ishise, H., Carre, A. L., Nishimoto, S., Longaker, M., & Lorenz, H. P. (2011). Calcium-based nanoparticles accelerate skin wound healing. *PLoS One*, 6(11). https://doi.org/10.1371/journal.pone.0027106

Konop, M., Damps, T., Misicka, A., & Rudnicka, L. (2016). Certain aspects of silver and silver nanoparticles in wound care: A minireview. In *Journal of Nanomaterials* (Vol. 2016). Hindawi Limited. https://doi.org/10.1155/2016/7614753

Kwan, K. H. L., Liu, X., To, M. K. T., Yeung, K. W. K., Ho, C. ming, & Wong, K. K. Y. (2011). Modulation of collagen alignment by silver nanoparticles results in better mechanical properties in wound healing. *Nanomedicine: Nanotechnology, Biology, and Medicine*, 7(4), 497–504. https://doi.org/10.1016/j.nano.2011.01.003

Lansdown, A.B.G. (2002). Calcium: A potential central regulator in wound healing in the skin. *Wound Repair and Regeneration*, 10(5), 271–285.

Laschke, M. W., Augustin, V. A., Sahin, F., Anschütz, D., Metzger, W., Scheuer, C., Bischoff, M., Aktas, C., & Menger, M. D. (2016). Surface modification by plasma etching impairs early vascularization and tissue incorporation of porous polyethylene (Medpor®) implants. *Journal of Biomedical Materials Research Part B: Applied Biomaterials*, 104(8), 1738–1748. https://doi.org/10.1002/jbm.b.33528

Liu, T., Liu, Y., Liu, M., Wang, Y., He, W., Shi, G., Hu, X., Zhan, R., Luo, G., Xing, M., & Wu, J. (2018). Synthesis of graphene oxide-quaternary ammonium nanocomposite with synergistic antibacterial activity to promote infected wound healing. *Burns & Trauma*, 6. https://doi.org/10.1186/s41038-018-0115-2

Macneil, S. (2008). Biomaterials for tissue engineering of skin. *Materials today*, 11(5), 26–35.

Moeini, A., Pedram, P., Makvandi, P., Malinconico, M., & Gomez d'Ayala, G. (2020). Wound healing and antimicrobial effect of active secondary metabolites in chitosan-based wound dressings: A review. *Carbohydrate Polymers*, 233, 115839. https://doi.org/10.1016/j.carbpol.2020.115839

Nikbakht, M., Karbasi, S., Rezayat, S. M., Tavakol, S., & Sharifi, E. (2019). Evaluation of the effects of hyaluronic acid on poly (3-hydroxybutyrate)/chitosan/carbon nanotubes electrospun scaffold: Structure and mechanical properties. *Polymer-Plastics Technology and Materials*, 58(18), 2031–2040. https://doi.org/10.1080/25740881.2019.1602645

Ninan, N., Muthiah, M., Park, I. K., Wong, T. W., Thomas, S., & Grohens, Y. (2015). Natural polymer/inorganic material based hybrid scaffolds for skin wound healing. *Polymer Reviews*, 55(3), 453–490. https://doi.org/10.1080/15583724.2015.1019135

O'Donoghue, J. M., O'Sullivan, S. T., Beausang, E. S., Panchal, J. I., O'Shaughnessy, M., & O'Connor, T. P. (1997). Calcium alginate dressings promote healing of split skin graft donor sites. *Acta Chirurgiae Plasticae*, 39(2), 53–55.

Oliver, L. C., & Blaine, G. (n.d.). *Hemostasis with Absorbable Alginates in Neurosurgical Practice. British Journal of Surgery*, 37(147), 307–310.

Osmani, R. A. M., Singh, E., Jadhav, K., Jadhav, S., & Banerjee, R. (2021). Biopolymers and biocomposites: Nature's tools for wound healing and tissue engineering. In *Applications of Advanced Green Materials* (pp. 573–630). Elsevier. https://doi.org/10.1016/B978-0-12-820484-9.00023-4

Parani, M., Lokhande, G., Singh, A., & Gaharwar, A. K. (2016). Engineered nanomaterials for infection control and healing acute and chronic wounds. In *ACS Applied Materials and Interfaces* (Vol. 8, Issue 16, pp. 10049–10069). American Chemical Society. https://doi.org/10.1021/acsami.6b00291

Park, D. U., Park, J., Yang, K. W., Park, J. H., Kwon, J. H., & Oh, H. Bin. (2020). Properties of polyhexamethylene guanidine (PHMG) associated with fatal lung injury in Korea. *Molecules*, 25(14). https://doi.org/10.3390/molecules25143301

Qi, L., Xu, Z., Jiang, X., Hu, C., & Zou, X. (2004). Preparation and antibacterial activity of chitosan nanoparticles. *Carbohydrate Research*, 339(16), 2693–2700. https://doi.org/10.1016/j.carres.2004.09.007

Qian, W., Hu, X., He, W., Zhan, R., Liu, M., Zhou, D., Huang, Y., Hu, X., Wang, Z., Fei, G., Wu, J., Xing, M., Xia, H., & Luo, G. (2018). Colloids and surfaces B : Biointerfaces Polydimethylsiloxane incorporated with reduced graphene oxide (rGO) sheets for wound dressing application : Preparation and characterization. *Colloids and Surfaces B: Biointerfaces*, 166, 61–71. https://doi.org/10.1016/j.colsurfb.2018.03.008

Rahman, M. A., Islam, M. S., Haque, P., Khan, M. N., Takafuji, M., Begum, M., Chowdhury, G. W., Khan, M., & Rahman, M. M. (2020). Calcium ion mediated rapid wound healing by nano-ZnO doped calcium phosphate-chitosan-alginate biocomposites. *Materialia*, 13. https://doi.org/10.1016/j.mtla.2020.100839

Rangaraj, A., Harding, K., & Leaper, D. (2011). Role of collagen in wound management. *Clinical Review Wounds UK*, 7(2), 54–63.

Rigo, C., Ferroni, L., Tocco, I., Roman, M., Munivrana, I., Gardin, C., Cairns, W. R. L., Vindigni, V., Azzena, B., Barbante, C., & Zavan, B. (2013). Active silver nanoparticles for wound healing. *International Journal of Molecular Sciences*, 14(3), 4817–4840. https://doi.org/10.3390/ijms14034817

Shalumon, K. T., Anulekha, K. H., Nair, S. V., Nair, S. V., Chennazhi, K. P., & Jayakumar, R. (2011). Sodium alginate/poly(vinyl alcohol)/nano ZnO composite nanofibers for antibacterial wound dressings. *International Journal of Biological Macromolecules*, 49(3), 247–254. https://doi.org/10.1016/j.ijbiomac.2011.04.005

Sharifi, F., Nazir, I., Asim, M. H., Jahangiri, M., Ebrahimnejad, P., Matuszczak, B., & Bernkop-Schnürch, A. (2019). Zeta potential changing self-emulsifying drug delivery systems utilizing a novel Janus-headed surfactant: A promising strategy for enhanced mucus permeation. *Journal of Molecular Liquids*, 291. https://doi.org/10.1016/j.molliq.2019.111285

Shoulders, M. D., & Raines, R. T. (2009). Collagen structure and stability. *Annual Review of Biochemistry*, 78(1), 929–958. https://doi.org/10.1146/annurev.biochem.77.032207.120833

Siritienthong, T., Ratanavaraporn, J., & Aramwit, P. (2012). Development of ethyl alcohol-precipitated silk sericin/polyvinyl alcohol scaffolds for accelerated healing of full-thickness wounds. *International Journal of Pharmaceutics*, *439*(1–2), 175–186. https://doi.org/10.1016/j.ijpharm.2012.09.043

Suarato, G., Bertorelli, R., & Athanassiou, A. (2018). Borrowing from nature: Biopolymers and biocomposites as smart wound care materials. In *Frontiers in Bioengineering and Biotechnology* (Vol. 6, Issue OCT). Frontiers Media S.A. https://doi.org/10.3389/fbioe.2018.00137

Subagio, A., Umiati, N. A. K., & Gunawan, V. (2020). Growth of collagen-nanosilver (Co-AgNP) biocomposite film with electrospinning method for wound healing applications. *Journal of Physics: Conference Series*, *1524*(1). https://doi.org/10.1088/1742-6596/1524/1/012032

Sulaiman, F. A., Adeyemi, O. S., Akanji, M. A., Oloyede, H. O. B., Sulaiman, A. A., Olatunde, A., Hoseni, A. A., Olowolafe, Y. V., Nlebedim, R. N., Muritala, H., Nafiu, M. O., & Salawu, M. O. (2015). Biochemical and morphological alterations caused by silver nanoparticles in Wistar rats. *Journal of Acute Medicine*, *5*(4), 96–102. https://doi.org/10.1016/j.jacme.2015.09.005

Venkataprasanna, K. S., Prakash, J., Vignesh, S., Bharath, G., Venkatesan, M., Banat, F., Sahabudeen, S., Ramachandran, S., & Devanand Venkatasubbu, G. (2020). Fabrication of Chitosan/PVA/GO/CuO patch for potential wound healing application. *International Journal of Biological Macromolecules*, *143*, 744–762. https://doi.org/10.1016/j.ijbiomac.2019.10.029

Xiao, J., Zhu, Y., Liu, Y., Liu, H., Zeng, Y., Xu, F., & Wang, L. (2008). Vaterite selection by chitosan gel: An example of polymorph selection by morphology of biomacromolecules. *Crystal Growth and Design*, *8*(8), 2887–2891. https://doi.org/10.1021/cg701233y

Yildirimer, L., Thanh, N. T. K., & Seifalian, A. M. (2012). Skin regeneration scaffolds: A multimodal bottom-up approach. In *Trends in Biotechnology* (Vol. 30, Issue 12, pp. 638–648). https://doi.org/10.1016/j.tibtech.2012.08.004

Yokota, J., & Kyotani, S. (2018). Influence of nanoparticle size on the skin penetration, skin retention and anti-inflammatory activity of non-steroidal anti-inflammatory drugs. *Journal of the Chinese Medical Association*, *81*(6), 511–519. https://doi.org/10.1016/j.jcma.2018.01.008

Zeb, A., Arif, S. T., Malik, M., Shah, F. A., Din, F. U., Qureshi, O. S., Lee, E. S., Lee, G. Y., & Kim, J. K. (2019). Potential of nanoparticulate carriers for improved drug delivery via skin. In *Journal of Pharmaceutical Investigation* (Vol. 49, Issue 5, pp. 485–517). Springer Netherlands. https://doi.org/10.1007/s40005-018-00418-8

Zhong, S. P., Zhang, Y. Z., & Lim, C. T. (2010). Tissue scaffolds for skin wound healing and dermal reconstruction. In *Wiley Interdisciplinary Reviews: Nanomedicine and Nanobiotechnology* (Vol. 2, Issue 5, pp. 510–525). https://doi.org/10.1002/wnan.100

Chapter 15

Nanocomposites in 3D Bioimplants and Fluorescent Bioimaging

*Nancy Jaswal, Vijay Bahadur, Ali Raza,
Arbind Prasad, and Pramod Kumar*

15.1 INTRODUCTION

Recently, the field of nanotechnology has gained immense recognition. It has become the current focal point of scientific research. A plethora of new opportunities and applications in a variety of fields have been made possible by the ability to modify and engineer materials at the nanoscale level. One of the core aspects of this interdisciplinary field is the study of nanomaterials and their intriguing properties. Materials with structural characteristics at the nanoscale, usually between 1 and 100 nanometers, are referred to as nanomaterials. At nano scale, materials exhibit distinctive properties owing to quantum mechanical effects and surface phenomena (Kumar et al., 2023). Nanomaterials possess a large surface-to-volume ratio, which significantly influences their behavior, reactivity, and performance due to their smaller size. Considering the quantum confinement effect, where electrons are confined to a restricted space, nanomaterials often display altered physical, chemical, and optical properties compared to their bulk counterparts. For instance, nanoparticles may exhibit different melting points, electrical conductivity, and even magnetic properties. Furthermore, manipulating the size, shape, and composition of nanomaterials allows for the creation of customized applications in a variety of disciplines due to their unique features (Chen & Yin, 2014).

Nanomaterials come in various forms, each with its own characteristic properties. Nanoparticles, nanowires, nanotubes, and nanocomposites are just a few examples of the wide range of nanomaterials available. The composition of nanomaterials spans across elements, ceramics, semiconductors, and polymers, amplifying the array of potential applications. Furthermore, the incorporation of different materials within a nanostructure can lead to synergistic effects, enhancing the properties of nanomaterials and opening up exciting avenues for novel technologies (S. Kumar et al., 2020). Another intriguing aspect of nanomaterials is their high surface area, which profoundly influences their chemical reactivity. Nanoparticles, due to their large surface-to-volume ratio, possess an increased number of surface atoms, enabling greater interaction with their

DOI: 10.1201/9781003470311-15

surroundings. This property is particularly crucial in catalysis, where nanomaterials exhibit enhanced catalytic activity, specific selectivity, and improved stability. Understanding and harnessing these surface properties can revolutionize fields such as energy conversion, environmental remediation, and pharmaceuticals (S. Kumar et al., 2018). The remarkable properties of nanomaterials have led to the emergence of several applications across various domains. Nanomaterials have made it possible for electronics to become smaller, faster, and more effective by facilitating the process of shrinking. In medicine, nanomaterials offer potential solutions for targeted drug delivery and imaging, enhancing the efficacy and precision of medical interventions. Moreover, nanomaterials find applications in energy storage, environmental monitoring, and even in the development of sustainable materials.

Fluorescence (and phosphorescence) imaging has piqued the interest of researchers due to the sensitivity, selectivity, contrast-rich, and versatility of these. Over the past 20 years, there has also been a notable development in resolution, approaching the single nanometer scale. First, two distinct types of fluorescence imaging are identifiable. The original technique for imaging was to use inherently fluorescent bio-chemical species. The second section describes imaging techniques for fluorescently labeled samples or cells, as well as nanoparticles, nanosensors, labels, or artificial fluorescent probes. Such probes are required to identify species (like pH) that are unsuitable for direct fluorometric imaging, but using them also carries the risk of the probe or the material introduced disrupting a particular species (Li & Zhu, 2013; Wolfbeis, 2015). Three methods can be identified when working with bioimaging that uses artificial fluorescent probes and nanoparticles. (a) The simplest involves imaging cells after internalizing fluorescent nanoparticles or a strong fluorophore. The aim of these fluorophores along with nanomaterials is to induce fluorescence in cells or tissues. They aren't meant to have any affinity for a specific site, therefore they are unresponsive to any sort of chemical species like specific ions or organic molecules. (b) The second method is referred to as "targeted bioimaging". It works similarly to fluorescence in situ hybridization or immunostaining in that it identifies particular species or domains. In order to do this, the specific counterpart is recognized by fluorophores or nanoparticles with appropriately functionalized surfaces, such as ligands, receptors, antibodies, or oligomers. Targeting amyloidic plaques in Alzheimer's tissue, mitochondria, genes, tumor indicators, and membranes are a few examples. (c) The third method makes use of nanomaterials and sensing probes. This makes it possible to image (bio) chemical entities that lack intrinsic fluorescence. As an illustration, consider imaging the distribution of chemical species in live and metabolizing cells, as opposed to cancerous cells or cells subjected to potential medications, such as pH values, glucose, calcium (II), or oxygen. This group also includes temperature nano sensors. This chapter aims to provide a comprehensive

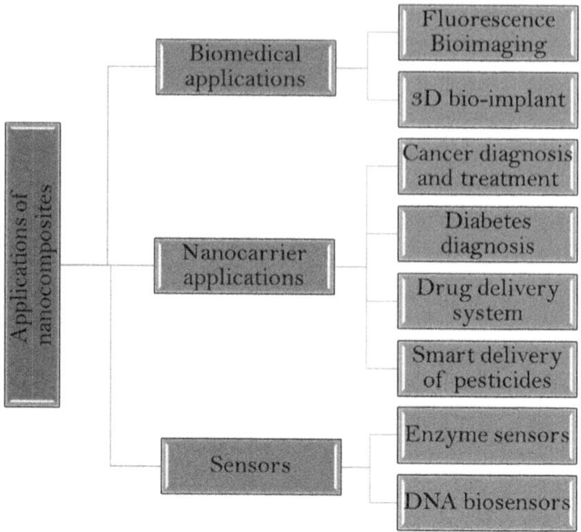

Figure 15.1 Applications of nanocomposites (S. Kumar et al., 2018).

understanding of nanomaterials, exploring their properties and shedding light on their potential implications in bioimplants and fluorescent imaging area (Kolahalam et al., 2019; Zhang et al., 2014).

15.2 NANOCOMPOSITES IN BIOIMPLANTS

Nanocomposites market production is increasing dramatically to meet global demand. 138,389 metric tons of nanocomposites were consumed globally in 2011 at a cost of $920 million, according to market research. From 2016 to 2021, the projected growth rate for this market share is a compound annual growth rate (CAGR) of 26.7%, generating $5.3 billion in revenue. Accordingly, it is anticipated that the market for polymer nano-composites alone will reach $11,549 million by 2022. The development of new, high-performing nanocomposites has been facilitated by ongoing technical innovation and creative processing methods. There are various types of nanomaterials utilized in 3D bioimplants, such as nanoparticles, nanofibers, and nanosheets. Additionally, nanocomposites, consisting of two or more nanomaterials, offer a hybrid platform that exploits the advantages of each component. There are various types of nano materials used in bioimplants. Metallic nanoparticles can be incorporated into dental implants to improve antimicrobial properties (Kandavalli et al., 2021). Carbon nanotubes can be utilized in orthopedic implants for bone tissue engineering applications due to their excellent mechanical properties. Nanocomposites are materials consisting of a matrix material reinforced with nanoparticles or nanofibers. For example, polymer-based nanocomposites can be used as coatings on cardiovascular devices to enhance blood compatibility and reduce thrombogenicity (Lee et al., 2021). The applications of nano materials in bioimplants are vast and diverse. In orthopedic implants, nanostructured coatings can be applied to enhance the osseointegration process, leading to improved implant stability. Dental implants can benefit from nano materials through the incorporation of nanoparticles or nanotubes to promote antibacterial activity and accelerate bone regeneration. Cardiovascular devices such as stents can be coated with nanostructured materials to prevent restenosis and promote endothelialisation (Kandavalli et al., 2021; Thu et al., 2023). Moreover, nanomaterials enable controlled drug release systems within bioimplants, allowing for targeted delivery of therapeutic agents directly to the desired site. The use of nano materials in bioimplant technology brings numerous benefits. Firstly, their small size allows for better interaction with biological systems at the cellular and molecular level. This results in improved biocompatibility and reduced immune response compared to conventional implant materials. Secondly, nano materials offer enhanced drug delivery capabilities due to their large surface area-to-volume ratio, enabling precise control over release kinetics. Additionally, these materials exhibit excellent mechanical properties such as high strength and flexibility, contributing to increased durability and longevity of bioimplants (Q. Wang et al., 2020).

However, there are also challenges associated with using nano materials in bioimplants that need consideration. One concern is the potential toxicity or adverse effects associated with certain types of nanoparticles or nanomaterials when released into the body. Careful evaluation of biocompatibility is essential during the design and fabrication process. Furthermore, standardization protocols should be established to ensure consistent quality control and regulatory compliance across different manufacturing processes (Ansarian et al., 2019).

Recent advancements have been made in utilizing nano materials for bioimplant applications. Researchers are exploring new strategies for surface modification using nanotechnology techniques to improve tissue integration and reduce bacterial colonization (Kandavalli et al., 2021; Q. Wang et al., 2020). Moreover, the development of biodegradable nano materials holds promise for temporary implants or devices that can be gradually replaced by natural tissues In the future, we can expect further advancements and innovations in this field. The integration of nanotechnology with emerging fields such as 3D printing and regenerative medicine may lead to the development of personalized bioimplants tailored to the individual patients' needs and anatomies. Additionally, ongoing research aims to optimize the fabrication techniques and improve the scalability of nanostructured bioimplants for widespread clinical applications (Poon et al., 2020; Yang et al., 2017).

Hence, nano materials have revolutionized bioimplant technology by offering unique properties and capabilities. Different types of nano materials such as nanoparticles, nanotubes, and nanocomposites are utilized in various applications including orthopedic implants, dental implants, and cardiovascular devices. The use of nano materials brings numerous benefits such as improved biocompatibility, enhanced drug delivery systems, increased durability, among others (M. Kumar et al., 2021). However, challenges related to toxicity and regulatory compliance need careful consideration. Recent trends indicate a promising future for utilizing nano materials in bioimplant technology with potential developments in surface modification techniques and personalized implant fabrication methods.

15.3 MATERIALS AND METHODS

Three distinct methodologies can be used to synthesize nanomaterials: chemical, physical, and biological processes.

15.3.1 Hydrothermal Method

High pressure and temperature are applied to the solutions in this method. Creating better crystals while retaining composition control is the key advantage offered by this technique. The divalent and trivalent transition metal salts have a mole ratio of 1:2. Stir the aforementioned solution continuously as you add the organic solvent to achieve a homogenous mixture. After that, the solutions are put inside an autoclave, which is a sealed container. Because of the autogenous pressure increase brought on by heating, the boiling points of solvents are immediately raised. Depending on the kind of nanoparticle to be created, different temperature and time changes are needed. (Kundu et al., 2017) synthesized PANI intercalated V_2O_5 xerogel hybrid nanocomposites hydrothermally. (Zhao et al., 2014) described the synthesis of $Mn0.6Zn0.4Fe_2O_4$-CNTs/polyaniline nanocomposites hydrothermally that exhibit excellent magnetic properties, followed by in situ polymerization. Hydrothermal routes were used to create fluorescent carbon dot-reinforced molecularly imprinted polymer (MIP) nanocomposites that shows high selectivity, which highlight their potential use in novel f biosensors. Coating the organic layer of MIPs on the nanomaterial surface can result in the formation of polymer nanocomposites; however, under intense UV light, this process can swiftly destroy organic layers. (Deng et al., 2014) used a sol-hydrothermal method to create $MIP-TiO_2/SiO_2$ nanocomposites. These nanocomposites showed good reusability and molecular recognition due to their inorganic structure. By matching the solubility of $BaTiO_3$ nanoparticles with the composition of the polymer, the dispersion of these particles can be enhanced via the hydrothermal approach. Moreover, phase segregation can be produced by employing block polymers to prevent nanoparticle aggregation in a polymer matrix. Rubbery butadiene moieties must be used since the glassy character of block copolymers may restrict the titanium precursor's mobility during the synthesis process.

15.3.2 Template Synthesis

The use of templates in the fabrication of heterogeneous nanocomposites has been widely and successfully used. This technique has been consistently used by various scientists due to its ease of use and diverse field applicability. (Ma et al., 2016) demonstrated the synthesis of a 3DrGO/PANI nanowire composite using this technique. The p-conjugated structures and hydrophobicity of rGO sheets evolve as the chemical process of template creation progresses. This enhances graphene oxide sheet cross-linking and p-p stacking. Using the template method, (Takeuchi et al., 2017) created polypropylene-silicon nanocomposites. Supercritical CO_2 was used to penetrate the polypropylene and introduce silicon alkoxide. The shape of an amorphous polypropylene film was modified by varying the quenching temperatures.

15.3.3 Melt Intercalation Technique

An eco-friendly method called melt intercalation entails heating polymeric material, adding filler, and then compressing the product to produce a homogeneous distribution. The temperature range for melt intercalation procedure used in the production of nanocomposites is 190–220 degrees Celsius. The melt intercalation approach is superior to alternative synthesis processes in terms of formulation flexibility, cost, compatibility, and suitability for industrial productivity. (Normand et al., 2017) described a melt mixing method for producing polypropylene-based nanocomposites. The dispersion efficiency of the nanocomposite was compared among three organoclays. The two other surfactants had double long alkyl tails, whereas Cloisite 30 B surfactants had a single alkyl tail. Cloisite 30 B was only advised for polar polymers due to its distinct affinity; for non-polar polymers, cloisite 20 and dellite 67 G were recommended. For example, maximum dispersibility of the shydrophobic organoclays reinforced with unsaturated polyester (UPE)-resin was discovered (S. Kumar et al., 2018).

15.4 SURFACE MODIFICATION TECHNIQUES

Surface modification plays a pivotal role in enhancing the biocompatibility of nanomaterial bioimplants. A non-biocompatible surface can lead to adverse effects such as inflammation, infection, and rejection by the host's immune system (Fernández-Lizárraga et al., 2022). By modifying the surface characteristics of these implantable devices through various techniques, it becomes possible to improve their interactions with biological systems and reduce the risk of complications. The surface modification of nanocomposites has become a focus of research in order to prevent nanoparticle agglomeration caused by specific volume and surface area effects. The modification techniques can aid in the improvement of particle–matrix and particle–particle interactions. Surface modification of nanocomposites can be accomplished in two ways: 1) Surface absorption and/or reaction with coupling agents and 2) grafting polymeric molecules via covalent or non-covalent bonding. The hydrophobicity and dispersion stability of the nanofillers were modified using modification techniques. These techniques specifically increased interfacial adhesion in nanocomposites via chemical bonding. A wide range of biocompatible materials can be utilized to modify the surfaces of nanomaterial bioimplants. These materials often possess inherent characteristics that facilitate cellular interactions while reducing adverse responses from host tissues. Examples include hydroxyapatite coatings for orthopedic implants to enhance osseointegration (Fernández-Lizárraga et al., 2022), titanium oxide films with antibacterial properties to minimize infection risks (Singh Sidhu et al., 2022) and biodegradable polymers for controlled drug release within tissue engineering scaffolds. The choice of biocompatible material depends on factors such as the intended application, desired functionality, mechanical compatibility with host tissues, degradation kinetics, and long-term performance requirements. Several techniques can be employed to modify the surface of nanomaterial bioimplants and enhance their biocompatibility. Chemical treatments, such as plasma etching or acid-base reactions, can alter the chemical composition of the implant's surface (Fernández-Lizárraga et al., 2022). Coating techniques, such as magnetron sputtering or electrochemical deposition, involve depositing a thin layer of biocompatible material onto the implant's surface. Physical modifications, including laser ablation or micro structuring, can create specific surface topographies that promote cellular adhesion and tissue integration. Each technique has its own principles, advantages, and limitations. For instance, chemical treatments offer simplicity and versatility but may affect bulk properties of the materials. Coating techniques provide excellent control over surface properties but might face challenges in terms of stability and durability. Physical modifications enable precise control over topographical features but require specialized equipment and expertise.

Several successful case studies demonstrate the positive impact of surface modifications in enhancing biocompatibility for nanomaterial bioimplants. For example, (Fernández-Lizárraga et al., 2022) evaluated metal oxide coatings applied by magnetron sputtering as potential bifunctional surface modifications for orthopedic implants. The study demonstrated improved osteogenic properties and enhanced biocompatibility compared to unmodified surfaces. These case studies emphasize that effective surface modifications can lead to reduced host responses, improved tissue integration, and increased implant longevity.

15.5 CHARACTERIZATION TECHNIQUES

To evaluate the effectiveness of surface modifications, various characterization techniques are employed. These techniques provide insights into the biocompatibility improvements achieved through surface modifications. Common methods include scanning electron microscopy (SEM) to visualize the surface morphologies, X-ray photoelectron spectroscopy (XPS) to analyse chemical compositions and bonding states, and atomic force microscopy (AFM) to measure surface roughness and topographical features.

15.6 NANOCOMPOSITES FOR ENHANCED IMPLANT PERFORMANCE

15.6.1 Functional Nanomaterials for Enhanced Sensing and Monitoring

Incorporation of nano sensors into bioimplants enables real-time monitoring of physiological indicators, facilitating early detection of implant failure or awareness of surrounding tissue conditions. Nanomaterial-based sensing platforms offer improved sensitivity, selectivity, and dynamic range, providing valuable information for clinicians. Functional nanomaterials have revolutionized the field of chemistry by enabling innovative sensing and monitoring applications. In particular, the development of bioimplants made of nanomaterials has significantly advanced the capabilities of sensors and monitoring devices in various domains. This portion aims to provide a comprehensive overview of functional nanomaterials for sensing and monitoring, discussing their unique properties, functionalization process, applications in sensing and monitoring, as well as challenges, limitations, and future perspectives. Functionalizing nanomaterials plays a significant role in enhancing their sensing and monitoring capabilities. The process involves modifying the surface properties or attaching biomolecules onto the nanomaterial surface to enable selective detection or interaction with target analytes or biomarkers. Various methods can be employed for functionalization purposes such as surface modification techniques including chemical functionalization through covalent bonding or physical adsorption (Erdem & İşcan, 2021). These modifications not only improve sensor selectivity but also enhance stability and biocompatibility. The application potential of bioimplants made from functional nanomaterials is vast within both sensing and continuous monitoring aspects. In terms of sensing applications, these bioimplants find utility in detecting different analytes or biomarkers (Viswambari Devi et al., 2015). For instance, glucose monitoring is a critical application where nanomaterial-based sensors have shown significant promise. By embedding these sensors in bioimplants, continuous and real-time glucose monitoring can be achieved, providing valuable information for diabetic patients. Furthermore, functional nanomaterials have been used to detect specific diseases by identifying disease-specific biomarkers.

Bioimplants made from functional nanomaterials enable continuous data collection and analysis within biological systems. They play a vital role in real-time physiological parameter monitoring such as heart rate, body temperature, or blood pressure. Additionally, nanomaterial-based bioimplants can also be employed for drug delivery monitoring purposes. By incorporating drug-loaded nanoparticles into the implant, the release kinetics of the drug can be monitored accurately. However, the utilization of functional nanomaterial-based bioimplants does come with challenges and limitations. One major concern is related to toxicity since some nanomaterials may pose potential risks to human health. This aspect necessitates thorough assessments and evaluations before their applications in clinical settings. Additionally, stability issues need to be addressed as well, since exposure to various environmental conditions may affect the performance of these implants (Erdem & İşcan, 2021). Moreover, bio compatibility often poses a challenge an immune response against implanted nanomaterials may occur.

Looking towards future perspectives, the development of functional nanomaterial-based bioimplants for sensing and monitoring holds immense potential. Advancements are expected through multidisciplinary collaborations between chemists, physicists, and biologists (Alamgir et al., 2023). Emerging technologies such as 3D printing could enable more precise fabrication techniques for designing complex sensor architectures (Amin et al., 2016) Furthermore, research efforts should focus on enhancing the stability, bio-compatibility, and long-term functionality of these devices. Thus, functional nanomaterials have opened up new opportunities in the field of sensing and monitoring. Bioimplants made from these nanomaterials offer improved sensitivity, selectivity, and real-time data collection capabilities for a wide range of applications. Although challenges such as toxicity concerns, stability issues, and compatibility with biological systems exist, the advancements in functional nanomaterials hold great promise for future developments. By addressing these challenges and exploring emerging technologies, we can expect further enhancements in the performance of bioimplants made from functional nanomaterials for sensing and monitoring purposes.

15.6.2 Principles of Fluorescence Bioimaging

Fluorescence bioimaging is a technique that utilizes fluorescent molecules or probes to visualize biological structures or processes within living organisms. The principles behind this technique involve excitation of fluorophores by absorbing photons at one wavelength followed by emission at a longer wavelength. When excited by light energy above a certain threshold known as the excitation energy level, electrons in fluorophores undergo an electronic transition from ground state to higher energy levels. Subsequently, these excited electrons return back to lower energy levels via non-radiative relaxation processes including internal conversion and vibrational relaxation. However, in some cases they release excess energy via fluorescence emission where they return back to the ground state by emitting a photon (Chen & Yin, 2014; Zhang et al., 2014).

15.6.3 Types of Nanocomposites Used in Fluorescence Bioimaging

Several types of nanocomposites have been utilized in fluorescence bioimaging applications. One example is the use of squaraines, which are two-photon absorbing dyes that exhibit strong fluorescence emission. These dyes have been employed for imaging cellular structures and monitoring biological processes due to their enhanced photostability and brightness (Chang et al., 2019). Another type of nanocomposite commonly used in fluorescence bioimaging is BODIPY-pyridyl hydrazone probe. This probe exhibits a turn-on response upon binding with Fe^{3+} ions, making it suitable for detecting this metal ion in biological systems (Nootem et al., 2021). Furthermore, gold nanoparticles biofunctionalized by tryptophan and riboflavin have demonstrated enhanced resonance energy transfer for improved bioimaging applications (Pajović et al., n.d).

15.6.4 Synthesis Methods for Nanocomposites in Fluorescence Bioimaging

Various synthesis methods have been employed to fabricate nanocomposites specifically designed for fluorescence bioimaging purposes. These methods include sol–gel method, hydrothermal synthesis, chemical vapor deposition, and self-assembly techniques. The advantage of sol–gel method lies in its ability to produce highly uniform nanoparticles with precise control over size and composition. Hydrothermal synthesis provides the opportunity to fabricate nanocomposites under high temperature and pressure conditions, resulting in unique properties such as enhanced stability and crystallinity.

15.6.5 Applications of Nanocomposites in Fluorescence Bioimaging

Nanocomposites have found successful applications in advancing fluorescence bioimaging techniques. For instance, Eu^{3+}/Gd^{3+} co-doped fluoroapatite nanocrystals synthesized through hydrothermal synthesis exhibited excellent photoluminescent properties that enabled efficient fluorescence imaging both in vitro and in vivo (Gedara et al., 2022). These nanocrystals were used for imaging bone tissue regeneration, demonstrating them potential for tissue-specific imaging and diagnosis. Similarly, gold nanoparticles difunctionalized by tryptophan and riboflavin have been utilized as contrast agents for improved bioimaging of tumor cells, showcasing the enhanced targeting capabilities conferred by nanocomposites.

15.7 NANOCOMPOSITES IN 3D BIOIMPLANTS

There is an exponential increase in demand for tissue engineering to replace or repair damaged organs or tissue due to chronic diseases and an ageing population. Since polymeric nanocomposites have biodegradable kinetics and are biocompatible, they are of tremendous interest in tissue engineering research. Consequently, research on the potential applications of nanocomposites has been conducted in numerous medical domains, including bone regeneration and nerve tissue repair. The textile and packaging industries may find it difficult to use synthetic polymers due to their high cost in the current business environment. Nevertheless, the creation of novel polymers with predictable mechanical properties and biodegradability ought to benefit from large-scale polymer manufacturing carried out under controlled circumstances. Tissue engineering is a technique used to repair damaged tissues that combines molecular biology and material engineering. In tissue engineering, scaffolds are built on a transient artificial matrix that offers a three-dimensional scaffold for cell seeding, proliferation, and the creation of new tissue (Pajović et al., n.d; X. Wang et al., 2017).

The scaffolds must give implants a substantial amount of mechanical support in order to maintain stresses and loadings over the afflicted tissue or organ. In order to replicate the natural extracellular matrix (ECM) surrounding bone tissue, 3D porous scaffold structures are intended to be osteoinductive and osteoconductive. They should also have the capacity to induce pluripotent cells that have been transferred from a non-osseous environment and differentiate them into osteoblasts (Balint et al., 2014; Luo et al., 2016).

Fukushima et al. used a free radical polymerization technique to create CNT/polymer nanocomposites. They consequently observed a 120-fold

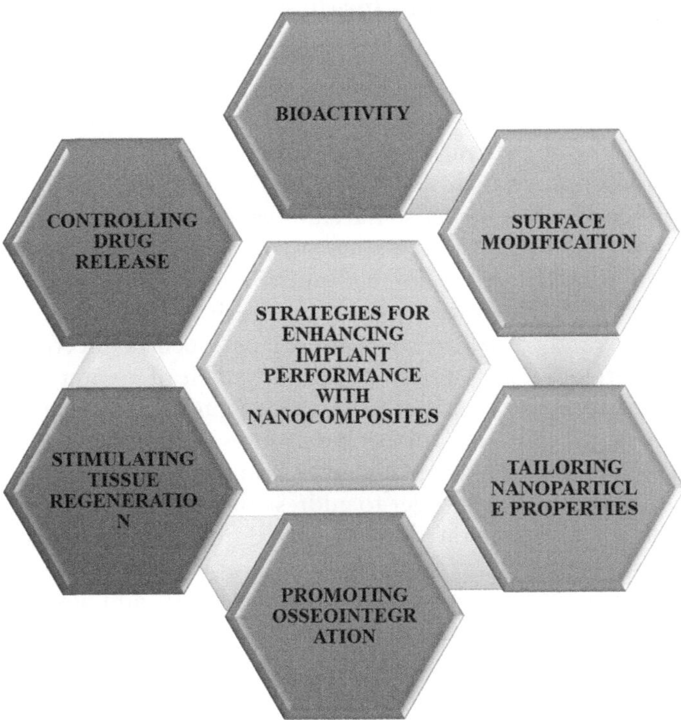

Figure 15.2 Strategies for enhancing the performance of medical implants with nano-composites (S. Kumar et al., 2018).

rise in Young's modulus at 7 weight percent CNT addition. According to Velasco-Santos et al., adding chemically functionalized MWCNTs (1 wt%) raised the polymer matrix's storage modulus by 1135%.

The characteristics of nanocomposites can be influenced by a number of additional factors in addition to the quantity of CNTs incorporated into the polymer matrix. Therefore, CNT-coated polymer nanofibrous-based scaffolds are suggested as an interesting field of study for neural tissue engineering applications including cell transplantation. Metallic nanoparticles add a lot of surface area and potent antibacterial action to polymer nanocomposites. In order to effectively regulate the surface wettability and roughness of the polymer nanocomposites, metallic nanoparticles should therefore drastically increase the rate of degradation. 3D-printed oligomeric poly(propylene fumarate) (PPF) scaffolds were created by Luo et al. L929 murine fibroblasts and human mesenchymal stem cells both demonstrated no toxicity towards these 3D-manufactured PPF scaffolds. In contrast, the main drawback of porosity scaffolds is that PLA-based nanocomposites have a lower hydrophilicity than biological polymers, which results in a lower affinity for cell seeding (Baker et al., 2014; Fukushima et al., 2006).

15.7.1 Recent Advances in Medical Implants

The availability of efficient and minimally invasive therapies for a variety of medical conditions made possible by medical implants has revolutionized modern healthcare. They have developed into vital tools for millions of people worldwide, helping to manage chronic conditions, regain physical function, and improve their quality of life. Medical implants come with a number of benefits, but they also have drawbacks and challenges related to their creation, application, and manufacturing. One major issue with medical implants is the potential for malfunction or failure, which can cause issues and have detrimental impacts on health (Arjmandi & Ramezani, 2019a; Sevost'yanov et al., 2018). Many factors, such as infection, mechanical wear, corrosion, and tissue rejection, can lead to implant failures. These issues can arise even with the most sophisticated implant designs and materials, necessitating further procedures and implant replacements. Researchers are looking into how nanocomposites might help medical implants function better in order to address these problems. Nanoparticles or nanofillers are incorporated into a matrix material, such a polymer or metal, to form materials referred to as nanocomposites. These materials have unique properties such high strength, flexibility, and biocompatibility that make them perfect for use in medical implant applications. Despite being in its early stages, the use of nanocomposites in medical implants has advanced significantly in recent years. Diverse nanocomposites have been developed by researchers for use in orthopedic implants, cardiac stents, and dental implants, among other medical implant uses (Davoodi et al., 2021; Giordano et al., 2017). The enhanced mechanical strength, wear resistance, and biocompatibility of these materials can help lower implant failure rates and enhance patient satisfaction.

15.7.2 Types of Medical Implants

15.7.2.1 Orthopedic Implants

Devices called orthopedic implants are used to replace or fix fractured bones and joints. They are often used to treat degenerative joint issues, arthritis, and fractures. These implants include knee and hip replacements, bone plates, fracture-healing screws and pins, and cartilage implants for those with osteoarthritis. Orthopedic implants have many benefits, but they can also fail for a number of reasons, including infection, mechanical wear, and implant loosening (Saeidi et al., 2019).

15.7.2.2 Cardiovascular Implants

Medical devices called cardiovascular implants are used to treat conditions related to the heart, including arrhythmias, heart failure, and coronary artery disease. These implants include heart valves, pacemakers, defibrillators, and stents. The goals of cardiovascular implants are to improve blood flow, control cardiac rhythm, and provide mechanical support for the heart. It is frequently used to increase blood flow, reduce the risk of a heart attack, and treat chest pain. Conversely, there are several reasons why cardiovascular implants could malfunction, such as thrombosis, infection, and mechanical failure (Arjmandi et al., 2018). The performance of cardiovascular stents has been greatly enhanced by the use of nanocomposite materials, particularly in terms of biocompatibility and hemocompatibility. Improved biocompatibility and hemocompatibility are benefits of biodegradable polymeric nanocomposites, including poly(lactic-co-glycolic acid) (PLGA) supplemented with nanoparticles like hydroxyapatite or bioactive glass. These nanocomposites have strong mechanical qualities in addition to strong biocompatibility and bioactivity (Bressloff, 2014; Ono & Varma, 2017).

15.7.2.3 Dental Implants

Dental implants serve as a replacement for lost teeth. Usually made of titanium or other biocompatible materials, they are surgically inserted into the mandible. Dental restorations like crowns, bridges, and dentures have a sturdy and long-lasting base thanks to dental implants. Implant loosening, implant fracture, or infection are the possible causes of these implant failures

15.7.2.4 Neurological Implants

Neurological disorders such as chronic pain, Parkinson's disease, and epilepsy are to be treated by neurological implants. Among these implants are spinal cord stimulators, vagus nerve stimulators, and deep brain stimulators. The purpose of neurological implants is to alter brain circuit activity in order to lessen symptoms and enhance quality of life. Lead fracture, mechanical malfunction, and infection are the primary causes of neurological implant failure (Elsanadidy et al., 2022).

15.7.2.5 Breast Implants

Breast implants are used for breast augmentation and reconstruction. They are surgically implanted into the breast tissue and are typically made of silicone or silicone shells filled with saline. Breast implants are intended to address breast asymmetry, restore breast volume following a mastectomy, and enhance the appearance of the breasts. Implant rupture, capsular contracture, and infection are three reasons why breast implants can malfunction (Arjmandi & Ramezani, 2019b; Mostakhdemin et al., 2021).

15.7.3 Types of Nanocomposites for Bioimplants

15.7.3.1 Metal-based Nanocomposites

Orthopedic and dental implants are among the many medical implant applications for which metal-based nanocomposites are being researched. Nanoparticles of titanium dioxide (TiO_2) scattered throughout titanium alloys are one instance. TiO_2 can enhance the biocompatibility and corrosion resistance of titanium alloys, which are frequently utilized in dental and orthopedic implants (Liu et al., 2016). TiO_2 is also well-known for its photocatalytic capabilities, which can be used to create antimicrobial implant coatings that can lessen the risk of infections linked to implants. Another illustration would be the application of silver nanoparticles to stainless steel, which can give the metal antibacterial qualities and lower the risk of infections related to implants. Many medical gadgets have included silver, a well-known antibacterial ingredient, to ward against infections (Govindaraj et al., 2017).

15.7.3.2 Polymer-based Nanocomposites

Carbon nanotube-reinforced polyetheretherketone (PEEK) is one type of polymer-based nanocomposite that is utilized in medical implants. Dental and spinal cage implants are among the many medical implants made with PEEK, a biocompatible polymer. PEEK's mechanical qualities, such as strength and stiffness, can be strengthened and its wear resistance increased by adding CNTs. CNTs are well-known for having exceptional mechanical qualities, including high stiffness and tensile strength, and combining them with PEEK can produce a nanocomposite that performs better mechanically. Furthermore, CNTs can give the polymer electrical conductivity, which may be advantageous for some implant applications (Sahu et al., 2021).

15.7.3.3 Ceramic-based Nanocomposites

For a variety of medical implant applications, including orthopedic and dental implants, ceramic-based nanocomposites are being investigated. Ceramics containing alumina (Al_2O_3) and zirconia (ZrO_2) nanoparticles are one example. Because of its biocompatibility and ability to improve alumina ceramics' mechanical strength, fracture toughness, and wear resistance, ZrO_2 is a good material for medical applications (Ramezani & Ripin, 2023).

15.8 FUTURE PERSPECTIVES AND POTENTIAL DEVELOPMENTS

Despite these challenges, the field of fluorescence bioimaging continues to advance rapidly. There are several potential developments on the horizon that may address current limitations. For instance, advancements in surface modification techniques can lead to improved biocompatibility and stability of nanocomposites. Emerging trends include the development of multifunctional nanocomposites that combine imaging capabilities with other functionalities such as drug delivery or therapeutic agents. Furthermore, the integration of artificial intelligence (AI) algorithms into fluorescence bioimaging systems holds promise for enhancing image analysis and interpretation. In conclusion, nanocomposites have demonstrated great potential in fluorescence bioimaging applications due to their unique properties. Their synthesis methods allow precise control over size, composition, and functionalization. Through various types of nanocomposites, such as squaraine dyes, BODIPY-pyridyl hydrazone probes, gold nanoparticles difunctionalized by tryptophan, and Eu^{3+}/Gd^{3+} co-doped fluoroapatite nanocrystals, fluorescence bioimaging techniques have been enhanced with improved sensitivity, resolution, targeting capabilities, and tissue-specific imaging. Nonetheless, challenges such as toxicity and stability issues must be addressed to ensure safe and effective utilization of nanocomposites in biological systems. Future developments may include advancements in surface modification techniques, multifunctional nanocomposites. Thus, nanocomposites hold great promise for the advancement of biomedical imaging techniques, enabling us to unlock deeper insights into complex biological processes.

15.9 CONCLUSION

Through the integration of nanomaterials, advancements in 3D bioimplants have opened up new possibilities in the field of biomedical engineering. By capitalizing on the unique properties and functionalities of nanomaterials, researchers have successfully improved biocompatibility, achieved targeted drug delivery, and enhanced the overall performance of bioimplants. However, challenges such as long-term safety and scale-up production need to be addressed before widespread clinical implementation can occur. Further research and collaboration across multiple disciplines, including materials science, biology, and medicine, are essential to advance this technology and ensure its successful utilization in patient care. As nanotechnology continues to evolve, it holds enormous potential in transforming healthcare and improving the quality of life for countless individuals.

REFERENCES

Alamgir, Md., Panchal, M., Mallick, A., Nayak, G. C., & Kumar Singh, S. (2023). Introduction of metal nanoparticles, dental applications, and their effects. In *Nanoparticles Reinforced Metal Nanocomposites* (pp. 23–52). Springer Nature Singapore. https://doi.org/10.1007/978-981-19-9729-7_2

Amin, R., Knowlton, S., Hart, A., Yenilmez, B., Ghaderinezhad, F., Katebifar, S., Messina, M., Khademhosseini, A., & Tasoglu, S. (2016). 3D-printed microfluidic devices. In *Biofabrication* (Vol. 8, Issue 2). Institute of Physics Publishing. https://doi.org/10.1088/1758-5090/8/2/022001

Ansarian, I., Shaeri, M. H., Ebrahimi, M., & Minárik, P. (2019). Tribological characterization of commercial pure titanium processed by multi-directional forging. *Acta Metallurgica Sinica (English Letters)*, 32(7), 857–868. https://doi.org/10.1007/s40195-019-00877-4

Arjmandi, M., & Ramezani, M. (2019a). Finite element modelling of sliding wear in three-dimensional textile hydrogel composites. *Tribology International*, 133, 88–100. https://doi.org/10.1016/j.triboint.2019.01.011

Arjmandi, M., & Ramezani, M. (2019b). Mechanical and tribological assessment of silica nanoparticle-alginate-polyacrylamide nanocomposite hydrogels as a cartilage replacement. *Journal of the Mechanical Behavior of Biomedical Materials*, 95, 196–204. https://doi.org/10.1016/j.jmbbm.2019.04.020

Arjmandi, M., Ramezani, M., Bolle, T., Köppe, G., Gries, T., & Neitzert, T. (2018). Mechanical and tribological properties of a novel hydrogel composite reinforced by three-dimensional woven textiles as a functional synthetic cartilage. *Composites Part A: Applied Science and Manufacturing*, 115, 123–133. https://doi.org/10.1016/j.compositesa.2018.09.018

Baker, B. A., Pine, P. S., Chatterjee, K., Kumar, G., Lin, N. J., McDaniel, J. H., Salit, M. L., & Simon, C. G. (2014). Ontology analysis of global gene expression differences of human bone marrow stromal cells cultured on 3D scaffolds or 2D films. *Biomaterials*, 35(25), 6716–6726. https://doi.org/10.1016/j.biomaterials.2014.04.075

Balint, R., Cassidy, N. J., & Cartmell, S. H. (2014). Conductive polymers: Towards a smart biomaterial for tissue engineering. In *Acta Biomaterialia* (Vol. 10, Issue 6, pp. 2341–2353). Elsevier Ltd. https://doi.org/10.1016/j.actbio.2014.02.015

Bressloff, N. W. (2014). Multi-objective design of a biodegradable coronary artery stent. In *Studies in Mechanobiology, Tissue Engineering and Biomaterials* (Vol. 15, pp. 1–28). Springer. https://doi.org/10.1007/8415_2013_164

Chang, Z., Liu, F., Wang, L., Deng, M., Zhou, C., Sun, Q., & Chu, J. (2019). Near-infrared dyes, nanomaterials and proteins. *Chinese Chemical Letters*, 30(10), 1856–1882. https://doi.org/10.1016/j.cclet.2019.08.034

Chen, M., & Yin, M. (2014). Design and development of fluorescent nanostructures for bioimaging. In *Progress in Polymer Science* (Vol. 39, Issue 2, pp. 365–395). https://doi.org/10.1016/j.progpolymsci.2013.11.001

Davoodi, E., Montazerian, H., Esmaeilizadeh, R., Darabi, A. C., Rashidi, A., Kadkhodapour, J., Jahed, H., Hoorfar, M., Milani, A. S., Weiss, P. S., Khademhosseini, A., & Toyserkani, E. (2021). Additively manufactured gradient porous Ti-6Al-4V hip replacement implants embedded with cell-laden gelatin methacryloyl hydrogels. *ACS Applied Materials and Interfaces*, 13(19), 22110–22123. https://doi.org/10.1021/acsami.0c20751

Deng, F., Liu, Y., Luo, X., Wu, S., Luo, S., Au, C., & Qi, R. (2014). Sol-hydrothermal synthesis of inorganic-framework molecularly imprinted TiO_2/SiO_2 nanocomposite and its preferential photocatalytic degradation towards target contaminant. *Journal of Hazardous Materials*, 278, 108–115. https://doi.org/10.1016/j.jhazmat.2014.05.088

Elsanadidy, E., Mosa, I. M., Hou, B., Schmid, T., El-Kady, M. F., Khan, R. S., Haeberlin, A., Tzingounis, A. V., & Rusling, J. F. (2022). Self-sustainable intermittent deep brain stimulator. *Cell Reports Physical Science*, *3*(10). https://doi.org/10.1016/j.xcrp.2022.101099

Erdem, B., & İşcan, K. B. (2021). Multifunctional magnetic mesoporous nano-composites towards multiple applications in dye and oil adsorption. *Journal of Sol-Gel Science and Technology*, *98*(3), 528–540. https://doi.org/10.1007/s10971-021-05528-8

Fernández-Lizárraga, M., García-López, J., Rodil, S. E., Ribas-Aparicio, R. M., & Silva-Bermudez, P. (2022). Evaluation of the biocompatibility and osteogenic properties of metal oxide coatings applied by magnetron sputtering as potential biofunctional surface modifications for orthopedic implants. *Materials*, *15*(15). https://doi.org/10.3390/ma15155240

Fukushima, T., Kosaka, A., Yamamoto, Y., Aimiya, T., Notazawa, S., Takigawa, T., Inabe, T., & Aida, T. (2006). Dramatic effect of dispersed carbon nanotubes on the mechanical and electroconductive properties of polymers derived from ionic liquids. *Small*, *2*(4), 554–560. https://doi.org/10.1002/smll.200500404

Gedara, S. M. K., Ding, Z. Y., Balasooriya, I. L., Han, Y., & Wickramaratne, M. N. (2022). Hydrothermal synthesis and in vivo fluorescent bioimaging application of Eu3+/Gd3+ co-doped fluoroapatite nanocrystals. *Journal of Functional Biomaterials*, *13*(3). https://doi.org/10.3390/jfb13030108

Giordano, M., Schmid, S., Arjmandi, M., & Ramezani, M. (2017). Wear evaluation of three-dimensionally woven materials for use in a novel cartilage replacement. *Wear*, *386–387*, 179–187. https://doi.org/10.1016/j.wear.2017.06.012

Govindaraj, D., Rajan, M., Munusamy, M. A., Alarfaj, A. A., & Suresh Kumar, S. (2017). Mineral-substituted hydroxyapatite reinforced poly(raffinose-citric acid)-polyethylene glycol nanocomposite enhances osteogenic differentiation and induces ectopic bone formation. *New Journal of Chemistry*, *41*(8), 3036–3047. https://doi.org/10.1039/C7NJ00398F

Kandavalli, S. R., Wang, Q., Ebrahimi, M., Gode, C., Djavanroodi, F., Attarilar, S., & Liu, S. (2021). A brief review on the evolution of metallic dental implants: history, design, and application. In *Frontiers in Materials* (Vol. 8). Frontiers Media S.A. https://doi.org/10.3389/fmats.2021.646383

Kolahalam, L. A., Kasi Viswanath, I. V., Diwakar, B. S., Govindh, B., Reddy, V., & Murthy, Y. L. N. (2019). Review on nanomaterials: Synthesis and applications. *Materials Today: Proceedings*, *18*, 2182–2190. https://doi.org/10.1016/j.matpr.2019.07.371

Kumar, H., Justa, P., Jaswal, N., Pani, B., & Kumar, I. (2023). Biomimetic and bioinspired composite processing for biomedical applications. In *Advanced Materials and Manufacturing Techniques for Biomedical Applications* (pp. 211–239). John Wiley & Sons, Inc. https://doi.org/10.1002/9781394166985.ch9

Kumar, M., Kumar, R., & Kumar, S. (2021). Synergistic effect of carbon nanotubes and nano-hydroxyapatite on mechanical properties of polyetheretherketone based hybrid nanocomposites. *Polymers and Polymer Composites*, *29*(9), 1365–1376. https://doi.org/10.1177/0967391120969503

Kumar, S., Nehra, M., Kedia, D., Dilbaghi, N., Tankeshwar, K., & Kim, K. H. (2020). Nanotechnology-based biomaterials for orthopaedic applications: Recent advances and future prospects. In *Materials Science and Engineering C* (Vol. 106). Elsevier Ltd. https://doi.org/10.1016/j.msec.2019.110154

Kumar, S., Sarita, Nehra, M., Dilbaghi, N., Tankeshwar, K., & Kim, K. H. (2018). Recent advances and remaining challenges for polymeric nanocomposites in healthcare applications. In *Progress in Polymer Science* (Vol. 80, pp. 1–38). Elsevier Ltd. https://doi.org/10.1016/j.progpolymsci.2018.03.001

Kundu, S., Satpati, B., Mukherjee, M., Kar, T., & Pradhan, S. K. (2017). Hydrothermal synthesis of polyaniline intercalated vanadium oxide xerogel hybrid nanocomposites: Effective control of morphology and structural characterization. *New Journal of Chemistry, 41*(9), 3634–3645. https://doi.org/10.1039/c7nj00372b

Lee, J., Lee, J. B., Yun, J., Rhyu, I. C., Lee, Y. M., Lee, S. M., Lee, M. K., Kim, B., Kim, P., & Koo, K. T. (2021). The impact of surface treatment in 3-dimensional printed implants for early osseointegration: A comparison study of three different surfaces. *Scientific Reports, 11*(1). https://doi.org/10.1038/s41598-021-89961-3

Li, J., & Zhu, J. J. (2013). Quantum dots for fluorescent biosensing and bio-imaging applications. In *Analyst* (Vol. 138, Issue 9, pp. 2506–2515). Royal Society of Chemistry. https://doi.org/10.1039/c3an36705c

Liu, C., Chan, K. W., Shen, J., Liao, C. Z., Yeung, K. W. K., & Tjong, S. C. (2016). Polyetheretherketone hybrid composites with bioactive nanohydroxyapatite and multiwalled carbon nanotube fillers. *Polymers, 8*(12). https://doi.org/10.3390/polym8120425

Luo, Y., Dolder, C. K., Walker, J. M., Mishra, R., Dean, D., & Becker, M. L. (2016). Synthesis and biological evaluation of well-defined poly(propylene fumarate) oligomers and their use in 3D printed scaffolds. *Biomacromolecules, 17*(2), 690–697. https://doi.org/10.1021/acs.biomac.6b00014

Ma, C., Peng, L., Feng, Y., Shen, J., Xiao, Z., Cai, K., Yu, Y., Min, Y., & Epstein, A. J. (2016). Polyfurfuryl alcohol spheres template synthesis of 3D porous graphene for high-performance supercapacitor application. *Synthetic Metals, 220*, 227–235. https://doi.org/10.1016/j.synthmet.2016.06.008

Mostakhdemin, M., Nand, A., & Ramezani, M. (2021). Articular and artificial cartilage, characteristics, properties and testing approaches—a review. In *Polymers* (Vol. 13, Issue 12). MDPI AG. https://doi.org/10.3390/polym13122000

Nootem, J., Sattayanon, C., Daengngern, R., Kamkaew, A., Wattanathana, W., Wannapaiboon, S., Rashatasakhon, P., & Chansaenpak, K. (2021). Bodipy-pyridylhydrazone probe for fluorescence turn-on detection of fe3+ and its bioimaging application. *Chemosensors, 9*(7). https://doi.org/10.3390/chemosensors9070165

Normand, G., Mija, A., Pagnotta, S., Peuvrel-Disdier, E., & Vergnes, B. (2017). Preparation of polypropylene nanocomposites by melt-mixing: Comparison between three organoclays. *Journal of Applied Polymer Science, 134*(28). https://doi.org/10.1002/app.45053

Ono, M., & Varma, N. (2017). Remote monitoring to Improve long-term prognosis in heart failure patients with implantable cardioverter-defibrillators. In *Expert Review of Medical Devices* (Vol. 14, Issue 5, pp. 335–342). Taylor and Francis Ltd. https://doi.org/10.1080/17434440.2017.1306438

Pajović, J. D., Dojčilovi´dojčilović, R. J., Kaščáková, S., Réfrégiers, M., Božanić, D. K., Djoković(n.d). Enhanced resonance energy transfer in gold nanoparticles bifunctionalized by tryptophan and riboflavin and its application in fluorescence bioimaging . https://ssrn.com/abstract=4384285

Poon, W., Kingston, B. R., Ouyang, B., Ngo, W., & Chan, W. C. W. (2020). A framework for designing delivery systems. In *Nature Nanotechnology* (Vol. 15, Issue 10, pp. 819–829). Nature Research. https://doi.org/10.1038/s41565-020-0759-5

Ramezani, M., & Ripin, Z. M. (2023). An overview of enhancing the performance of medical implants with nanocomposites. In *Journal of Composites Science* (Vol. 7, Issue 5). MDPI. https://doi.org/10.3390/jcs7050199

Saeidi, M., Ramezani, M., Kelly, P., Neitzert, T., & Kumar, P. (2019). Preliminary study on a novel minimally invasive extra-articular implant for unicompartmental knee osteoarthritis. *Medical Engineering and Physics*, 67, 96–101. https://doi.org/10.1016/j.medengphy.2019.02.016

Sahu, G., Rajput, M. S., & Mahapatra, S. P. (2021). Polylactic acid nanocomposites for biomedical applications: effects of calcium phosphate, and magnesium phosphate nanoparticles concentration. *Plastics, Rubber and Composites*, *50*(5), 228–240. https://doi.org/10.1080/14658011.2021.1871818

Sevost'yanov, M. A., Nasakina, E. O., Baikin, A. S., Sergienko, K. V., Konushkin, S. V., Kaplan, M. A., Seregin, A. V., Leonov, A. V., Kozlov, V. A., Shkirin, A. V., Bunkin, N. F., Kolmakov, A. G., Simakov, S. V., & Gudkov, S. V. (2018). Biocompatibility of new materials based on nano-structured nitinol with titanium and tantalum composite surface layers: Experimental analysis in vitro and in vivo. *Journal of Materials Science: Materials in Medicine*, *29*(3). https://doi.org/10.1007/s10856-018-6039-3

Singh Sidhu, V. P., Marchi, J., Borges, R., & Naghizadeh Raeisi, E. (2022). Surface modification of metallic orthopedic implants for anti-pathogenic characteristics. *Journal of Composites and Compounds*, 4(10), 51–60. https://doi.org/10.52547/jcc.4.1.6

Takeuchi, K., Maira, B., Terano, M., & Taniike, T. (2017). Templated synthesis of nano-sized silica in confined amorphous space of polypropylene. *Composites Science and Technology*, *140*, 1–7. https://doi.org/10.1016/j.compscitech.2016.12.025

Thu, M. K., Kang, Y. S., Kwak, J. M., Jo, Y. H., Han, J. S., & Yeo, I. S. L. (2023). Comparison between bone–implant interfaces of microtopographically modified zirconia and titanium implants. *Scientific Reports*, *13*(1). https://doi.org/10.1038/s41598-023-38432-y

Viswambari Devi, R., Doble, M., & Verma, R. S. (2015). Nanomaterials for early detection of cancer biomarker with special emphasis on gold nanoparticles in immunoassays/sensors. In *Biosensors and Bioelectronics* (Vol. 68, pp. 688–698). Elsevier Ltd. https://doi.org/10.1016/j.bios.2015.01.066

Wang, Q., Zhou, P., Liu, S., Attarilar, S., Ma, R. L. W., Zhong, Y., & Wang, L. (2020). Multi-scale surface treatments of titanium implants for rapid osseointegration: A review. In *Nanomaterials* (Vol. 10, Issue 6, pp. 1–27). MDPI AG. https://doi.org/10.3390/nano10061244

Wang, X., Jiang, M., Zhou, Z., Gou, J., & Hui, D. (2017). 3D printing of polymer matrix composites: A review and prospective. In *Composites Part B: Engineering* (Vol. 110, pp. 442–458). Elsevier Ltd. https://doi.org/10.1016/j.compositesb.2016.11.034

Wolfbeis, O. S. (2015). An overview of nanoparticles commonly used in fluorescent bioimaging. In *Chemical Society Reviews* (Vol. 44, Issue 14, pp. 4743–4768). Royal Society of Chemistry. https://doi.org/10.1039/c4cs00392f

Yang, F., Chen, C., Zhou, Q., Gong, Y., Li, R., Li, C., Klämpfl, F., Freund, S., Wu, X., Sun, Y., Li, X., Schmidt, M., Ma, D., & Yu, Y. (2017). Laser beam melting 3D printing of Ti6Al4V based porous structured dental implants: Fabrication, biocompatibility analysis and photoelastic study. *Scientific Reports, 7.* https://doi.org/10.1038/srep45360

Zhang, X., Zhang, X., Tao, L., Chi, Z., Xu, J., & Wei, Y. (2014). Aggregation induced emission-based fluorescent nanoparticles: Fabrication methodologies and biomedical applications. In *Journal of Materials Chemistry B* (Vol. 2, Issue 28, pp. 4398–4414). Royal Society of Chemistry. https://doi.org/10.1039/c4tb00291a

Zhao, J., Xie, Y., Li, M., Xu, F., Le, Z., Qin, Y., Zhou, D., Wang, Z., Xu, H., Pan, J., & Ling, Y. (2014). Preparation of magnetic-conductive Mn0.6Zn0.4Fe2O4-CNTs/PANI nanocomposites through hydrothermal synthesis coupled with in situ polymerization. *Composites Science and Technology, 99,* 147–153. https://doi.org/10.1016/j.compscitech.2014.05.023

Challenges and Perspectives of Polymeric Nanocomposites for Biomedical Applications

Milad Heidari, Sulaiman Al Hasani,
Sivasakthivel Thangavel, and Ashwani Kumar

16.1 INTRODUCTION

Polymeric nanocomposites have emerged as innovative materials in the field of biomedical applications by presenting as a versatile platform for addressing complex challenges. These nanocomposites consist of a combination of polymeric matrices and nanoscale fillers which exhibits unique and customizable properties that make them highly suitable for a range of biomedical purposes. The incorporation of nanofillers, such as nanoparticles or nanotubes, into polymer matrices has paved the way for improved mechanical strength, controlled drug release, and enhanced biocompatibility. The ability to precisely adjust the composition and structure of these materials allows for precise customization, enabling researchers and engineers to design platforms tailored to specific biomedical needs. Polymeric nanocomposites have demonstrated exceptional versatility in their applications ranging from advanced drug delivery systems to tissue engineering scaffolds and diagnostic imaging agents. Their nanoscale dimensions facilitate molecular-level interactions and targeted delivery minimizing side effects and optimizing therapeutic outcomes. Moreover, the integration of nanocomposites in diagnostic imaging has revolutionized detection and imaging modalities pushing the boundaries of precision and sensitivity. As we explore the challenges and perspectives surrounding these materials, it becomes clear that the unique properties of polymeric nanocomposites hold great promise for overcoming obstacles in biomedical research and clinical applications. This chapter aims to provide a comprehensive exploration of the challenges and perspectives associated with harnessing the potential of polymeric nanocomposites while shedding light on their transformative role in shaping the future of biomedical technologies [1–3].

The significance of polymeric nanocomposites in contemporary biomedical research is emphasized by their unparalleled ability to overcome long-standing challenges and pave the way for new frontiers in medical applications. These advanced materials have become key players due to their unique combination of polymer matrices with nanoscale fillers, thus surpassing the properties of traditional materials. One of the crucial

DOI: 10.1201/9781003470311-16

aspects contributing to their significance is their inherent adjustability. The precise tailoring of nanofiller composition, size, and distribution within the polymeric matrix allows for precise control over mechanical, thermal, and biological properties. This adjustability is essential in designing materials that can seamlessly integrate with biological systems; offering improved biocompatibility and reduced toxicity.

Polymeric nanocomposites play a crucial role in the development of next-generation drug delivery systems by leveraging their controlled release capabilities to provide a strategic advantage. By utilizing the unique surface properties and biodegradability of polymeric matrices, these nanocomposites enable sustained and targeted drug delivery while minimizing side effects and maximizing therapeutic efficacy. Furthermore, their application extends to tissue engineering where the design of biomimetic scaffolds with enhanced mechanical strength and biocompatibility is vital for successful tissue regeneration. The versatility of polymeric nanocomposites is evident in their role in diagnostic imaging. With the integration of nanofillers; these materials can function as contrast agents, enhancing imaging modalities, and offering clinicians unprecedented precision in diagnostics. This is particularly crucial in early disease detection, improving patient outcomes, and treatment efficacy [4, 5].

In addition to their practical applications, the significance of polymeric nanocomposites is also evident in their contribution to scientific comprehension. These materials serve as a connection between nanotechnology, materials science, and biomedicine, fostering interdisciplinary collaboration. Their investigation not only advances technological applications but also provides valuable insights into the fundamental interactions between nanomaterials and biological systems.

As we navigate the complexities of contemporary healthcare challenges, the importance of polymeric nanocomposites becomes increasingly apparent. Their capacity to address multifaceted issues, from controlled drug delivery to tissue regeneration and advanced imaging, positions them as indispensable tools in the pursuit of innovative and effective biomedical solutions. This chapter delves into the numerous facets of challenges and perspectives associated with polymeric nanocomposites while shedding light on their pivotal role in shaping the landscape of biomedical engineering.

The aim of this chapter is to provide a comprehensive exploration of the challenges and perspectives surrounding polymeric nanocomposites in biomedical applications. It aims to clarify the unique properties of these advanced materials, their significance in addressing critical biomedical issues, and the evolving landscape of research in this field. The scope encompasses an in-depth analysis of the fundamental aspects, diverse applications, and emerging trends in polymeric nanocomposites. By offering insights into the challenges faced and innovative solutions, this chapter serves as a valuable resource for researchers, practitioners, and students seeking a deeper understanding of the dynamic intersection between nanotechnology and biomedical engineering.

16.2 FUNDAMENTALS OF POLYMERIC NANOCOMPOSITES

The fundamentals of polymeric nanocomposites lay the groundwork for understanding their transformative role in biomedical applications. These materials, characterized by the integration of nanoscale fillers within polymer matrices, exhibit distinctive properties critical for their success. Exploring their definition, types, and key characteristics unveils the versatile nature of polymeric nanocomposites. Understanding their unique attributes, such as enhanced mechanical strength and controlled release capabilities, provides a foundation for their application in drug delivery systems, tissue engineering, and diagnostic imaging. Delving into the fundamentals is paramount for appreciating the tailored design possibilities that make polymeric nanocomposites integral to advancements in biomedical technologies [2, 6].

16.2.1 Types of Polymeric Nanocomposites

Polymeric nanocomposites, an advanced material class at the forefront of contemporary research, are characterized by the integration of nanoscale fillers within polymer matrices. This amalgamation imparts distinctive and customizable properties to the resulting nanocomposites by making them versatile for a variety of applications. The classification of polymeric nanocomposites is nuanced and dependent on the nature of the polymer matrix and the nanofiller. This section presents a comprehensive academic and professional discourse on the types of polymeric nanocomposites by elucidating their unique characteristics and applications.

16.2.1.1 Organoclay-based Nanocomposites

Organoclay-based nanocomposites are created by incorporating modified clay minerals, such as montmorillonite, into a polymer matrix. The modification process involves intercalating organic molecules into the clay layers, thus enhancing compatibility with the polymer. This type of nanocomposite exhibits improved mechanical strength, thermal stability, and gas barrier properties. Common polymer matrices include polyethylene, polypropylene, and polyamide. Organoclay-based nanocomposites find applications in packaging materials, automotive components, and flame-retardant systems.

16.2.1.2 Carbon-based Nanocomposites

Carbon-based nanocomposites involve the incorporation of carbonaceous nanofillers like carbon nanotubes (CNTs) and graphene into polymer matrices. These nanocomposites exhibit exceptional mechanical, thermal, and electrical properties due to the unique structure of carbon allotropes. CNT-reinforced nanocomposites, for instance, demonstrate remarkable tensile strength and electrical conductivity while making them suitable for applications in structural materials, sensors, and conductive polymers. The dispersion and alignment of carbon nanofillers significantly impact the overall performance of these nanocomposites.

16.2.1.3 Metal-based Nanocomposites

Metal-based nanocomposites incorporate metallic nanoparticles, such as silver, gold, or magnetic nanoparticles within a polymer matrix. These nanocomposites often exhibit enhanced antimicrobial properties, making them valuable in medical applications, such as wound dressings and drug delivery systems. Additionally, magnetic nanoparticles contribute to responsive materials for targeted drug delivery and imaging applications. The interaction between the metallic nanoparticles and the polymer matrix influences the overall properties and functionalities of these nanocomposites.

16.2.1.4 Polymer–Clay Nanocomposites

Polymer–clay nanocomposites involve the integration of layered clay minerals, such as kaolinite or smectite, into a polymer matrix. Unlike organo-clay-based nanocomposites, polymer–clay nanocomposites may not involve organic modifications of the clay. The layered structure of the clay imparts improved barrier properties, flame resistance, and mechanical strength to the polymer matrix. These nanocomposites find applications in packaging materials, coatings, and flame-retardant polymers.

16.2.1.5 Silica-based Nanocomposites

Silica-based nanocomposites involve the incorporation of silica nanoparticles or nanosilicates into polymer matrices. The unique properties of silica, such as high surface area and optical transparency, contribute to the enhanced mechanical, thermal, and barrier properties of the resulting nanocomposites. Common polymer matrices include epoxy, polyurethane, and silicone. Silica-based nanocomposites are utilized in coatings, adhesives, and electronic devices due to their improved mechanical and thermal stability.

16.2.1.6 Biopolymer-based Nanocomposites

Biopolymer-based nanocomposites utilize natural polymers, such as chitosan, cellulose, or starch, as the matrix material combined with nanofillers. These nanocomposites are of particular interest in biomedical applications due to their biocompatibility and sustainability. The incorporation of nanofillers enhances the mechanical strength, thermal stability, and biodegradability of biopolymer matrices. Biopolymer-based nanocomposites find applications in drug delivery, tissue engineering, and environmentally friendly packaging materials.

16.2.2 Key Properties Influencing Biomedical Applications

The Table 16.1 and Figure 16.1 provide a structured overview of the key properties influencing biomedical applications of polymeric nanocomposites while offering a quick reference for researchers and practitioners in the field.

16.3 BIOMEDICAL APPLICATIONS

Polymeric nanocomposites have garnered significant attention and promise in the realm of biomedical applications by offering a multifaceted approach to address complex challenges in healthcare (Figure 16.2). Their unique properties, stemming from the integration of nanoscale fillers into polymer matrices, make them particularly well-suited for a diverse array of applications [7].

16.3.1 Drug Delivery Systems

Polymeric nanocomposites play a pivotal role in revolutionizing drug delivery systems. Their controlled release capabilities allow for precise modulation of drug release kinetics, thereby ensuring therapeutic agents are delivered in a targeted and sustained manner. This not only enhances the efficacy of treatments but also minimizes side effects, a critical consideration in developing patient-centric pharmaceutical solutions. Polymeric nanocomposites have considerable potential in drug delivery, but several challenges need to be addressed for their optimal use. The delicate balance between therapeutic effectiveness and safety necessitates careful evaluation of potential immune responses due to concerns about biocompatibility and toxicity. Achieving precise drug release profiles for various therapeutic regimens is challenging due to controlled release kinetics, which are influenced by the choice of polymer and environmental factors. Maintaining stability over long periods is essential, and issues such as polymer degradation and

Table 16.1 Key properties influencing biomedical applications of polymeric nanocomposites

Key property	Explanation	Impact on biomedical applications
Biocompatibility	The ability to interact harmoniously with biological systems without causing toxicity or immune responses.	Essential to prevent adverse reactions, immune responses, and ensure compatibility in medical applications.
Mechanical Strength	The resistance to deformation or rupture is critical for structural support in applications like tissue engineering.	Crucial in tissue engineering where scaffolds need to mimic natural tissues and provide mechanical integrity.
Controlled Release	The ability to regulate the release kinetics of therapeutic agents.	Critical in drug delivery systems to achieve precise and targeted therapeutic outcomes.
Surface Chemistry	The chemical composition of the nanocomposite surface impacts cellular adhesion and bioactivity.	Influences interactions with biological entities, modulates bioactivity, and facilitates targeted applications.
Degradation Rate	The rate at which the nanocomposite degrades over time.	Important for biodegradable implants and drug delivery systems to align with therapeutic timelines and prevent unnecessary persistence.
Thermal Stability	The ability to withstand elevated temperatures during processing or exposure ensuring structural integrity.	Crucial during manufacturing and sterilization processes to maintain structural integrity.
Imaging Contrast	The nanocomposite's ability to act as a contrast agent in imaging modalities enhancing visualization.	Significant in diagnostic imaging for clearer visualization of tissues or targeted areas.
Electrical Conductivity	The capacity to conduct electrical currents often conferred by carbon-based nanofillers.	Essential for applications requiring electrical conductivity, such as neural interfaces or sensors.

nanofiller aggregation need to be addressed to ensure consistent performance in complex biological environments [8–10].

To translate these findings into clinical applications, rigorous regulatory scrutiny is necessary focusing on the safety, scalability, and reproducibility of results. Collaboration among researchers, industry partners, and regulatory bodies is crucial to bridge the gap between successful preclinical

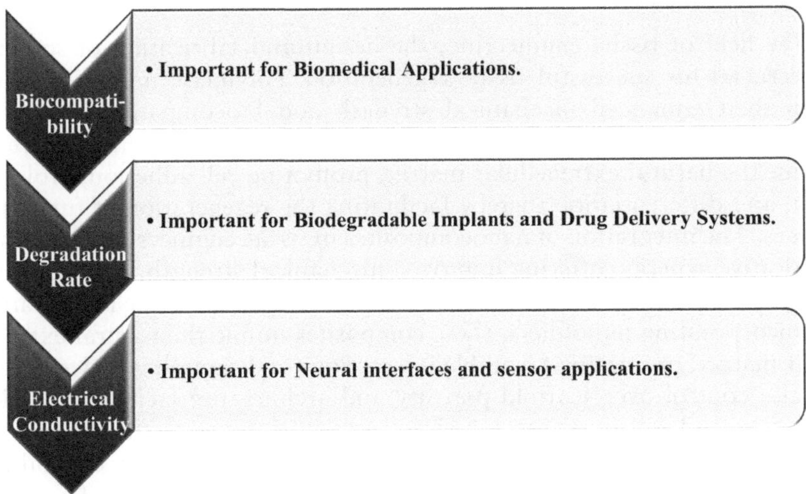

Figure 16.1 Three key properties of polymeric nanocomposites.

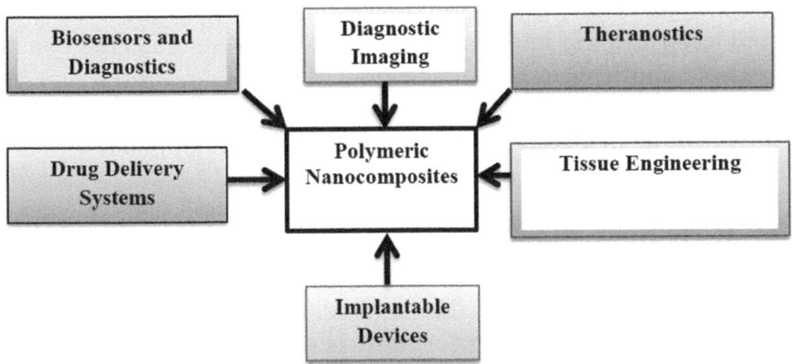

Figure 16.2 Different applications of polymeric nanocomposites.

outcomes and clinical implementation. Designing innovative strategies is necessary to address the formidable challenges of achieving targeted drug delivery, minimizing off-target effects, and optimizing nanocomposites' responses to biological cues. Large-scale manufacturing also poses challenges in terms of reproducibility, batch consistency, and cost-effectiveness. Interactions with complex biological environments add another layer of complexity to drug delivery applications, requiring a nuanced understanding and mitigation of influences from proteins, enzymes, and other biological components. Addressing these challenges collectively is essential to unlock the full potential of polymeric nanocomposites in advancing drug delivery systems.

16.3.1.1 Tissue Engineering

In the field of tissue engineering, the design and fabrication of scaffolds are crucial for successful tissue regeneration. Polymeric nanocomposites, with their enhanced mechanical strength and biocompatibility, provide an ideal platform for constructing biomimetic scaffolds. These scaffolds mimic the natural extracellular matrix, promoting cell adhesion, proliferation, and differentiation thereby facilitating the regeneration of functional tissues. The integration of nanocomposites in tissue engineering presents an innovative synergy, offering improved mechanical strength, enhanced biocompatibility, and controlled drug delivery for optimal tissue regeneration. By incorporating nanofillers, these composites mimic the natural extracellular matrix, promoting favorable interactions and signaling between cells. Precise control over scaffold porosity and architecture facilitates nutrient diffusion and cell ingrowth which are critical for successful tissue development. Additionally, some nanocomposites have imaging capabilities, allowing real-time monitoring of tissue regeneration progress. Their anti-inflammatory and antimicrobial properties contribute to minimizing complications during the regeneration process [11, 12].

However, challenges such as long-term biocompatibility, potential toxicity of nanomaterials, and regulatory considerations must be carefully addressed to ensure the safety and efficacy of tissue-engineered constructs. Despite these challenges, the integration of nanocomposites represents a transformative approach in regenerative medicine providing a versatile toolkit to advance the field and enable innovative clinical applications.

16.3.1.2 Diagnostic Imaging

In diagnostic imaging, polymeric nanocomposites serve as versatile contrast agents. Their unique optical, magnetic, or acoustic properties enhance imaging contrast thus allowing for more accurate and thorough visualization of anatomical structures or pathological conditions. This capability improves accuracy in medical diagnostics and facilitates the early detection of diseases.

By leveraging the unique characteristics of nanomaterials, the integration of nanocomposites for enhanced medical imaging is transforming the field of medical diagnostics. These materials act as highly effective contrast agents by enhancing visibility in various imaging techniques such as Magnetic Resonance Imaging (MRI), Computed Tomography (CT), and fluorescence imaging. The functionalization of nanocomposites allows for targeted imaging by attaching specific ligands to selectively bind to cells or tissues thus improving specificity and enabling early detection of diseases. Additionally, nanocomposites have the potential to enable multimodal imaging by combining different techniques to provide more comprehensive diagnostic insights. The ability to monitor in real-time and integrate nanocomposites into theranostic platforms, which combine diagnostic imaging with therapy, further contributes to personalized medicine [13, 14].

For example, in the case of MRI, superparamagnetic iron oxide nanoparticles (SPIONs) are often used as contrast agents due to their superparamagnetic properties, which significantly enhance the contrast by affecting the relaxation times of nearby water protons and therefore resulting in a higher signal-to-noise ratio (SNR). This enhancement allows for clearer delineation of anatomical structures and pathologies [15]. Additionally, Gadolinium-based nanomaterials are considered contrast agents in MR imaging due to their paramagnetic properties. They enhance the relaxation rate of water protons in their vicinity, leading to increased signal intensity in T1-weighted images [16]. When it comes to CT imaging, which uses X-ray, gold nanoparticles (AuNPs) and other high atomic number materials are used as contrast agents due to their high X-ray attenuation coefficients. These materials provide significant contrast by efficiently absorbing X-rays, thus enhancing the visibility of the target tissues or organs. The enhanced contrast is directly related to the high density and atomic number of the nanocomposite components, which increases the X-ray attenuation compared to surrounding tissues [17].

In fluorescence imaging, lanthanide-doped nanoconstructs (LDNCs) and quantum dots (QDs) are utilized for their ability to emit bright fluorescence upon excitation. LDNCs can emit in the near-infrared (NIR) range, offering deeper tissue penetration and reduced autofluorescence for clearer imaging. The mechanism involves upconversion and downconversion processes where the absorption of photons leads to emission at a different wavelength facilitating the use of these materials in bioimaging applications [18]. Quantum dots' size-tunable fluorescence and high photostability make them ideal for long-term imaging and multiplexing applications thus enabling the tracking of multiple targets simultaneously [19].

With these enhancements, there are challenges to consider for the safe clinical implementation of nanocomposites such as biocompatibility, potential toxicity, and long-term effects. Despite these challenges, ongoing advancements in nanotechnology show great promise in reshaping diagnostic imaging, providing a versatile toolkit to overcome limitations and improve the accuracy and effectiveness of medical diagnostics.

16.3.1.3 Implantable Devices

In the field of implantable medical devices, polymeric nanocomposites with tailored properties and biocompatibility play a crucial role. These materials offer improved integration with host tissues, reduced risk of rejection, and enhanced durability for various applications including orthopedic implants and cardiovascular stents. The controlled degradation of certain nanocomposites aligns with the natural healing process, making them suitable for temporary implants.

16.3.1.4 Biosensors and Diagnostics

Polymeric nanocomposites also contribute to the development of highly sensitive biosensors for diagnostic purposes. Their ability to interact with biological molecules and possess electrical conductivity or optical properties makes them valuable in creating biosensing platforms. This is especially important for the rapid and accurate detection of biomarkers associated with different diseases.

16.3.1.5 Theranostics

The integration of therapeutic and diagnostic capabilities, known as theranostics, is an advanced application of polymeric nanocomposites. These materials can deliver therapeutic agents while providing real-time imaging feedback. This comprehensive approach allows for personalized and precise treatment strategiesthus leading to advancements in individualized medicine.

16.4 CHALLENGES IN POLYMERIC NANOCOMPOSITES FOR BIOMEDICAL APPLICATIONS

The use of polymeric nanocomposites in biomedical applications presents unprecedented opportunities ranging from drug delivery systems to tissue engineering. However, this field is not without its challenges, and a thorough exploration is necessary to fully harness the potential of polymeric nanocomposites in healthcare. This includes considerations of biocompatibility and toxicity as achieving a delicate balance between utilizing the unique properties of nanomaterials and ensuring compatibility with biological systems is crucial. The introduction of nanofillers can introduce foreign elements thus raising concerns about potential adverse reactions and cytotoxicity.

16.4.1 Biocompatibility and Toxicity Concerns

Biocompatibility and toxicity are critical considerations in the utilization of polymeric nanocomposites for biomedical purposes. The attainment of a delicate equilibrium between harnessing the distinctive properties of nanomaterials and ensuring their compatibility with biological systems is of utmost importance. The incorporation of nanofillers can introduce foreign elements therefore giving rise to concerns regarding potential adverse reactions and cytotoxicity. In essence, biocompatibility refers to the ability of polymeric nanocomposites to interact harmoniously with living tissues without eliciting detrimental responses. To ensure the safe integration of these materials in biological environments, comprehensive evaluations of their biocompatibility are essential. This involves assessing the impact on cellular viability, potential inflammatory responses, and systemic effects ensuring that nanocomposites do not compromise the health of the host organism [20, 21].

Simultaneously, the issue of toxicity emphasizes the need to discern any harmful effects arising from the presence of nanomaterials. Evaluating the toxicity of polymeric nanocomposites entails understanding their fate within biological systems, potential long-term effects, and the intricate dynamics of interactions with cellular components. Thorough investigations are necessary to mitigate risks and establish the foundation for the responsible and ethical use of polymeric nanocomposites in biomedical applications. As researchers navigate the frontiers of nanotechnology, addressing biocompatibility and toxicity concerns becomes pivotal for advancing the transformative potential of polymeric nanocomposites in healthcare.

16.4.2 Long-term Stability and Degradation

Long-term stability and controlled degradation are crucial aspects in the successful application of polymeric nanocomposites for biomedical purposes. These materials must withstand the dynamic and often harsh biological environment while maintaining their structural integrity over extended periods. The challenge lies in striking a balance between the need for stability and the controlled degradation required for specific applications. Polymeric nanocomposites used in implants or drug delivery systems, for instance, must exhibit a gradual and predictable degradation rate aligned with therapeutic timelines. Achieving this balance is essential to prevent premature material breakdown or persistent presence beyond the required duration [22, 23].

Understanding the degradation mechanisms of the polymer matrix and nanofillers, as well as their interactions with biological fluids and tissues, is crucial. Factors such as environmental conditions, pH variations, and enzymatic activity influence the degradation process. Tailoring the composition and design of nanocomposites to achieve the desired degradation characteristics requires a nuanced approach, considering both short-term functionality and long-term biocompatibility.

Maintaining the right balance between stability and controlled degradation ensures that polymeric nanocomposites retain their functionality throughout the intended duration of use, avoiding potential complications or adverse effects associated with uncontrolled degradation. Researchers and engineers in the field of biomedical materials continuously explore innovative strategies to optimize the long-term performance of polymeric nanocomposites, facilitating their safe and effective integration into therapeutic and diagnostic applications.

16.4.3 Regulatory Challenges

Navigating regulatory challenges poses a formidable task in the integration of polymeric nanocomposites into biomedical applications. The transition from promising laboratory research to clinical translation involves a complex regulatory landscape that requires meticulous adherence to safety standards and thorough documentation.

Manufacturing and scalability challenges are significant obstacles to the widespread use of polymeric nanocomposites in biomedical applications. The transition from small-scale laboratory synthesis to large-scale production requires careful attention to reproducibility, batch consistency, and cost-effectiveness. Achieving scalability involves addressing the complexities of nanocomposite manufacturing such as controlling particle size, distribution, and polymer-nanofiller interactions. This must be done without compromising the quality of the material. Collaboration between researchers, engineers, and industry experts is crucial in developing scalable manufacturing processes. Additionally, the economic feasibility of large-scale production must be considered to make polymeric nanocomposites commercially viable. Overcoming these challenges requires interdisciplinary collaboration, technological advancements, and a commitment to developing scalable processes [24, 25].

The evolving nature of nanotechnology introduces an additional layer of complexity to regulatory frameworks, thereby prompting regulatory bodies to adapt and refine guidelines continually. As the field progresses, it is crucial to establish clear and harmonized regulatory pathways to fully utilize the potential of polymeric nanocomposites in improving healthcare outcomes. Researchers and regulatory professionals play a crucial role in shaping this landscape, by ensuring that innovative biomedical applications meet the necessary safety and effectiveness standards for successful clinical implementation.

16.4.4 Manufacturing and Scalability Challenges

The widespread adoption of polymeric nanocomposites for biomedical applications faces significant challenges in terms of manufacturing and scalability. Moving from small-scale laboratory synthesis to large-scale production requires meticulous attention to reproducibility, batch consistency, and cost-effectiveness, therefore necessitating innovative approaches to overcome inherent challenges.

Achieving scalability involves dealing with manufacturing complexities related to nanocomposite production. The incorporation of nanofillers requires precise control over parameters such as particle size, distribution, and interactions between polymers and nanofillers. Scaling up these intricate processes without compromising the quality and characteristics of the nanocomposite material requires advanced manufacturing technologies and process optimization. Additionally, the economic feasibility of large-scale production is a critical consideration. The cost-effectiveness of manufacturing processes, raw material expenses, and equipment investments must be carefully balanced to ensure that polymeric nanocomposites are commercially viable for biomedical applications. Collaboration between researchers, engineers, and industry experts becomes crucial in developing scalable manufacturing processes. Continuous innovation in manufacturing techniques, such as advanced mixing methods and continuous flow synthesis, is essential to streamline production and enhance reproducibility [26, 27].

As the field advances, addressing manufacturing and scalability challenges will be pivotal in realizing the transformative potential of polymeric nanocomposites in healthcare. Overcoming these hurdles requires interdisciplinary collaboration, technological advancements, and a commitment to developing scalable processes that ensure the reliable and cost-effective production of nanocomposites for widespread biomedical applications.

16.4.5 Clinical Translation Challenges

Clinical translation of polymeric nanocomposites for biomedical applications poses a range of challenges that create a divide between promising preclinical outcomes and practical implementation in patient care. These challenges include regulatory complexities, safety concerns, and the need for rigorous clinical validation. To ensure compliance with regulations, strict adherence to safety standards and comprehensive documentation are essential. The dynamic nature of nanotechnology requires regulatory bodies to continuously adapt guidelines to accommodate innovations in the application of polymeric nanocomposites. Safety concerns, such as potential toxicity and long-term effects, necessitate thorough evaluation in rigorous clinical trials. Understanding the fate of nanocomposites in different patient populations and predicting their responses are crucial aspects of clinical translation. Closing the knowledge gap between preclinical research and human trials is vital for the responsible introduction of nanocomposites in clinical settings. Large-scale studies are needed for clinical validation to assess efficacy, safety, and long-term outcomes. This requires collaboration among researchers, clinicians, and industry partners. Addressing these challenges in clinical translation is crucial for unlocking the full potential of polymeric nanocomposites and integrating them seamlessly into healthcare practices for the benefit of patients. The multidimensional nature of these challenges requires a collective effort from the scientific community, regulatory bodies, and healthcare stakeholders to bridge the translational gap and harness the true clinical impact of polymeric nanocomposites [28–33].

16.5 PERSPECTIVES AND INNOVATIONS

Recent advancements in polymeric nanocomposites have propelled the field forward by opening up innovative possibilities in various domains including healthcare and electronics. Notably, progress has been made in refining fabrication techniques, thus allowing for precise control over the structures and properties of nanocomposites. Advanced synthesis methods, such as electrospinning, emulsion polymerization, and in-situ polymerization, contribute to the production of nanocomposites with tailored characteristics such as controlled size, distribution, and functionality of nanofillers. In the biomedical realm, the design of polymeric nanocomposites for drug delivery systems has seen significant advancements. Researchers are exploring stimuli-responsive nanocomposites that release therapeutic agents in response to specific triggers, such as changes in pH, temperature, or enzymatic activity in the body. This improves the precision of drug delivery, minimizing side effects, and maximizing therapeutic efficacy. Furthermore, the integration of polymeric nanocomposites in regenerative medicine and tissue engineering has made notable progress. The enhanced mechanical properties, biocompatibility, and controlled degradation of these nanocomposites contribute to the development of scaffolds that closely mimic the natural extracellular matrix. This facilitates cell adhesion, proliferation, and differentiation, which are crucial for successful tissue regeneration.

In the field of electronics, advancements in conductive polymeric nanocomposites have led to the development of flexible and lightweight materials with excellent electrical conductivity. These materials find applications in flexible electronics, wearable devices, and sensors, thus paving the way for the next generation of electronic technologies. Additionally, the incorporation of nanocomposites in energy storage devices, such as batteries and supercapacitors, has gained attention. Nanocomposite materials enhance the performance, stability, and energy storage capacity of these devices, contributing to the development of more efficient and sustainable energy storage solutions [34–38].

However, challenges persist, particularly in scaling up production processes and ensuring the long-term biocompatibility and safety of polymeric nanocomposites in clinical applications. Nevertheless, recent advancements underscore the transformative potential of polymeric nanocomposites, driving interdisciplinary research and fostering collaborations that promise to revolutionize various industries and improve the quality of life. As these innovations continue to unfold, the future holds exciting prospects for the widespread integration of polymeric nanocomposites in diverse fields. The Table 16.2 highlights pivotal emerging trends in biomedical application.

Table 16.2 Emerging trends in biomedical applications [39–43]

Trend	Description
Drug Delivery Innovations	Advanced drug delivery systems including stimuli-responsive nanocomposites, targeted drug carriers, and personalized medicine approaches are revolutionizing the precision and efficacy of therapeutic interventions.
3D Printing in Tissue Engineering	Integration of 3D printing technologies for creating complex tissue scaffolds with precise architectures facilitates tissue engineering and regenerative medicine.
Nanomedicine for Diagnostics	Development of nanoscale contrast agents and imaging probes, enhancing diagnostic capabilities through improved imaging contrast, and real-time monitoring of physiological processes.
Immunotherapy Advancements	Advancements in immunotherapy, utilizing nanocarriers for targeted delivery of immunomodulatory agents, enhance the immune system's response against diseases, particularly in cancer treatment.
Bioelectronic Medicine	Emergence of bioelectronic devices and neuromodulation techniques for personalized medicine by leveraging electronic interfaces with biological systems for therapeutic interventions.
Gene Editing and Nanogenomics	Integration of nanotechnology in gene editing tools and nanogenomics enables precise manipulation of genetic material for potential therapeutic interventions and personalized medicine.

16.5.1 Innovative Approaches to Address Challenges

In the dynamic field of polymeric nanocomposites for biomedical applications, the resolution of challenges has sparked a surge of innovative approaches that collectively redefine the landscape of healthcare technologies. The multifaceted challenges, encompassing concerns regarding biocompatibility, controlled release kinetics, scalability issues, and regulatory complexities have incited inventive solutions at various levels of material design, manufacturing, and translational research. Precision engineering emerges as a prominent strategy to augment biocompatibility. Surface modifications, including biomimetic coatings and biofunctionalization, enable customized interactions with biological entities, mitigating unfavorable reactions and cytotoxicity. Simultaneously, advancements in manufacturing technologies, such as continuous flow synthesis and microfluidics, address scalability challenges thus ensuring large-scale production while preserving the integrity of nanocomposite properties.

To address controlled release kinetics, intelligent nanocomposites have surfaced. These materials respond to specific stimuli, permitting precise control over drug release, and optimizing therapeutic effectiveness while minimizing side effects. The development of multifunctional nanocomposites is another notable advancement; integrating diagnostic and therapeutic functionalities for real-time treatment monitoring, contributing to the paradigm of personalized medicine. Navigating regulatory challenges requires innovative strategies, including early engagement with regulatory agencies, comprehensive safety profile documentation, and proactive collaboration between researchers and regulatory bodies. Additionally, bioinformatics and computational models offer insights into nanocomposite behavior within biological systems thereby expediting the design process. Collaborative interdisciplinary research plays a crucial role in finding holistic solutions by bringing together expertise from materials science, biology, engineering, and regulatory affairs. This collaborative approach ensures a comprehensive understanding of challenges from various perspectives. Furthermore, a patient-centric design philosophy is reshaping the approach to polymeric nanocomposites. Customizing materials to meet specific patient needs, considering individual variations in responses, and incorporating feedback from end-users contribute to more effective and personalized biomedical applications [44–47].

16.6 FUTURE DIRECTIONS

16.6.1 Anticipated Developments in the Field

The field of polymeric nanocomposites for biomedical applications is on the verge of transformative developments with anticipated advancements poised to reshape healthcare technologies. One area of anticipation involves refining nanomaterial design to enhance biocompatibility, mechanical properties, and functionality. Molecular-level tailoring is expected to result in breakthroughs that closely mimic biological structures thus ushering in a new era in materials science.

The integration of artificial intelligence (AI) is projected to play a pivotal role in the field's evolution. By incorporating AI into design and optimization processes, material development can be expedited through the analysis of vast datasets. These algorithms have the potential to predict nanocomposite behaviors, optimize formulations, and contribute to the creation of materials with enhanced therapeutic efficacy and safety profiles. Precision in targeted drug delivery is another focus of anticipated developments. Smart nanocomposites that respond to specific cellular or environmental cues are expected to redefine drug delivery systems, minimizing side effects and maximizing treatment efficiency. The movement towards personalized medicine is gaining momentum with the anticipation that polymeric nanocomposites can be tailored based on individual patient characteristics. This shift is likely to optimize treatment outcomes by considering variations in patient responses and fostering more effective and patient-centric healthcare solutions.

The integration of theranostic platforms, which combine diagnostic and therapeutic functions in a single nanocomposite, is on the horizon. These platforms are expected to redefine disease management strategies, particularly in fields such as oncology and chronic conditions, through real-time monitoring, feedback mechanisms, and responsive interventions. Sustainability is also emerging as a prominent theme with a focus on the development of biodegradable nanocomposites. This shift aligns with a broader commitment to environmentally friendly solutions while ensuring that materials effectively serve their purpose while minimizing their impact on the environment over time. Lastly, there is an anticipated emphasis on seamless clinical translation and commercialization. To streamline the pathway from laboratory success to practical applications, close collaboration between researchers, industry stakeholders, and regulatory bodies will be essential. This collaboration will ensure that the anticipated advancements effectively contribute to improving patient outcomes and the overall landscape of healthcare technologies [48–50].

16.6.2 Potential Interdisciplinary Collaborations

Potential interdisciplinary collaborations in the field of polymeric nanocomposites for biomedical applications are crucial for transformative advancements. These collaborations bring together experts from various scientific disciplines to address the multifaceted challenges in this field thus fostering innovation and ensuring the practical applicability of polymeric nanocomposites in healthcare.

Integration of materials science and engineering is a cornerstone of these collaborations. By combining the expertise of materials scientists and engineers, a synergy is established to design and manufacture polymeric nanocomposites with enhanced properties. This collaboration bridges the gap between theoretical advancements and practical scalability which enables the production of materials that are not only advanced in theory but also feasible for large-scale production.

Collaborations between biologists and nanomedicine experts are essential for understanding the complex interactions between nanocomposites and biological systems. This interdisciplinary approach focuses on optimizing biocompatibility, minimizing toxicity, and unraveling the complexities of nanomaterial behavior within living organisms, ensuring the safe and effective application of polymeric nanocomposites in healthcare. The involvement of computational modelers and data scientists in interdisciplinary collaborations contributes to predictive modeling of nanocomposite behavior. By utilizing advanced computational techniques and analyzing extensive datasets, these collaborations expedite the design process and facilitate the development of optimized nanocomposites. The collaboration between researchers and regulatory affairs experts is crucial for navigating the intricate regulatory landscape. This partnership ensures that polymeric nanocomposites meet stringent safety and efficacy standards required for clinical translation. Clinicians provide valuable insights and offers a practical perspective on the applicability of these materials in real-world healthcare settings. Incorporating patient advocacy groups and ethicists into interdisciplinary collaborations ensures a holistic approach. By considering patient perspectives and ethical considerations from the outset, these collaborations contribute to the responsible development and deployment of polymeric nanocomposites. This inclusive approach aligns technological advancements with societal values thus ensuring that ethical considerations are integral to the research process [51, 52].

16.7 CONCLUSION

To conclude, this chapter extensively explores the pivotal role of polymeric nanocomposites in advancing biomedical technologies by providing a comprehensive overview of their applications, challenges, and prospects. The integration of nanoscale fillers into polymer matrices has endowed these materials with unique properties thereby positioning them as transformative agents across diverse healthcare domains.

Polymeric nanocomposites have played a pivotal role in the advancement of drug delivery systems by offering controlled release capabilities that enhance treatment efficacy while minimizing side effects. Despite the challenges related to biocompatibility and regulatory considerations, the precision afforded by these nanocomposites in modulating drug release kinetics represents a significant step forward in patient-centric pharmaceutical solutions. In the field of tissue engineering, polymeric nanocomposites are notable for their enhanced mechanical strength and biocompatibility thus making them an ideal platform for constructing biomimetic scaffolds. These scaffolds, which mimic the extracellular matrix, contribute to the regeneration of functional tissues. Although there are challenges in terms of long-term biocompatibility and regulatory considerations, the integration of nanocomposites offers a transformative approach in the field of regenerative medicine.

Polymeric nanocomposites have proven to be versatile contrast agents in diagnostic imaging which leads to improved accuracy in medical diagnostics and enabling early disease detection. Despite the challenges related to biocompatibility and potential toxicity, the ongoing advancements in nanotechnology hold the promise of reshaping diagnostic imaging and providing more accurate and comprehensive insights into physiological conditions. In the realm of implantable medical devices, polymeric nanocomposites play a crucial role by offering improved integration with host tissues, reduced rejection risks, and enhanced durability. Moreover, these materials contribute to the development of highly sensitive biosensors for diagnostic purposes by showcasing their versatility in various biomedical applications.

The chapter skillfully addresses the challenges faced by polymeric nanocomposites including issues of biocompatibility, long-term stability, regulatory scrutiny, manufacturing, and clinical translation. However, the narrative takes an optimistic approach, emphasizing innovative strategies such as precision engineering, smart nanocomposites, and interdisciplinary collaborations to overcome these challenges and propel the field forward.

Expected advancements in the field include improved nanomaterial design, the integration of artificial intelligence, precise targeted drug delivery, and a shift toward personalized medicine. Sustainability emerges as a prominent theme with a focus on developing biodegradable nanocomposites. The chapter underscores the significance of seamless clinical translation and commercialization through close collaboration between researchers, industry stakeholders, and regulatory bodies.

In summary, the chapter highlights that polymeric nanocomposites are at the forefront of biomedical innovation. Their transformative potential lies not only in addressing current challenges but also in pioneering solutions that have the potential to revolutionize patient care, diagnostics, and regenerative medicine. As these materials continue to evolve, they hold the exciting prospect of being seamlessly integrated into a wide range of biomedical applications which ultimately leads to improved healthcare outcomes and enhances the overall quality of human life.

REFERENCES

1. A. P. Meera*, Reshma R. Pillai, P. B. Sreelekshmi. (2023). Novel polymer nanocomposites: Synthesis. *Designing and Cost-effective Biomedical Applications* (17), 56–72, https://doi.org/10.2174/9789815080179123010006
2. Olaf Holderer, Anne-Caroline Genix, Margarita Kruteva, Julian Oberdisse. (2023). Editorial: Nanocomposites with interfaces controlled by grafted or adsorbed polymers. *Frontiers in Physics*, 10, https://doi.org/10.3389/fphy.2022.1117549
3. Shahrzad Rahmani, Mahshid Maroufkhani, Sanaz Mohammadzadeh-Komuleh, Zahra Khoubi-Arani. (2022). *Chapter 7 - Polymer Nanocomposites for Biomedical Applications, Fundamentals of Bionanomaterials*. Elsevier, Pages 175–215, ISBN 9780128241479
4. Pooja Chawla, Viney Chawla, Sumel Ashique, Aakash Upadhyay, Monica Gulati, Dilpreet Singh. (2023). One-dimensional polymeric nanocomposites in drug delivery systems. *Current Nanoscience*, https://doi.org/10.2174/1573413719666230110110706
5. Idrees Khan, Ibrahim Khan, Khalid Saeed, Mohammed Salim Akhter. (2022). Polymer nanocomposites: An overview. *Smart Polymer Nanocomposites*, https://doi.org/10.1016/B978-0-323-91611-0.00017-7

6. Leng Shi-liang. (2023). Preparation and application of polymer nanocomposites. *Nanomaterials*, https://doi.org/10.3390/nano13040657, 13(4), 657.
7. Lara Wiedmann. (2023). Polymer nanocomposite technologies designed for biomedical applications, https://doi.org/10.2174/9789815080179123010005
8. T. R. Athira, K. Selvaraju, N. L. Gowrishankar. (2023). Biodegradable polymeric nanoparticles: The novel carrier for controlled release drug delivery system. *International Journal of Science and Research Archive*, https://doi.org/10.30574/ijsra.2023.8.1.0103
9. Mohammed Elmowafy, Khaled Shalaby, Mohammed H. Elkomy, Omar Awad Alsaidan, Hesham A. M. Gomaa, Mohamed A. Abdelgawad, Ehab M. Mostafa. (2023). Polymeric nanoparticles for delivery of natural bioactive agents: Recent advances and challenges. *Polymers*, https://doi.org/10.3390/polym15051123
10. Pooja Chawla, Viney Chawla, Sumel Ashique, Aakash Upadhyay, Monica Gulati, Dilpreet Singh. (2023). One-dimensional polymeric nanocomposites in drug delivery systems. *Current Nanoscience*, https://doi.org/10.2174/1573413719666230110110706
11. Feng Han, Qingchen Meng, En Xie, Kexin Li, Jie Hu, Qianglong Chen, Jiaying Li, Fengxuan Han. (2023). Engineered biomimetic micro/nano-materials for tissue regeneration. *Frontiers in Bioengineering and Biotechnology*, https://doi.org/10.3389/fbioe.2023.1205792
12. Jie Cui, Xiao Yu, Yihong Shen, Binbin Sun, Wanxin Guo, Mingyue Liu, Yujie Chen, Li Wang, Xingping Zhou, Muhammad Shafiq, Xiumei Mo. (2023). Electrospinning inorganic nanomaterials to fabricate bionanocomposites for soft and hard tissue repair. *Nanomaterials*, https://doi.org/10.3390/nano13010204
13. Xinyu Xie. (2023). Application of nanomedicine in diagnostic technology. *Highlights in Science, Engineering and Technology*, https://doi.org/10.54097/hset.v40i.6577
14. Jeladhara Sobhanan, Abdulaziz Anas, Vasudevanpillai Biju. (2023). Nanomaterials for fluorescence and multimodal bioimaging. *Chemical Record*, https://doi.org/10.1002/tcr.202200253
15. J. Weinstein, C. Varallyay, E. Dósa, S. Gahramanov, B. Hamilton, W. Rooney, L. Muldoon, E. Neuwelt. (2010). Superparamagnetic iron oxide nanoparticles: Diagnostic magnetic resonance imaging and potential therapeutic applications in neurooncology and central nervous system inflammatory pathologies, a review. *Journal of Cerebral Blood Flow & Metabolism*, 30, 15–35. https://doi.org/10.1038/jcbfm.2009.192.
16. Y. Zeng, H. Li, Z. Li, Q. Luo, H. Zhu, Z. Gu, H. Zhang, Q. Gong, K. Luo. (2020). Engineered gadolinium-based nanomaterials as cancer imaging agents. *Applied Materials Today*, 20, 100686. https://doi.org/10.1016/j.apmt.2020.100686.
17. N. Aslan, B. Ceylan, M. Koç, F. Findik. (2020). Metallic nanoparticles as X-ray computed tomography (CT) contrast agents: A review. *Journal of Molecular Structure*, 1219, 128599. https://doi.org/10.1016/j.molstruc.2020.128599.
18. J. Xu, A. Gulzar, P. Yang, H. Bi, D. Yang, S. Gai, F. He, J. Lin, B. Xing, D. Jin. (2019). Recent advances in near-infrared emitting lanthanide-doped nanoconstructs: Mechanism, design and application for bioimaging. *Coordination Chemistry Reviews*. https://doi.org/10.1016/J.CCR.2018.11.014.

19. S. Ghaderi, B. Ramesh, A. Seifalian. (2011). Fluorescence nanoparticles "quantum dots" as drug delivery system and their toxicity: A review. *Journal of Drug Targeting*, 19, 475–486. https://doi.org/10.3109/1061186X.2010.526227.

20. Shilpa Bhandi. (2023). Biocompatibility of restorative materials- a review. *Texila International Journal of Public Health*, https://doi.org/10.21522/tijph.2013.11.02.art014

21. Altun Buse Karakullukçu, Emel Taban, Olatunji Oladimeji Ojo. (2023). Biocompatibility of biomaterials and test methods: A review. *MP Materialpruefung - MP Materials Testing*, https://doi.org/10.1515/mt-2022-0195

22. Karan Malhotra, Richard Fuku, Balmiki Kumar, David A. Hrovat, J. Van Houten, Paul A. E. Piunno, Patrick T. Gunning, Ulrich J. Krull. (2022). Unlocking long-term stability of upconversion nanoparticles with biocompatible phosphonate-based polymer coatings. *Nano Letters*, https://doi.org/10.1021/acs.nanolett.2c00437

23. Traian Zaharescu, T. Borbáth, Marius Maris, I. Borbáth, Mihaela Maris. (2022). The stability consequences promoted by doping metallic atoms on the degradation of poly (ε-Caprolactone). *Macromol*, https://doi.org/10.3390/macromol2030025

24. Nayanika Mookherjee. (2023). Scale-up of nanoparticle manufacturing process. *AAPS Introductions in the Pharmaceutical Sciences*, https://doi.org/10.1007/978-3-031-31380-6_12

25. M.N. Subramaniam. (2022). Grand challenges in fabrication of nanocomposite hollow fiber membranes. *Journal of Applied Membrane Science & Technology*, https://doi.org/10.11113/amst.v26n3.251

26. Lara Wiedmann. (2023). Polymer nanocomposite technologies designed for biomedical applications, https://doi.org/10.2174/9789815080179123010005

27. Amaresh Kumar Sahoo. (2023). Polymeric nanocomposites: Synthesis, characterization, and recent applications. *Nanomaterials*, https://doi.org/10.1007/978-981-19-7963-7_10.

28. Atanu Kumar Paul, Arbind Prasad, Ashwani Kumar. (2022). Review on artificial neural network and its application in the field of engineering. *Journal of Mechanical Engineering: PRAKASH*, 1(1), 53–61, https://doi.org/10.56697/JMEP.2022.1107.

29. Gourhari Chakraborty, Vivek Pandey, Arbind Prasad, Ashwani Kumar. (2023). Introduction to sustainable manufacturing for industries 4.0. In *Sustainable Smart Manufacturing Processes in Industry 4.0*, Ramesh Kumar, Arbind Prasad, Ashwani Kumar, Editors. CRC Press: Boca Raton, FL, Chapter 01, pp. 01–17. https://doi.org/10.1201/9781003436072-1.

30. Subhash Singh, Sanjay K. Behura, Ashwani Kumar, Kartikey Verma. (2022). *Nanomanufacturing and Nanomaterials Design: Principles and Applications.* Taylor & Francis (CRC Press), ISBN: 9781032081687, ISBN: 9781003220602, https://doi.org/10.1201/9781003220602.

31. Ashwani Kumar, Yatika Gori, Nitesh Dutt, Yogesh Kumar Singla, Ambrish Maurya. (2021). *Advanced Computational Methods in Mechanical and Materials Engineering.* Taylor & Francis (CRC Press), ISBN: 9781032052915, https://doi.org/10.1201/9781003202233.

32. Ashwani Kumar, Mangey Ram, Yogesh Kumar Singla. (2022). *Advanced Material for Biomechanical Applications.* Taylor & Francis (CRC Press), ISBN: 9781032054490, https://doi.org/10.1201/9781003286806.

33. Arbind Prasad, Ashwani Kumar, Kishor Kumar Gajrani. (2022). *Biodegradable Composites for Packaging Application.* Taylor & Francis (CRC Press), ISBN: 978103231511, https://doi.org/10.1201/9781003227908.

34. Ashwani Kumar, Yatika Gori, Avinash Kumar, Chandan Swaroop Meena, Nitesh Dutt. (2022). *Advanced Materials for Biomedical Applications.* Taylor & Francis (CRC Press), ISBN: 9781003344810, https://doi.org/10.1201/9781003344810.

35. Arbind Prasad, Ashwani Kumar, Manoj Gupta. (2023). *Advanced Materials and Manufacturing Techniques in Biomedical Applications.* Wiley Scrivener, ISBN: 9781394166190, https://doi.org/10.1002/9781394166985.

36. Anka Datta, Avinash Kumar, Ashwani Kumar, Abhishek Kumar, Varun Pratap Singh. (2022). Advanced materials in biological implants and surgical tools. In *Advanced Materials for Biomedical Applications.* CRC Press (Taylor & Francis), ISBN: 9781003344810, https://doi.org/10.1201/9781003344810-2.

37. Ashwani Kumar, Arun Kumar Singh Gangwar, Avinash Kumar, Chandan Swaroop Meena, Varun Pratap Singh, Nitesh Dutt, Arbind Prasad, Yatika Gori. (2022). Biomedical study of femur bone fracture and healing. In *Advanced Materials for Biomedical Applications.* CRC Press (Taylor & Francis), ISBN: 9781003344810, https://doi.org/10.1201/9781003344810-14.

38. Arbind Prasad, Gourhari Chakraborty, Ashwani Kumar. (2022). Bio-based environmentally benign polymeric resorbable materials for orthopedic fixation applications. In *Advanced Materials for Biomedical Applications.* CRC Press (Taylor & Francis), ISBN: 9781003344810, https://doi.org/10.1201/9781003344810-15.

39. Arbind Prasad, Gourhari Chakraborty, Ashwani Kumar, Kishor Kumar Gajrani. (2022). Introduction to biodegradable polymers. In *Biodegradable Composites for Packaging Applications.* CRC Press (Taylor & Francis), ISBN: 978103227908, https://doi.org/10.1201/9781003227908-1.

40. Gourhari Chakraborty, Arbind Prasad, Ashwani Kumar. (2022). Processing of biodegradable composites. In *Biodegradable Composites for Packaging Applications.* CRC Press (Taylor & Francis), ISBN: 978103227908, https://doi.org/10.1201/9781003227908-3.

41. Ramesh Kumar, Arbind Prasad, Ashwani Kumar. (2023). *Sustainable Smart Manufacturing Processes in Industry 4.0.* Taylor & Francis (CRC Press), ISBN: 9781003436072, https://doi.org/10.1201/9781003436072.

42. Ramesh Kumar, Ashwani Kumar, Laxmi Kant, Arbind Prasad, Sandeep Bhoi, Chandan Swaroop Meena, Varun Pratap Singh, Aritra Ghosh. (2023). Experimental and RSM-based process-parameters optimisation for turning operation of EN36B steel. *Materials,* 16, 339, https://doi.org/10.3390/ma16010339.

43. Sandeep Bhoi, Ashwani Kumar, Arbind Prasad, Chandan Swaroop Meena, Rudra Bubai Sarkar, Bidyanand Mahto, Aritra Ghosh. (2022). Performance evaluation of different coating materials in delamination for micro- milling applications on high-speed steel substrate. *Micromachines,* 13, 1277. https://doi.org/10.3390/mi13081277.

44. Sandeep Bhoi, Arbind Prasad, Ashwani Kumar, Rudra Bubai Sarkar, Bidyanand Mahto, Chandan Swaroop Meena, Chandan Pandey. (2022). Experimental study to evaluate the wear performance of UHMWPE and XLPE material for orthopedics application. *Bioengineering*, 9, 676, https://doi.org/10.3390/bioengineering9110676.

45. Ashwani Kumar, Yatika Gori, Sachin Rana, Neelesh Kumar Sharma, Brijesh Yadav. (2022). FEA of humerus bone fracture and healing. In *Advanced Materials for Biomechanical Applications*. CRC Press (Taylor and Francis), ISBN: 9781032054490, https://doi.org/10.1201/9781003286806-14.

46. Ashwani Kumar, Deepak Prasad Mamgain, Himanshu Jaiswal, Pravin P. Patil. (2015). Modal analysis of hand arm vibration (Humerus Bone) for biodynamic response using varying boundary conditions based on FEA. In *Springer Book Series: Advances in Intelligent Systems and Computing* (Vol. 308, pp. 169–176), https://doi.org/10.1007/978-81-322-2012-1_18. Series ISSN-2194-5357.

47. Arun Kumar Singh Gangwar, P. Sudhakar Rao, Ashwani Kumar. (2021). Biomechanical design and analysis of femur bone. *Materials Today: Proceedings*, 44, Part 1, 2179–2187, ISSN 2214-7853, https://doi.org/10.1016/j.matpr.2020.12.282.

48. Arun Kumar Singh Gangwar, P. Sudhakar Rao, Ashwani Kumar, Pravin P. Patil. (2019). Design and analysis of femur bone: biomechanical aspects. *Journal of Critical Reviews*, 6(4), 133–139, ISSN-2394-5125.

49. Arbind Prasad, Sudipto Datta, Ashwani Kumar, Manoj Gupta. (2023). Introduction to next-generation materials for biomedical applications. In *Advanced Materials and Manufacturing Techniques for Biomedical Applications*, Arbind Prasad, Ashwani Kumar, Manoj Gupta, Editors. John Wiley & Sons, Chapter 01, pp. 01–24, https://doi.org/10.1002/9781394166985.ch1.

50. Sriparna De, Dipankar Das, Arbind Prasad, Ashwani Kumar, Dipankar Chattopadhyay. (2023). Insights into multifunctional smart hydrogels in wound healing applications. In *Advanced Materials and Manufacturing Techniques for Biomedical Applications*, Arbind Prasad, Ashwani Kumar, Manoj Gupta, Editors. John Wiley & Sons, Chapter 03, pp. 37–60, https://doi.org/10.1002/9781394166985.ch3

51. Avinash Kumar, Mohit Byadwal, Abhishek Kumar, Ashwani Kumar, Francis Luther King M. (2023). Laser micromachining in biomedical industry. In *Laser-based Technologies for Sustainable Manufacturing*, Avinash Kumar, Ashwani Kumar, Abhishek Kumar, Editors. CRC Press: Boca Raton, FL, Chapter 08, pp. 169–206, https://doi.org/10.1201/9781003402398-8.

52. Avinash Kumar, Anka Datta, Ashwani Kumar, Abhishek Kumar. (2022). Recent advancements and future trends in next-generation materials for biomedical applications. In *Advanced Materials for Biomedical Applications*. CRC Press (Taylor & Francis), ISBN: 9781003344810, https://doi.org/10.1201/9781003344810-1.

Index

Acetic acid, 281–282, 284, 286, 288
Acrylic-acid, 203–206
Adhesion, 278
Adsorbent, 196, 198, 200, 201, 204, 205, 208
Adsorption, 196, 198–205, 207, 208
Alginate, 197, 198, 206, 208–209
Alumina, 3
Amylopectin, 95, 96, 99, 103
Amylose, 95, 96, 99, 101, 103
Angiogenic, 278
Anthropogenic, 278
Antibacterial, 28, 98, 104, 234–240, 244–246, 278, 280–282, 284–285, 287, 290
Anticancer activity, 247
Antidiabetic activity, 246
Anti-fungal, 282, 285
Antimicrobial activity, 245, 282, 285–286, 288–290
Antioxidants, 101, 105
Apoptosis assay, 179–180
Applications, 196–198, 209
Atomic force microscopy, 32, 35, 36
Atom transfer radical polymerization (ATRP), 172

Bacterial, 39, 40, 42, 50, 281–282, 287, 289
Beads, 202, 206, 208, 209
Bio absorbable materials, 5
Bioactive, 278, 290
Bioactive glass, 12
Bio-based, 39–41, 43, 45, 47, 49–50
Biocompatibile/ity, 2, 7, 27, 28, 40, 42, 43, 47, 48, 198, 209, 278, 280, 282, 284–285, 290

Biocomposites, 278, 280, 282, 286–288, 290–291
Biodegradable/ity, 25, 36, 41, 44, 50, 196–198
Biological, 40, 45–48, 50, 233, 235, 237–239, 241–243, 250
Biomaterials, 40, 50, 278, 280, 287, 289–290
Biomedical, 39, 50
Biomedical engineering, 2, 3, 5, 6, 10, 11, 15, 16, 19–20
Bio-nanocomposite, 39, 200, 202, 203, 205, 207, 208, 234, 235, 244–246
Biopolymeric, 39, 50
Biopolymers, 25–27, 29, 36, 197, 198, 205
Biosensors, 39, 48, 51
Biphasic calcium phosphates (BCP), 13
Blood, 280
Bone engineering, 236, 238–241
Bone regeneration, 39, 43

Calcium, 287–290
Calcium carbonate, 12
Calcium phosphates, 11
Calcium sulfate, 12
Capacity, 196, 201, 205, 207, 208
Carbonate apatite, 12
Carbon-dots, 195, 200, 202, 203, 205, 207–209
Carbon nanotube (CNT) nanocomposites, 171
Carbon nanotubes, 25, 27, 34
Catalyst, 199, 200
Cell adhesion, 42, 43
Cell proliferation assays, 178

Cellular, 287
Cellulose, 25, 26, 28, 30, 33, 36, 39, 41, 42, 50–51, 197, 198, 203, 205–207
Cell viability assays, 176–178
Ceramic-matrix nanocomposites (CMNCs), 173
Ceramic nanocomposites, 172, 173
Ceramics, 3, 10–12
Chitin, 40, 50
Chitosan, 26–28, 30, 31, 40, 41, 45, 49–51, 197, 200–203, 206, 281–290
Chitosan and biosilica, 241
Chitosan–copper nanocomposites, 238
Chitosan–gold nanocomposites, 237
Chitosan–silver nanocomposites, 236
Chitosan–titanium oxide nanocomposites, 239
Chitosan–zinc oxide nanocomposites, 240
Chromium, 195, 202, 203, 207
Clay–polymer nanocomposites, 171
Collagen, 41, 43, 278, 280–281, 287
Composite materials, 4
Composites, 196, 198, 201–205, 207–209
Conductivity, 25
Copolymer, 284
Cross-linker, 201, 203
Cytotoxicity, 175

Degradation, 200, 203
Desorption, 200, 201, 204, 208
Detection, 196, 197, 202, 203, 205, 207–209
Diagnostics, 237, 243
Dicalcium phosphate, 12
Dispersed, 25, 27, 28, 33, 34
Drug delivery, 39, 49–51
Ductility, 284–285

E. coli, 290
Efficiency, 200–205, 208
Elasticity, 287
Electrochemiluminescence, 47
Electrons, 32, 33, 35, 36
Electrospinning
    machine, 283, 289
    process, 283
    set-up, 281
Electrostatic, 201, 205
Emission, 34

Environment, 44, 195, 196, 199, 201, 208
Equilibrium, 201–203, 205
Exfoliation, 198–200
Extracellular, 281
Extraction, 202, 203

Fibrotic, 278
Fibrous, 41
Flexibilty, 284–285, 287, 290
Fluorescence, 34, 44–46, 48, 49
Fluorescent, 202, 203, 207
Food packaging, 26–28, 36
Freundlich, 204

Gelatin, 12, 41, 43, 50, 278
Gentamicin, 285–287, 290
Glycerophosphate, 238
Gold, 45, 48, 51
Graphene, 5, 27, 34, 46, 51, 283–285
Graphitic, 45, 51

Haemostasis, 279–280
Hazardous, 195, 196
Heavy metal, 195, 196, 198, 209
Hemicellulose, 26
Hydrogel, 202–204, 206, 207
Hydrophobic, 44, 50
Hydrothermal, 203
Hydroxyapatite, 3, 11, 12, 40, 42, 236, 237, 240

Imaging, 39, 40, 43–49, 51
Industries, 39, 41, 50
Infection, 278–282, 289–290
Inflammation, 279–280, 287, 290
Initial corrosion, 8
Ion release, 8, 13
Ions, 195–198, 201–209
Iron, 6, 12, 20
Iron oxide, 39, 47, 51
In situ polymerization, 29
Isotherms, 200–202, 204
In vitro, 40, 43, 48, 49, 51
In vivo, 40, 45, 47–49

Langmuir, 201, 202, 204
Lignin, 26
Limit of detection, 203, 205, 207, 209
Living organisms, 39
Luminescence, 46–49, 51

Magnesium, 6–9, 12
Magnetic, 39, 44, 45, 47, 49, 51, 200,
        201, 203, 204, 206, 207
Material, 280–282, 284–288
Matrix, 25, 27–31, 33–35, 281,
        287–289
Medical devices, 3, 4, 11, 19
Melt processing, 29, 30, 36
Mercury, 195, 205
Mesenchymal stem cells, 237, 238
Mesoporous silica nanoparticles, 238
Metal ions, 195–198, 200–206
Metal-matrix nanocomposites
        (MMNCs), 173
Metal-organic frameworks, 47, 51
Metals, 3, 5
Method, 280–284, 286–288
Methylene blue, 205, 206
Microorganisms, 281, 287, 290
Modalities, 46, 47, 49, 51
Modified graphene oxide (mGO), 284
Molybdenum, 7
Morphological analysis, 179
MTT, 175–178
Multimodal imaging, 47, 49
Multi-walled carbon nanotubes
        (MWCNTs), 172

Nanocomposites, 27, 28, 30–35, 39–
        51, 196–200, 202, 204, 206,
        207, 209, 233–242, 244–251,
        278, 285, 290
Nanofibres, 26, 30, 33
Nanofibrous, 282–283, 285, 289–290
Nanofillers, 25, 26, 29, 36
Nanomaterials, 39, 46, 234, 236, 248
Nanoparticles, 39, 41, 44, 45, 48, 49,
        51, 196, 201, 203, 205–209,
        280–283, 285–290
Nano-sensor, 209
Nanostructured, 50
Nanotechnology, 233, 250
Nano-tubes, 201, 206, 208
Natural polymers, 170
Near-infrared, 46, 48
Necrosis assays, 179–180
Nickel, 196, 200, 208, 209
Non-covalent drug delivery, 182–183

Optical imaging, 46
Organoclays, 31
Osteocalcin genes, 237, 238
Osteoinductive capabilities, 237

Packaging, 94, 95, 99–106
Phagocytosis, 8
pH-induced drug delivery, 184–185
Phonons, 47
Photoacoustic imaging, 44, 46
Photocatalytic activity, 234
Photodynamic therapy, 50, 51
Photothermal, 44, 45, 48, 50
Plasticizer, 98, 100, 104, 106
Pollutants, 195, 204, 208
Poly (lactic-co-glycolic acid), 4, 15
Polyamide, 94
Polycaprolactone, 41
Polyepoxide, 233
Polyester, 27, 31, 102
Polyetherimide, 233
Polyethylene, 94, 99, 102, 104
Polyethylene oxide (PEO), 282–283
Polyhexamethylene guanidine
        (PHMG), 284–285
Polyhydroxyalkanoates, 27
Polyhydroxyl butyrate, 25
Polylactic acid, 4, 15, 25
Polymer/s, 4, 5, 10, 15–20, 25–36,
        196–200, 203, 205,
        208–209, 234, 241, 242,
        280, 282–288, 290
Polymer nanocomposites (PNCs), 170
Polypropylene, 94, 101, 102
Polysaccharide/s, 25, 27, 28, 30, 95,
        101, 106, 197
Polystyrene, 94, 101
Polyvinyl alcohol (PVA), 281,
        284–285, 289
Polyvinyl alcohol/chitosan
        (PVA/CS), 284
Polyvinyl alcohol/chitosan/modified
        graphene oxide (PVA/CS/
        mGO), 284, 290
Porphyrins, 44, 51
Proliferation, 278–280, 290
Proteins, 25, 28, 32, 33, 35
Pseudomonas aeruginosa, 290

Raman imaging, 47
Regenerative medicine, 11, 15
Remodeling, 279–280, 290
Removal, 197, 198, 201–206,
        208–209
Renewable, 26
Resorbable, 1–7, 9, 11, 13–18, 20
Resorbable materials, 2, 4, 19
Reusability, 200, 201, 209

Salmonella Typhimurium, 39
Scaffold, 278, 282–283, 290
Scaffolding system, 238
Scarring, 290
Selectivity, 196, 203, 207–209
Sensitivity, 203, 207
Silver, 280–283, 285, 289–290
Skin, 278, 280, 282, 287–290
Sodium, 204, 206, 208, 209
Solvents, 199, 200, 203, 209
Staphylococcus aureus, 237, 290
Staphylococcus epidermidis, 237
Starch, 25, 26, 28, 30, 197, 203–206
Surgical, 279, 288
Sustainable, 36
Synthesis, 198–200, 203, 208

Temperature-induced drug delivery,
    185–187
Template, 196, 198–200
Thermal, 25, 27, 28, 30–32
Thermoplastic, 27, 36
Thermoset, 27
Three-dimensional, 41
Tissue, 278, 280, 283, 285,
    287–288, 290
Tissue engineering, 40–43, 50–51
Titanate, 202, 206, 208

Titanium, 233, 234, 236, 239, 240,
    243–245
Topical, 280
Toxic, 195–197, 209
Treatment, 280, 284, 288, 291
Tricalcium phosphate, 13
TUNEL assay, 179
Tungsten, 7

Upconversion luminescence, 48

Vibrations, 34

Waste-water, 195, 198, 207, 208
WAXD, 32
Whiskers, 26, 30
Wound acute, 279
Wound chronic, 278–280
Wound healing, 278–282, 285,
    287–290
Wound site, 280, 288, 290
Wound treatment, 280, 284,
    288, 291

Zinc, 6, 7, 12, 20, 234, 238–240,
    243–246, 249
Zinc oxide (ZnO), 282, 285,
    287–290